MW01028846

The CRC's Guide to Coordinating Clinical Research

Karen E. Woodin, Ph.D.

THOMSON
CENTERWATCH

22 Thomson Place · Boston, MA 02210
Phone (617) 856-5900 · Fax (617) 856-5901
www.centerwatch.com

THOMSON
CENTERWATCH

The CRC's Guide to Coordinating Clinical Research
by Karen E. Woodin, Ph.D.

Editor
Sara Gambrill

Design
Paul Gualdoni, Jr.

Printed in the United States.
2 3 4 5 07 06 05

For more information, contact CenterWatch, 22 Thomson Place, Boston, MA 02210. Or you can visit our Internet site at http://www.centerwatch.com.

ISBN 1-930624-46-8

Instructions for Obtaining Continuing Education Credit

Objectives

Upon completion of this activity, participants will be able to:

1. Determine the role of the Clinical Research Coordinator at a clinical study site by describing the general responsibilities associated with that role.
2. Identify the regulations governing clinical research.
3. Describe the drug development process.
4. Discuss Good Clinical Practices and how to apply them in clinical trials.
5. Organize a clinical practice to manage clinical trials successfully to their completion.

This continuing education offering is co-provided by Thomson American Health Consultants and Thomson CenterWatch. Thomson American Health Consultants is accredited as a provider of continuing education in nursing by the American Nurses Credentialing Center's Commission on Accreditation and by the California Board of Registered Nursing (provider number CEP 10864). Upon completion of the activity, participants may earn approximately 10 nursing contact hours. To complete the activity, the participant must earn a score of at least 70% on the online exam no later than August 1, 2007.

The online exam and instructions are available through the following web site: www.centerwatch.com/bookstore/pubs_profs_crcguide.html.

Financial Disclosure

Author Karen E. Woodin, Ph.D., reports no relationships with companies related to this field of study. The Editorial Board: Diane Butler, R.N., M.A.; Gail Conaway, R.N., CCRC, CIP; Paul W. Goebel, Jr., CIP; Louis Kirby, M.D.; and Joan Matusin report no relationships with companies related to this field of study. Peer reviewer Elizabeth E. Hill, R.N., MS, DNSc, reports no relationships with companies related to this field of study.

For Bob Assenzo, Pat Keelan, Art Hearron, and John Schultz, with thanks for the opportunities and support you gave me over the years, and for John, who makes it all worthwhile.

ACKNOWLEDGMENTS

The many CRCs I worked with throughout the years helped form the basis of my knowledge. Thank you all. Thanks to Diane Butler for her many comments and insights along the way, and to my sister, Peg McCann, who reviewed many of the chapters for me in advance of submitting the book for editing. Sara Gambrill, my editor at CenterWatch, was as helpful and easy to work with as one could ever hope; the changes were painless, Sara.

A special thanks to those who read and reviewed the book and made helpful comments:

Diane Butler, R.N., M.A.
Administrative Director
Westside Family Medical Center, P.C.
Research Department

Gail Conaway, R.N., CCRC, CIP
Senior Manager Site Relationships and Compliance
Chesapeake IRB

Paul W. Goebel, Jr., CIP
Vice President
Chesapeake Research Review
Guest Lecturer, Johns Hopkins University
Guest Lecturer, George Washington University

Elizabeth E. Hill, R.N., M.S., DNSc
Assistant Professor
Director, Clinical Research Management Program
Duke University School of Nursing

Louis Kirby, M.D.
Medical Director
Pivotal Research, LLC

Joan Matusin
Director Corporate Quality Assurance and Training
Essential Group

The book went more smoothly along the way because of the loving support and critical analysis from my other half, John Kapenga. Thank you, always.

TABLE OF CONTENTS

CHAPTER 1

The Clinical Research Coordinator (CRC)

The clinical research coordinator (CRC) is a specialized research professional working with, and under the direction of, the clinical investigator. Although the clinical investigator is legally responsible for the management of a clinical trial at a site, the CRC handles the bulk of daily clinical trial activities and plays a critical role in study conduct. In this chapter, we will discuss the knowledge and skills necessary to be a good CRC, as well as the duties and responsibilities of a CRC. The importance of the CRC to the efficient and effective operation of clinical trials cannot be over-emphasized; in fact, many sponsor companies will not place a trial at a study site that does not have a CRC working there.

Background and Training of the CRC

Although not required, most CRCs have been trained as nurses, physician assistants (PAs) or other medical professionals. If the CRC is a medical professional, he or she is better prepared to participate and be involved in study subject visits and care during the clinical trial. Medical personnel are more familiar with most of the settings where clinical trials are conducted, and therefore understand the language, the political interactions and the systems in those settings; this facilitates the ability to be effective within that system.

Many CRCs, however, are not medical professionals. They may have a science background and/or have worked their way up to their position through experience-based training in a physician's office. Many non-medical people have gained the appropriate knowledge to function effectively as a CRC.

There are many opportunities for CRCs to obtain training. The most common is informal training by another more experienced CRC, either at the same site or another site. If there is no experienced CRC on-site, an investigator may even send a new CRC to another research site for training.

Sponsor companies (the pharmaceutical, medical device and biotechnology companies that sponsor the conduct of clinical trials) also train CRCs, although this training is usually protocol- and study-specific, rather than covering the basics of the CRC job. Even investigator meetings, which are discussed later in this book, offer training opportunities for CRCs, both through the formal presentations and the informal interactions with the sponsor's clinical research associates (CRAs) and other CRCs who attend these meetings.

There are also books and other materials that are relevant for CRCs (including this book). There is a list of reference materials included in Appendix C.

There are formal training courses for CRCs, some offered by professional or other organizations, and some offered in university settings. Both the Association of Clinical Research Professionals (ACRP) and the Society for Clinical Research Associates (SoCRA) offer training, as well as certification programs for CRCs. The Drug Information Association (DIA) also offers training courses.

An increasing number of universities are offering undergraduate and graduate degrees in clinical research management. A formal education in this field enables CRCs to begin their career with the skills necessary for efficient and ethical management of clinical research, and provides them with knowledge and background needed to advance their career in clinical research management.

Certification for CRCs has been very well accepted over the past several years. There are prerequisites for taking the ACRP and SoCRA certification examinations, including at least two years of experience. Becoming certified is an excellent choice for an experienced CRC, as it shows a commitment to the position, and adds to the CRC's overall credentials. Details of each certification program may be found on each organization's web site at www.acrpnet.org and www.socra.org.

Personality and Skills

The CRC job is multi-faceted, with a mix of administrative, business, medical and patient duties. With such a wide range of responsibilities, CRCs must possess many skills. CRCs must have extremely good organizational skills, including the ability to handle a number of different tasks simultaneously. They must be detail-oriented (being picky and a perfectionist is helpful) in order to handle the paperwork aspects of the job well.

CRCs must also be people-oriented, as they must interact with patients, sponsor companies and others on a regular basis. CRCs must be self-confident, flexible and adaptable to change. They must also be focused, manage time well and follow through on problems and commitments. And perhaps most of all, CRCs need to have a high energy level—they are usually very busy people.

Where Do CRCs Work?

There are many types of investigative sites conducting studies, and CRCs work in all of them. It is useful for a CRC to have an understanding of these different organizations when looking for and assessing potential places to work. Some of the more common investigative site organizational types are listed below.

Part-Time Sites

Investigators at part-time sites participate in research studies but also maintain their regular medical practice. Sometimes these investigators do only one or two studies at a time, while others may participate in research to a greater degree, depending on their interest and the resources they have for doing studies. Most sponsors like this kind of site because there is greater potential for having study subjects readily available and because the physicians chosen for a study will become familiar with the drug, so that by the time it is marketed, they will be more likely to prescribe it to their patients. A CRC at a part-time site may only work part-time, or will be likely to have other responsibilities in addition to working on studies. There are other variations of the part-time site; for example, a large clinic may have a separate unit or department that does only studies, although the clinic as a whole sees non-study patients also. In this case, a CRC may work full-time as a CRC within the research unit.

Dedicated Sites

These sites are dedicated only to conducting studies; they do not have any other patients. They are generally very experienced, very productive, and have the advantage of being consistent in their practices. They tend also to be aware of which studies they can do successfully and are less apt to accept studies for which they do not think they can enroll sufficient subjects within the given time period. A CRC at a dedicated site will only work on studies and may be part of a team of CRCs.

Academic Sites

Academic sites are those located in universities and teaching hospitals. They tend to do a mix of investigator-initiated research and government-sponsored clinical trials, as well as industry-sponsored clinical trials. Often these organizations are headed by "thought leaders," the top specialists in their fields. Clinical trials may or may not be the academic site's primary interest. It is sometimes the industry trials that provide added funding to allow these sites to carry on other research. It is desirable for a sponsor to use some academic sites in their development programs. This allows thought leaders to become familiar with the new compounds and, hopefully, to become spokespersons in favor of the compound when it is marketed. Depending on the amount of research being done, an academic site may have anything from one part-time CRC to several CRCs.

Site Management Organizations (SMOs)

Site management organizations (SMOs) bring together a group of sites and organize them centrally to do studies. They standardize procedures across sites and often provide standardized materials (standard operating procedures (SOPs), study file procedures, source documents, etc.) to each site in the organization. Many SMOs also provide training for their sites and assist the site in compiling and submitting the required regulatory documents. They usually provide centralized services for marketing the sites (attracting clinical studies) and for subject recruitment. There are several types of SMOs, from those that own the sites in the group to those with other partnership agreements. Each practice within an SMO may have its own CRC(s) or they may be contracted from the SMO.

A variation of an SMO is the Coordinator Organization. This is usually a group of experienced study coordinators (CRCs) who have formed a business. They recruit investigators to do trials and then place an experienced CRC in the investigator's office to manage and help conduct the trial. These coordinators usually act as the interface with the sponsor/contract research organization (CRO) and manage the operational aspects of the trial; the physician is utilized for his or her medical expertise and patient base. In this case, the CRC is the main contact for all business aspects of the trial, including grant payments. (Note that the investigator is usually paid a fee by the coordinator organization.)

Regardless of how the physician's research practice is organized, the CRC will have the same general duties and responsibilities.

CRC Responsibilities

The CRC has multiple responsibilities. Although they may vary from site to site, the following list will show you the breadth of duties CRCs handle.

1. The CRC assists in evaluating new protocols for feasibility at the site. This includes:
   - Reviewing the protocol and other materials, such as the Investigator Brochure and informed consent form.
   - Looking at subject eligibility requirements and determining if those subjects would be available in the practice.
   - Assessing the ability to meet study timelines in light of other site commitments and overall feasibility.
   - Assessing the resources necessary to do the study, including people, physical space, materials, etc.
   - Assessing financial feasibility of performing the study (varies by site—CRC may or may not be involved).

2. The CRC prepares the site for conducting the study, including:
   - Training the people involved.
   - Setting up and organizing study files.
   - Creating or reviewing study-specific source documents (i.e., medical records, case report forms) and other study-related materials.
   - Disseminating information about the study to others in the institution and/or the community.
   - Creating advertising, if appropriate.
   - Preparing documents for submission to the institutional review board (IRB).
   - Collecting the documents needed to initiate the study and sending them to the sponsor.
   - Attending the investigator meeting, as appropriate.
   - Clarifying any necessary items with the sponsor.

3. The CRC participates in the informed consent process, which may include:
   - Assisting in writing consents.
   - Interacting with the sponsor and/or IRB on informed consent wording issues.
   - Presenting the informed consent form to potential subjects, discussing the consent and the study with them, and answering questions.
   - Obtaining subjects' signatures on the informed consent forms.
   - Ensuring that all necessary signatures and dates are on the informed consent forms.
   - Documenting, distributing and filing signed informed consent forms appropriately.
   - Ensuring that all amended consent forms are appropriately implemented and signed.

4. The CRC manages study conduct throughout the trial. This often includes:
   - Contacting and screening potential subjects for the study.
   - Recruiting subjects.
   - Scheduling subject and sponsor visits.
   - Preparing for each subject visit to ensure that all appropriate study procedures are done.
   - Assisting the investigator with study subject visits.
   - Ensuring that all necessary data are gathered and recorded in the appropriate source documents (i.e., patient charts) and the case report forms.
   - Reviewing case report form entries for completeness, correctness and logical sense. In addition, reviews the source documents and case report forms for adverse events that may have been missed.
   - Working with sponsor monitors (CRAs) during monitoring visits.
   - Making corrections to case report forms, if appropriate.
   - Resolving data queries.
   - Ensuring that study documents are complete, current and filed correctly.
   - Ensuring that test article accountability is done correctly for each subject and overall.
   - Managing laboratory procedures (drawing samples, processing, packaging and shipping).
   - Reordering study supplies as necessary.
   - Managing payments to study subjects, if appropriate.
   - Completing study closeout activities at the end of the study.

5. Other duties a CRC may have include:
   - Maintaining regular communications with sponsors and/or CROs, IRBs, and the institution, if the site is part of a larger institution such as a university or hospital. (Note: A contract research organization, CRO, is often retained by a sponsor company to perform some of the activities of a clinical program such as site monitoring.)
   - Collaborating with other departments (laboratory, pharmacy, etc.) as necessary.
   - Assisting the investigator with financial aspects of the trial, including budgeting and contracts.
   - Problem-solving.
   - Coordinating sponsor and/or regulatory audits.
   - Helping to recruit new studies.
   - Professionally representing the site to all people/organizations in the best possible light.

On top of all these responsibilities, the CRC must conduct all trial activities according to the appropriate federal and state regulations. Most important of all, the CRC must help to ensure the safety and well-being of all study subjects throughout the trial.

As you can see, being a CRC is a challenging position, but one filled with opportunities, with the added benefit of being involved in the process of bringing new drugs and therapies to people who will benefit from them.

Problems and Opportunities

One of the main problems sites have had to cope with over the past few years is the loss of one or more CRCs. Turnover among CRCs has a huge impact on site operations. A CenterWatch survey demonstrated that the number of CRCs who have been in their current position for less than three years rose from 40% in 1999 to 56% in 2002 and seems to have stabilized in 2003. It was also found that many CRCs were taking new jobs as clinical research associates (CRAs) for sponsors or CROs, or switching to careers outside of clinical research. The overall result is a decrease in the experience levels of CRCs. It appears that there are four common reasons for this CRC turnover: poor compensation, burnout due to heavy workload, personal life changes and competitive hiring by other sites.[1]

Table 1: Average Tenure with a Company

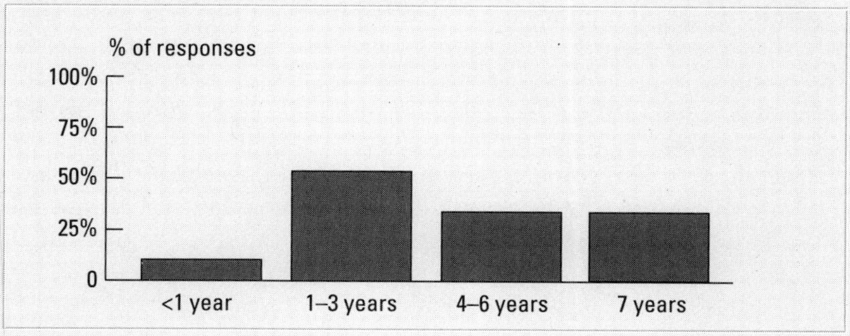

Source: CenterWatch analysis, 2003.

Since the loss of a good coordinator is devastating to a research site, sites are looking for ways to encourage their CRCs to stay. According to a recent CenterWatch survey, about 70% of CRCs make less than $49,000, about 25% make between $50,000 and $79,000, and a very small percentage make

1. "CRC Loss Tied to Heavy Workload." *The CenterWatch Monthly*, July 2004.

more than $80,000. Proactive sites are also looking for new solutions to improve retention and decrease turnover. Some sites have instituted flexible work schedules to allow their CRCs to adapt their work time for family schedules. Letting their CRCs know how much they are appreciated and needed also helps, so many sites work hard at acknowledging the contributions of their CRCs.

Table 2: Salary Ranges

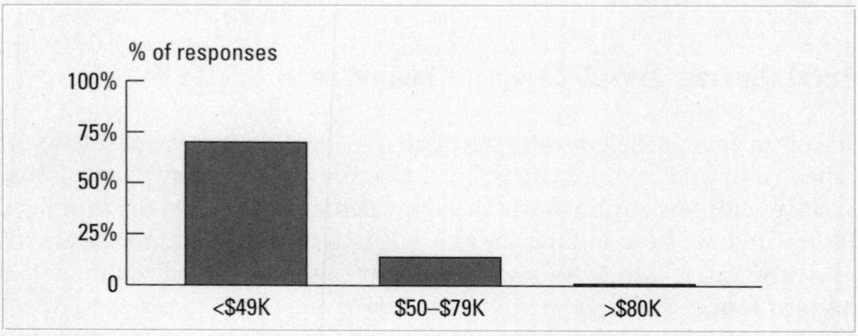

Source: CenterWatch analysis, 2003.

Burnout can be a real problem, so many sites are now trying to ensure that, with the exception of emergency situations, their CRCs work no more than 40 hours per week. They also work hard at providing extras—including such things as monthly lunches, team building seminars, laptops and computer training, and other opportunities for CRCs to develop new skills.

Sites are also becoming more selective in how they use their CRCs. Instead of using them for regulatory, recruitment and clerical tasks, they allow them to specialize in their main areas of responsibility and expertise, and funnel some of the other activities to ancillary personnel. This helps with the overtime and burnout problem.

Overall, sites have come to recognize the critical role that CRCs play in study success and are doing everything possible to retain and reward their CRCs. They are finding ways to better accommodate the professional and personal needs of study coordinators in order to improve retention and maintain the efficiency and effectiveness of their research operations.[2]

2. Ibid.

CHAPTER 2

Institutional Review Boards (IRBs)

Introduction

When conducting clinical trials, the safety of human subjects is paramount. The two main safeguards for human subjects are institutional review boards (IRBs) and the informed consent process. In this chapter, we'll discuss IRBs—what they are, their purpose and how they function. We will also discuss the interactions between IRBs and investigative sites.

The regulatory definition of an IRB (21 CFR § 56.102(g)) is: "any board, committee or group formally designated by an institution to review, approve the initiation of and to conduct periodic review of biomedical research involving human subjects. The primary purpose of such review is to assure the protection of the rights and welfare of the human subjects." Notice that an IRB must approve a study before it can start. Most research conducted with humans in the United States must be approved by an IRB. (21 CFR Part 56 contains the regulations that pertain to IRBs.) Note that "CFR" stands for the United States Code of Federal Regulations.

An investigator who is planning to do a trial must contact an IRB, submit the appropriate materials, including the proposed study protocol, and informed consent form, and wait for formal approval from the IRB before he or she may initiate the trial. Details about this process will appear later in the chapter. Interacting with and asking an IRB for approval are the responsibilities of the clinical investigator, not the pharmaceutical company that is sponsoring the research. On occasion a sponsor may send the protocol and study information for a multicenter trial directly to an independent IRB; however, the IRB must still interact with and approve the study for each individual investigator.

Types of IRBs

There are two types of IRBs, those affiliated with an institution ("local IRBs") and those that are not affiliated with a particular institution. The unaffiliated IRBs are called independent, central or national IRBs and can be used by any researcher who is not constrained by institutional policy to the use of a particular institutional review board.

If an investigator is affiliated with an institution (hospital or university, etc.) that has an IRB, and if that investigator is conducting the trial, or any part of the trial, at the institution, then he or she must usually use the institution's IRB. If the trial is being conducted at the investigator's private practice, and is not affiliated in any way with an institution, then he or she is not normally required to use the institution's IRB. If an investigator is doing a study at more than one institution (e.g., two hospitals) then IRB approval is required for each institution where the study will be conducted.

Independent IRBs, those not affiliated with a particular institution, are available to any investigator who is not affiliated with an institution, or who will not be conducting clinical trials at an institution, or whose institution does not have an IRB. Independent IRBs are frequently used for multi-center studies in non-hospitalized subjects. Study sponsors prefer to use independent IRBs when possible because, in general, they tend to act more quickly. The IRBs at some teaching hospitals, for example, can take three to six months to review a protocol, while most independent IRBs will have a review time of less than one month.

IRB Membership

An IRB must have at least five members, with varied backgrounds. Most IRBs also have alternate members, so that they will have a quorum if a regular member is unable to be present. The members must possess appropriate professional competence to review the diverse types of protocols that are received.

There must be at least one member who is not affiliated with the institution (and who has no immediate family member affiliated with the institution) other than his or her IRB membership. There must also be one member whose interests and background are non-scientific (i.e., a layperson). It's acceptable for one IRB member to fulfill both of these criteria. In addition, an IRB that reviews FDA-regulated products (drugs, biologics and devices) must have at least one member who is a physician.

IRB membership should be selected to assure appropriate diversity, including representation by multiple professions, multiple ethnic backgrounds and both genders, and must include both scientific and non-scientific members.

IRB Operations

IRBs are required by regulation to follow written procedures. IRBs are audited by regulatory authorities, and they will be held responsible for having appropriate written procedures and for following them. They must also carefully document their decisions and retain this documentation appropriately.

IRB Responsibilities

Whether the IRB is affiliated with a particular institution or not, its primary responsibility is to protect the rights and welfare of human subjects participating in clinical research. To fulfill this responsibility, the IRB will answer two basic questions:

1. Should the study be done at all?
2. If so, what constitutes adequate informed consent?

The Benefit vs. Risk Assessments

In determining whether or not the study should be done, the IRB must consider several items. The IRB members must have assurance that the study is scientifically valid, that is, that there is a properly designed protocol. The charge of an IRB is not to judge the scientific merit or worth of the trial. This means that it is not the function of an IRB to decide whether we need another drug for hypertension, for example, but rather to determine if the research methods being used to study that potential antihypertensive are valid.

Risks to the subjects must be minimized, so the IRB will look for a sound research design without unnecessary exposure to risk. They will also ascertain if the protocol uses procedures that would be performed on these patients, both diagnostically and for treatment, even if they were not in the study, insomuch as it is feasible to do. The idea is to treat patients in a study as closely as possible to how they would be treated if they were not in the study, adding, of course, those activities that are required to test the study hypothesis.

The IRB must determine whether the anticipated benefit to subjects and the overall knowledge to be gained from the research compares favorably to the risks. In this evaluation, the IRB considers only those risks and benefits that may result directly from the research, excluding the risks and benefits that the subjects would have encountered even if they had not been involved in the research (if they had just received the standard treatment for the condition). Remember that there are always risks involved in doing research. The compounds being studied are new and not much is known about them; that is why research to determine if they are safe and efficacious is being done.

The IRB will also want to know what the subject selection process is, in order to ensure that the selection is equitable, and that no groups of potential subjects are routinely excluded or included based on non-study-related characteristics. Depending on the particular study, some of these characteristics might include sex, race, ethnic background, weight, smoking, educational background, etc. In making this assessment, the IRB will consider the particular setting in which the research will be done, as well as the purposes of the research.

What Constitutes Adequate Informed Consent?

If the IRB determines that the benefits outweigh the risks and that it is acceptable to do the study, then they will consider the consent form submitted by the investigator. It is a regulatory requirement that informed consent be sought from each subject, or the subject's legally authorized representative, before that person may be enrolled in the research project. By regulation (21 CFR 50.27), informed consent must be documented, which is usually done by having the subject sign a hard copy of the informed consent document. Consents are discussed in detail in Chapter 3, Informed Consent.

Along with the hard copy of the informed consent, there must be provisions in the research plan for ongoing sponsor safety monitoring of the data, with the goal of ensuring the safety of the subjects during the research. It's not sufficient, for example, to have all the adverse event data looked at only at the completion of a trial—it must be regularly reviewed throughout the study period, in case problems arise as more is learned about the product under investigation.

The IRB will also determine whether or not there are adequate provisions in the research to protect the privacy of the research subjects, as well as to maintain the confidentiality of the data, where appropriate.

Payments to study subjects and advertising are considered by the U.S. Food and Drug Administration (FDA) and IRBs as part of the consent process, as they both might encourage a subject to enroll in a trial. If subjects are to be paid for their participation in the research, the IRB will review the planned compensation to ensure that it does not constitute an undue influence, or coercion, that could influence the subject's decision to participate. Ideally, subjects would not take the risks involved in study participation simply because of the compensation. An exception is phase I studies using healthy volunteers; in this case, subjects usually volunteer due, at least in part, to the compensation offered. The IRB's decision will be based not only on the amount subjects may receive for being in the study, but the setting in which the study will take place. An amount that may be coercive in one setting may not be so in another.

The IRB will also review any proposed advertising to ensure it does not make misleading or untruthful claims, and does not constitute undue influence. Glowing claims of success for a new treatment, for example, can also influence subjects to participate in a trial that they would not want to be involved with otherwise.

Vulnerable Subjects

Sometimes special, vulnerable populations are studied in research trials. Vulnerable subjects include children, pregnant women, prisoners, handicapped or mentally disabled people, people with acute or severe mental illness, people who are economically or educationally disadvantaged, and those who are vulnerable because they are institutionalized. If any of these categories of people are going to be included in the research, the IRB needs to determine whether or not there are sufficient additional safeguards to protect them from coercion or undue influence. There are a number of National Institutes of Health (NIH) regulations (45 CFR 46) regarding research in various vulnerable populations. 21 CFR 50 Subpart D (Additional Safeguards for Children in Clinical Investigations) contains regulations that must be taken into account when conducting clinical trials that involve children. If an investigator and his or her staff are involved in research with vulnerable populations, they should familiarize themselves with these regulations.

State and Local Regulations

The IRB must determine that the research does not violate any existing state or local laws or regulations, or any applicable institutional policies or practices. Some states, notably California and Massachusetts, have regulations that may exceed the federal regulations. People working in these states, and others, should be familiar with their state requirements for doing research. As an example, California has a patient bill of rights that must be provided to every study subject in a trial.

IRB Review of Proposed Research

An IRB considers each research project submitted for review separately. In order to determine if the research meets all the criteria discussed above, the IRB will review the investigator qualifications, the study protocol and supporting documents, the proposed consent form, and any subject compensation or advertising, if applicable.

Materials Submitted to the IRB by an Investigator

To ensure an adequate review, the investigator must submit a number of materials to the IRB for review, including the following:

1. A current CV that includes his or her qualifications for conducting the research, including education, training and experience.
2. The study protocol, which includes or addresses the following items, as applicable:
   - Title of the study.
   - Purpose of the study, including any expected benefits.
   - Sponsor of the study.
   - Results from previous related research.
   - Subject inclusion/exclusion criteria.
   - Study design, including a discussion of the appropriateness of the research methods.
   - Description and schedule of the procedures to be performed.
   - Provisions for managing adverse events.
   - Payment to subjects for their participation.
   - Compensation for injuries to research subjects.
   - Provisions for protecting subject privacy.
   - Extra costs to subjects for participation in the study.
   - Extra costs to third-party payers because of a subject's participation.
3. The investigator brochure or package insert, if applicable.
4. The proposed informed consent document, containing all appropriate elements.
5. All subject advertisements and recruitment procedures. In general, advertising includes anything that is directed toward potential research subjects and is designed for recruitment.
6. Form FDA 1572 (Statement of Investigator form), if applicable. This form is required for all FDA-regulated studies done under an Investigational New Drug Application (IND). Some IRBs do not require this, but many do. (See form in Appendix D.)
7. Grant application for federally funded research, if applicable.

8. Any other specific forms or materials required by the IRB, such as an application form.

At many, if not most, investigative sites, the clinical research coordinator is the one who actually assembles and submits the packet of information to an IRB. It helps to use a checklist so that nothing is forgotten; missing documents cause delays in IRB review. Some IRBs furnish investigators with a checklist that comprises all their particular requirements. If your IRB does not furnish you with one, it is good to make your own and have it ready for each study. There is an example of a checklist in Appendix D.

FAQ

Do I have to tell the IRB how much the site is being paid for doing the study?

No. However, if you are doing federally funded research, you must submit a copy of the grant proposal to the IRB with the other research materials. (With conflict of interest becoming more of an issue, this may change in the future.)

IRB Deliberations

After the complete documents are received from an investigator, an IRB will schedule the protocol for review. For the initial review of a protocol, the board will meet to decide whether or not to approve the proposed research. In order to make this decision, the board will review all the submitted materials and discuss the proposed research, followed by a vote. The IRB may approve the project, request changes or additional information in order to approve it, or disapprove it.

FAQ

The IRB chair notified us in person that our study has been approved. Can we start enrolling subjects now?

No. You must wait for the official written notification. Most sponsor companies will not send you the investigational drug or device until they have a copy of the IRB approval letter, but even if they have, you may not start until you have the written approval.

The IRB must notify the investigator in writing that the study is approved. If a study is disapproved, the IRB will also notify the investigator in writing of its action, and the reasons for disapproval, and must allow the investigator to address the IRB concerning the decision either in writing or in person.

Any planned advertising must be approved before use, although this does not have to be approved before the study begins. Advertising is often started after study initiation, especially when subject recruitment has not been as rapid as anticipated. We will discuss the specifics of advertising in Chapter 9, Working with Study Subjects.

Most importantly, IRB approval of the study and the consent form must be obtained prior to subject enrollment. It is most often the CRC who will be in contact with the IRB in order to check on the status of the approval and the official written notification of approval.

FAQ

If the IRB disapproves my study, can I take it to another IRB?

No. You should determine why the research was not approved and see if it is possible to modify it to make it acceptable. Note: there could be an exceptional circumstance where it might be ethical to submit the research to another IRB, but this is extremely rare, and the second IRB should be informed of the first disapproval and reasons for it.

Investigator Reporting Responsibilities

Throughout the study, the investigator must report any protocol changes or amendments to the IRB. Any change that would increase risk to subjects must be approved by the IRB prior to implementation and may require a change to the informed consent form. The only exception to this is when the change is necessary to eliminate an apparent immediate hazard to the safety and well-being of the subjects, in which case the change should be implemented immediately, followed by a timely notification and submission to the IRB. For example, if it were determined during a trial that taking a particular concomitant medication is unsafe, sites would be notified by the sponsor to immediately stop giving that particular medication to study patients. Sites would start doing this immediately, then notify their IRBs. These exceptions are relatively rare.

The investigator must also promptly report "immediately reportable" adverse events to the IRB. These usually include deaths and other serious medical events that are unexpected during the study. Occasionally deaths may be the expected outcome in a study; in this case, the reporting rules may change and deaths will not be reported as immediately reportable adverse events. This exception is also quite rare. (Adverse event reporting is discussed in detail in Chapter 11.)

The investigator must also promptly report to the IRB any unanticipated problems that arise during the research that involve risk to the study subjects or others.

The investigator is also required to submit periodic reports to the IRB, detailing the progress of the study. This will be submitted at least annually, and may be required on a more frequent basis. Although the investigator is the responsible person for these reports to the IRB, the reports are usually delegated to the CRC.

Continuing Review of a Research Study

The IRB will review each research project at least annually, although the IRB may require updates on a more frequent basis, such as quarterly, based on the degree of risk to which the subjects are exposed. At the continuing review, the IRB will ensure that the risk-to-benefit relationship remains acceptable, that the consent and study documents being used are still appropriate, and that the selection of subjects has been equitable.

To help in making these determinations, most IRBs will require the investigator to submit an IRB-specific form asking about the progress of the study, including enrollment figures and withdrawals, adverse events and unanticipated problems, protocol violations, etc., at each review period. The IRB may also want to see a copy of the currently used consent form, advertising and any other appropriate documents. The IRB will ask for any protocol amendments during the time period, especially if they were not previously reviewed by the IRB. This information allows the IRB to determine whether or not the research can continue. Many IRBs have a checklist to be used for periodic reporting; some IRBs provide these forms on their own web site. By obtaining this checklist in advance, the CRC can be prepared to submit these reports in a timely manner.

All research must be reapproved at least annually. The investigator will receive written notification of each formal reapproval. Re-review and reapproval continue throughout the entire research project, until such time as all subjects have completed their participation and the project is closed. If the study is not reapproved by the date that the last approval expired, it is out of compliance with the regulations. This is not a situation that an investigative site wants to be in; not only could it result in an unfavorable audit finding, but it reflects poorly on the organizational skills of the CRC and the investigator.

If an investigator has not submitted the required study updates to the IRB for review, the IRB has several options. The IRB may send the investigator a reminder that he or she is required to submit the update, with a deadline for receipt of the requested materials. If the reminder does not work, the IRB may put enrollment on hold until the updates are received and reviewed. In the worst case, the IRB may withdraw approval of the study. It is important to remember that each approval is good only for a specified time period. If reapproval is not received prior to the expiration date of the previous approval, the study is out of compliance with the regulations.

Expedited Review

Upon occasion, an IRB may utilize an expedited review process for minor changes in previously approved research; this may be done only during the time period for which the approval was authorized. Expedited review may be done by the IRB Chairperson, or by experienced members who are designated as expedited reviewers. Items may be approved by expedited review, but they cannot be disapproved. If the expedited reviewer(s) think something should be disapproved, it must go to the full board. The board must also be made aware of all expedited review decisions, which is usually done at the first regular meeting following the review.

Expedited review is never used in circumstances where the risk to human subjects increases. It cannot, in general, be used for the initial review of a research study. There are a few exceptions where initial review of a project can be done using expedited review, but these are not the kinds of studies in which CRCs would normally be involved; these exceptions are published in the Federal Register. A site should never expect to have an initial approval done by expedited review.

Conflict of Interest

No IRB member may participate in the initial or continuing review of any research project with which they have a conflicting interest. A person whose research is being reviewed may be present at the IRB meeting to answer questions and give information about the project, but he or she should not be present for the discussion leading to the vote, nor during the actual voting. The minutes of the meeting need to reflect that the person was not present, to alleviate any claim of conflict of interest.

An investigator may sit on an IRB, as may a CRC or other site staff. However, if your study is going to be reviewed, you need to leave the meeting during the discussion leading to the vote and during the actual vote, and this information must be included in the minutes. This resolves any conflict of interest situation.

FAQ

Can an investigator sit on an IRB?

Yes, but he or she can participate neither in the discussion leading to the vote nor in the voting for his or her own research. (Look under the section on conflict of interest.)

CRC Duties and Responsibilities

Usually the CRC is the one who puts together the submissions to the IRB, tracks their progress and maintains the appropriate files. This involves gathering together all the documents that are required, obtaining signatures from the investigator as needed and ensuring that appropriate copies go to the necessary people by the deadlines. It helps to use checklists, either those furnished by the IRB, or ones you have made yourself. It also involves maintaining good, organized files and keeping them current. Ensuring that IRB documentation is done appropriately helps keep your study in compliance and eliminates future problems. Sponsors are increasingly involved in this process and may want to see the documents being submitted to the IRB before they are actually sent.

Key Things to Remember

- IRBs are one of the primary safeguards for the protection of human subjects of research.
- CFR Part 56 contains the FDA regulations that pertain to IRBs.
- An IRB must approve a study and the informed consent document before the study can start.
- There are two types of IRBs, those affiliated with an institution and those that are independent.
- The IRB must make a risk vs. benefit assessment for each proposed project.
- There are special regulations concerning research in vulnerable subjects (children, pregnant women, prisoners, etc.).
- State and local research regulations must also be followed.
- IRBs must approve advertising prior to use.
- IRBs must approve any subject compensation.
- An investigator must report adverse events and study progress to the IRB at least annually.
- Continuing review of a study must be done at least annually.

- Expedited review may not be used for the initial review of a project, except in particular instances published in the Federal Register.
- IRB members may not vote if they have conflicts of interest.
- The CRC is the primary person who interacts with the IRB at most investigative sites.

CHAPTER 3

Informed Consent

Introduction

The decision each subject makes whether or not to participate in a study is not an easy one. A potential subject should not make a decision that is based purely on emotions such as fear and hope. Instead, everything possible must be done to provide complete information in a format that is comprehensive yet easy to comprehend, along with sufficient time to make an informed decision.

One of the main safeguards for the protection of human subjects in research is informed consent. In this chapter, we will discuss informed consents, including the regulations governing consent, the writing of consents and the administration of consents.

Defining Informed Consent

Informed consent is defined by the International Conference on Harmonisation (ICH) Guidelines for Good Clinical Practice as "*A process by which a subject voluntarily confirms his or her willingness to participate in a particular trial, after having been informed of all aspects of the trial that are rel-*

evant to the subjects decision to participate. Informed consent is documented by means of a written, signed and dated informed consent form."[1]

The two key words in this definition are "voluntarily" and "informed." These words form the cornerstone of ethical conduct in clinical research, and are in place to protect the rights and safety of the subjects who participate in research. Potential subjects of clinical research must understand what they are getting into, and must be free to decline to participate.

A proper informed consent process should leave the potential study subject the freedom to say "No" without feeling guilty or fearing repercussion. Many people have a certain reverence for their personal physicians; they want to please their physicians and will do as their doctor directs. This carries over into consenting to participate in a study and needs to be avoided by physicians involved in research. Investigators and CRCs must make every effort to help potential study subjects understand that it is entirely acceptable if they choose not to participate. People should understand that they are free to decline participation and that they will not lose any benefits of care if they decline.

Preparing the Informed Consent Document

Unless the consent for your study has been provided by the sponsor, preparing the informed consent document is one of the primary responsibilities of the investigator and CRC during a clinical trial. This is because it is so important ethically and because problems with consent forms are frequent deficiencies in clinical investigator inspections conducted by the FDA. The problem is not that the consent process is not done, but that it is not being done correctly. Common problems are:

- The timing is not correct, e.g., study procedures being done before the consent is signed.
- Proper signatures are not always obtained.
- The consent form is poorly written.
- There are missing required elements.

The first step in properly obtaining informed consent is to be familiar with the requirements, both for the document itself and the process. There are three basic requirements that a consent form must meet:

1. ICH Guideline for Good Clinical Practice, as published in the Federal Register May 9, 1997. Part I. Glossary.

- It must completely and accurately describe all of the activities required by the protocol and what the subject's participation will involve.
- It must be understandable by the study subjects.
- It must contain all the elements required by regulation (21 CFR, Part 50).

In other words, consents must inform, be comprehensible and comply with regulations. Let's look more closely at each of these requirements.

Activities and Participation

Potential study subjects need to be told about the study and their involvement in detail to be able to make an informed decision regarding their participation. Subjects need to know they will be participating in research, what is required of them and the potential benefits and risks they will face. The required elements of consent will be discussed later in this chapter. All the requirements (tests, procedures, activities, etc.) of the protocol must be described, including a description of how these various activities will have an impact on the subjects, both in terms of personal discomfort and any lifestyle changes. Subjects also need to know when each activity must be done, and how long it will take for each activity and study visit.

Readability and Comprehension

It is difficult to adequately inform potential subjects about a study without overwhelming them. A consent form may contain a very detailed description of protocol activities and consequences, but when it is a long, multiple-page document, a subject may not have a good feel for what will happen because the document is just too long and there is simply too much information to deal with.

The consent form needs to be technically correct, yet intelligible for non-medical people. Consent forms should be written at approximately the 6th to 8th grade levels according to most IRBs. This is a challenge in an industry filled with jargon, acronyms, medical terminology and highly educated people. In general, the shorter the sentences and the fewer syllables per word that there are in the text, the easier it will be to comprehend and understand. Make a conscious effort to use terminology such as "teaspoons" instead of "cubic centimeters or milliliters," or "sick to your stomach" instead of "nauseated." Here is an example of some text from an informed consent document that is written at different grade levels:

> *"If any significant new information about the study drug becomes available during your participation in the study, and that information might affect your willingness to continue in the study, the doctor in charge of the study will tell you about it."*

This paragraph is written at the 12th grade level, which is too high for an informed consent document.

> *"If we find out anything new about the study drug while you are in the study, we will let you know. This will help you to decide if you would like to continue."*

This is written at a 5th grade level and would be much more acceptable in a consent form.

Recent Findings

In a recent article,[2] the way grade levels are measured was called into question. Recent studies demonstrate that the way reading comprehension is tested varies to the point where it is impossible to compare the results. Mark Hochhauser, Ph.D., in his article "Informed Consent: Reading and Understanding Are Not the Same" contends that the Flesch-Kincaid formula in MicroSoft Word is "too unreliable and inaccurate to recommend or use since researchers cannot reliably verify the grade level of a consent form." Hochhauser also posits that testing a potential subject's reading comprehension with "true-false and multiple-choice questions are flawed because subjects can get a percentage of answers correct by guessing... Such methods for measuring subject comprehension may not be sufficiently sensitive to detect true understanding."

According to a study published in the *Journal of the American Information Association*,[3] potential subjects want features such as those listed in Table 1 in their informed consent forms. The same study found that IRB members and researchers made similar recommendations.

Table 1: Tips for an Improved Consent Form

- Provide a summary of highlights, with the details kept separate.
- Provide a glossary; define terms.
- Use lay language throughout.
- Provide information on the clinical trials in general.
- Use larger font for text.
- Emphasize what is important.
- Use graphics and video.

2. M. Hochhauser, "Informed Consent: Reading and Understanding Are Not the Same," *Applied Clinical Trials*, Vol. 13, Number 4, pp. 42–48, April 2004.
3. H. Jimison, P.P. Sher, R. Appleyard, Y. LeVernois, "The Use of Multimedia in the Informed Consent Process," *Journal of the American Information Association* 5(3) 245–256 (1998).

Elements

Finally, and by far the easiest of the three requirements for a proper consent form, is to make it compliant with federal regulations. 21 CFR Part 50.25, which contains the elements of informed consent, is one of the more straightforward regulations. It clearly lists the elements that must be present in a consent form (basic elements) and those additional elements, which are to be provided when appropriate.

Basic Elements of Consent[4]

The basic elements of consent, taken from the federal regulations, must be present in all consent forms. They are:

- A statement that *the study involves research*, the *purpose* of the research, *duration* of the subject's participation, a *description of procedures* to be followed, and identification of any *procedures that are experimental.*
- A description of any reasonably foreseeable *risks or discomfort* to the subjects.
- A description of any *benefits* to the subjects or others that can reasonably be expected from the research.
- A disclosure of appropriate *alternate procedures* or courses of treatment, if any, that might be advantageous to the subject.
- A statement describing the extent, if any, to which *confidentiality of records* identifying the subject will be maintained and that notes the possibility that the FDA may inspect the records.
- For research involving more than minimal risk, an explanation as to whether any *compensation* and an explanation as to whether any *medical treatments* are available if injury occurs and, if so, what they consist of, or where further information may be obtained.
- An explanation of *whom to contact* for answers to pertinent questions about the research and research subjects' rights, and whom to contact in the event of a research-related injury to the subject.
- A statement that participation is *voluntary*, that refusal to participate will involve no penalty or loss of benefits to which the subject is otherwise entitled, and that the subject may discontinue participation at any time without penalty or loss of benefits to which the subject is otherwise entitled.

Additional Elements of Consent

The additional elements of consent,[5] which should be included as appropriate, are:

---

4. 21 CFR 50.25.
5. 21 CFR 50.25.

- A statement that the particular treatment or procedure may involve risks to the subject (or to the embryo or fetus, if the subject is or may become pregnant) that are currently unforeseeable.
- Anticipated circumstances under which the subject's participation may be terminated by the investigator without regard to the subject's consent.
- Any additional costs to the subject that may result from participation in the research.
- The consequences of the subject's decision to withdraw from the research and procedures for orderly termination of participation of the subject.
- A statement that significant new findings developed during the course of the research that may relate to the subject's willingness to continue participation will be provided to the study subject.
- The approximate number of subjects involved in the study.

One way of ensuring that all the elements are present in a consent form is to have an explicit heading for subsections that address each element. In any case, it must be clear that each of the elements is addressed in the form, so the form will not be found deficient in an FDA review.

Table 2: Example of an Informed Consent Element Using a Heading

Purpose of the research
The purpose of this research study is to find out if the study drug is safe and works for patients with moderately high blood pressure. The study drug has the brand name ANTIACHE Tablets. It is not yet approved for sale, but this is not the first time it has been tested in people. (Grade level is 6.5.)

Some states and institutions also have requirements that may affect the content of the form. California, for example, has a one-page Patient Bill of Rights that must be attached to all consent forms.

Note that if the sponsor has provided you with an informed consent template, you should not change this consent without consulting the sponsor.

An increasing number of universities are offering undergraduate and ...te degrees in clinical research management. A formal education in this ... CRCs to begin their career with the skills necessary for efficient ...ment of clinical research, and provides them with knowl- ...eded to advance their career in clinical research

Obtaining Informed Consent

The investigator and/or the CRC are usually the people charged with obtaining consent from study subjects. Informed consent must be obtained from subjects at the proper time and in the proper manner. The first thing to remember is that no person may be involved as a research subject unless the person, or the person's legally authorized representative, has given consent. Secondly, a subject's consent must be obtained before the subject is involved in any study-related activity. Your sponsor CRA will always check consents for when they were signed when monitoring your study. The time of consent versus when the subject started the study is also almost always checked during FDA site inspections.

FAQ

The consent for our study was changed by the sponsor to reflect new information about adverse events. Nothing else changed—just the addition of two more possible adverse events to the list. Does the IRB need to approve the revised consent?

Yes. Any change in a consent that involves risk should be approved by an IRB before use. Most IRBs will want to approve any change to a consent form. The revised consent form should be dated appropriately to differentiate it from previous versions.

Who must sign the revised consent?

All new subjects enrolled after the revised consent became effective should sign it. Also, all subjects who are still in the trial should sign the revised consent form. Generally it is acceptable for those subjects to read and sign the new consent at their next regularly scheduled visit. Some IRBs allow sites to add the new material as a one-page addendum to the consent, and just ask their current subjects to review and sign the addendum; new subjects must have the full consent, of course.

There are two types of consent forms, the short form and the long form. Both must be approved by an IRB before use. Documentation of approval must be maintained by the site.

FAQ

Sometimes we're caught in the middle between the sponsor and the IRB when it comes to the preferred language for the consent form. Who has the ultimate responsibility for this decision?

This is always awkward—you can't do the study without IRB approval for the consent, and yet sometimes the sponsor will not budge on the wording they want, especially when it comes to indemnification language. Sometimes it works best to suggest direct contact between the IRB chairman and the sponsor; having everything go through the site is not very effective. If agreement can not be reached, you may not be able to participate in the study.

The Informed Consent—Short Form[6]

The short form consent may be used in circumstances when, in the best judgment of the investigator and with the concurrence of the IRB, it would be the most appropriate way for the subject to comprehend and give informed consent. The short form supplements and documents an oral presentation of the information that is provided to the study subject as part of the consent process. If this method is used:

- The form must state that all elements of consent required by regulation have been presented orally to the subject or subject's legally authorized representative.
- There must be a witness to the oral presentation.
- The IRB must approve a written summary of what is to be said to the subject or his or her representative.
- Only the short form itself is to be signed by the subject or his or her representative.
- The witness will sign both the short form and a copy of the written summary.
- The person obtaining the consent will sign a written copy of the summary.
- A copy of the short form and the summary will be given to the subject or his or her representative.

The Informed Consent—Long Form

This is the standard consent form and process and is the consent method of choice whenever possible. The main difference between the two forms is that the long form spells out in writing everything that is presented orally when

6. 21 CFR 50.27.

Table 3: Example of a California Patient's Bill of Rights for Study Subjects

Any person who is requested to consent to participate as a subject in a research study involving a medical experiment, or who is requested to consent on behalf of another, has the right to:

- Be informed of the nature and purpose of the experiment.
- Be given an explanation of the procedures to be followed in the medical experiment, and any drug or device to be used.
- Be given a description of any attendant discomforts and risks reasonably to be expected from the experiment, if applicable.
- Be given an explanation of any benefits to the subject reasonably to be expected from the experiment, if applicable.
- Be given a disclosure of any appropriate alternative procedures, drugs, or devices that might be advantageous to the subject, and their relative risks and benefits.
- Be informed of the avenues of medical treatment, if any, available to the subject after the experiment or if complications should arise.
- Be given an opportunity to ask any questions concerning the experiment or other procedures involved.
- Be instructed that consent to participate in the medical experiment may be withdrawn at any time, and the subject may discontinue in the medical experiment without prejudice.
- Be given a copy of a signed and dated written informed consent form when one is required.
- Be given the opportunity to decide to consent or not to consent to a medical experiment without the intervention of any element of force, fraud, deceit, duress, coercion, or undue influence on the subject's decision.

the short form is used; the subject reads the written long form. Consequently, no summary is needed. The subject signs and dates two copies, one to keep and one for the investigator. The only signature required on the long form is that of the subject; however, many IRBs also require investigator and/or witness signatures.

The Consent Process

As a CRC you will frequently be involved in the actual consent process. Here are some suggestions that can be used during the informed consent process:

- Have a site person read the consent form while the subject follows along. This usually improves comprehension and is helpful for subjects who may not read well.
- Have the presenter summarize what was read, emphasizing the more important activities.
- Always ask the subject if there are any questions. Answer them completely and truthfully.
- Never try to convince a subject to participate.
- Ask the subject some questions about the consent material to determine how well the subject understood what was presented. This will often generate additional questions from the subject.
- A video presentation of the consent form can be an effective tool. If the site has a person who is a particularly good presenter, this person could describe the study in the video. Camcorders are relatively inexpensive and can produce good quality recordings. In addition to ensuring that all subjects hear the same thing, the video documents what was said. The video, however, should never replace the involvement of the investigator, who should always be present to talk with subjects and to answer questions.
- The consent process should not be rushed. Subjects must be given ample time to assess, evaluate and discuss the information they have been given before having to make a decision. A subject may want to take the form home to discuss with family members before making a decision.
- The consent process should always be documented in the patient's chart.

Table 4: Example of a Chart Notation Documenting the Informed Consent Process

June 8, 2004
The informed consent document for the Acme Company protocol 1234/0012 was presented to Bill Smith at 2:15 p.m. This protocol is for an investigational drug (Drug 1234) vs. placebo in moderate hypertension. Details of the protocol procedures were discussed, as well as potential benefits and risks. Alternate therapies were presented. Mr. Smith read the consent (Version dated 4/3/2004), asked questions, discussed it with his wife, and decided to participate. He signed the consent at 3:25 p.m. 6/8/04. A signed copy of the consent form was given to the patient. His first study visit will take place on Thursday, June 10, 2004.

—Cynthia Rodgers, CRC

Exceptions from Consent

There are two situations in which exceptions to consent may be made for patients using investigational products. Since the use of consents is usually mandatory in clinical studies, these two situations are unique. The individual exception is for research involving the individual emergency use of a test article in a single individual, as provided for in 21 CFR 50.23. Chances are good that you will never be involved in an individual exception from consent, as these are quite rare. The emergency research exception involves entire studies in which, because of the expected circumstances, it is not generally feasible to obtain consent before patients must be treated (21 CFR 50.24). If you do studies in trauma patients, you may very well be involved in the exception to consent for emergency research. These exceptions are discussed below.

Individual Exceptions[7]

An occasional circumstance will arise where an investigator feels there is a subject who would benefit from the use of an investigational product, but who is not in a study or who would not qualify for the study. For example, there may be a patient who is near death from a severe infection, where all suitable marketed antibiotics have been tried, but the infective bacteria are all resistant to these drugs. The patient does not qualify for any on-going study. Under this exemption this patient may be treated with one of the new unapproved powerful antibiotics that might cure his infection. Although a physician may treat a patient with an investigational product in a case like this, he must follow the regulations discussed below.

According to the regulations, obtaining informed consent is feasible unless, before use of the investigational product, both the investigator and a physician who is not otherwise participating in the clinical investigation certify in writing all of the following:

- The human subject is confronted by a life-threatening situation necessitating the use of the test article.
- Informed consent cannot be obtained from the subject because of an inability to communicate with, or obtain legally effective consent from, the subject.
- Time is not sufficient to obtain consent from the subject's legally authorized representative.
- There is available no alternative method of approved or generally recognized therapy that provides an equal or greater likelihood of saving the life of the subject.

The exception to this is if immediate use of the test article is, in the investigator's opinion, required to preserve the life of the subject, and time is not

7. 21 CFR 50.23.

sufficient to obtain the independent determination in advance of using the test article. In this case, the determination of the clinical investigator shall be made and, within five working days after the use of the article, be reviewed and evaluated in writing by a physician who is not participating in the clinical investigation. The documentation required must be submitted to the investigator's IRB within five working days after the use of the test article.

These types of exceptions are rare. If the investigator wants to be able to use the product for this type of patient again in the future, then the investigator must submit a protocol to the IRB as for any study.

Exception From Informed Consent Requirements for Emergency Research Studies[8]

In some kinds of studies, obtaining informed consent from study subjects prior to their participation may not be possible. Examples of these studies are those in which the subject has a life-threatening trauma to the body, such as a head injury or a heart attack. Not only are the subjects in these studies not able to give consent prior to being treated, but there may not be time to identify and locate a subject's legally authorized representative before treatment must begin. Frequently, these studies have a relatively short window of opportunity for treatment; e.g., treatment must commence within two hours of the injury.

Exceptions or waivers from consent must be approved in advance of the study by the IRB. It is not the investigator or the sponsor who makes the determination of whether or not the exception is allowed. It must be approved by an IRB, with the agreement from a licensed physician who is not associated with the research project but who may or may not be a member of the IRB. In order for the IRB to make this determination, the following must be documented:

- The subjects are in a life-threatening situation, available treatments are unproven or unsatisfactory and the collection of valid scientific evidence is necessary to determine the safety and effectiveness of the particular intervention.
- Obtaining informed consent is not feasible because:
  - The subjects will not be able to give consent because of their medical condition.
  - The intervention under investigation must be administered before consent can be obtained from the subject's legally authorized representative.
  - There is no way to identify prospectively the individuals likely to become eligible for participation in the study.
  - Participation in the research may have direct benefit to the subject because:

8. 21 CFR 50.24.

- The subject is in a life-threatening situation that necessitates intervention.
- Previous research, both pre-clinical and/or clinical, provides supporting evidence of the potential for the intervention to provide a direct benefit to the subject.
- Risks associated with the intervention are reasonable in relation to what is known about the medical condition of the potential class of subjects, the risks and benefits of standard therapy, and what is known, if anything, about the risks and benefits of the experimental treatment or intervention.

- The clinical investigation could not practically be carried out without the waiver.
- The protocol defines the length of the therapeutic window based on scientific evidence and the investigator commits to attempting to contact the subject's legally authorized representative or family member within that window of opportunity and asking for consent, if feasible, rather than proceeding without consent. The investigator will summarize efforts to contact legally authorized representatives and provide this information to the IRB and the time of continuing review.
- The IRB has approved the consent form and process to be used when informing the subject, when possible, or the subject's legally authorized representative or a family member.
- Additional protections of the rights and welfare of the subjects will be provided to include:
  - Consultation with the community in which the study will be conducted and the subjects selected.
  - Public disclosure (in the community in which the study is to be conducted) prior to initiation of the study, including plans for the study and the risks and benefits associated with it.
  - Public disclosure following completion of the study of sufficient information to apprise researchers and the community of the study, including demographics of the study population and its results.
  - Establishment of an independent data monitoring committee to exercise oversight of the investigation.

The IRB also has a responsibility to see that the study subject is informed about the nature of the study and his or her involvement in it as soon as that can be done. If the subject remains incapacitated, then the legally authorized representative, or if not available, a family member, must be updated. The legally authorized representative (or family member) should also be told that he or she may request that the subject be removed from the study at any time without penalty or loss of benefit.

Conclusion

A primary safeguard for the rights, safety and well-being of human subjects of research is informed consent. The informed consent process is a complex and important part of conducting clinical research. CRCs must have a working knowledge of consent forms and processes so that deficiencies can be avoided. It is recommended that CRCs read the regulations governing informed consent (CFR 21 part 50). There is a checklist for reviewing informed consents in Appendix D.

Key Things to Remember

- Informed consent is a cornerstone of the ethical conduct of clinical research.
- Informed consent documents must be approved by the IRB before use.
- Informed consent must be obtained before a subject enters a study.
- Informed consent must be documented.
- Proper preparation of forms and conduct of the procedure is vital to insure truly informed consent.
- Informed consent is usually required for all subjects involved in a research project.
- There are exceptions to the informed consent process under certain circumstances.

CHAPTER 4

Regulations and Good Clinical Practices (GCPs)

Introduction

In this chapter, we will discuss the regulations and guidelines that are important for a CRC to be familiar with and understand. A CRC should read and have a working knowledge of the regulations pertaining to clinical research. We will also briefly discuss the Declaration of Helsinki and the Belmont Report, which are both documents important for the protection and well-being of human subjects in clinical trials.

Many people think they have a good working knowledge of the regulations when they actually don't. How can this happen? Very easily. Instead of reading the regulations for themselves, too many people rely on information they get by asking someone else, and that someone else may not have actually read them either. This leads to an increasing spiral of misinformation and self-perpetuating myths and legends.

FDA Regulations for Clinical Trials

As a CRC, you will want to ensure that you have a thorough understanding of the regulations. This will help you do a better job of helping your study sites stay in compliance. The regulations that CRCs should be familiar with are:

- 21 CFR Part 50—Protection of Human Subjects
- 21 CFR Part 54—Financial Disclosure by Clinical Investigators
- 21 CFR Part 56—Institutional Review Boards
- 21 CFR Part 312—Investigational New Drug Application

These four parts plus 21 CFR Part 314 (Applications for FDA Approval to Market a New Drug) of the Code of Federal Regulations form the basis of the regulations pertinent to conducting clinical trials in the United States.

The regulations tell us what is actually required by the U.S. Food and Drug Administration (FDA) when involved in doing clinical studies. They cover the responsibilities of sponsors, investigators and IRBs for conducting trials involving human subjects.

ICH Guidelines for Good Clinical Practice

In addition to the FDA regulations, CRCs must also be familiar with the ICH Guideline for Good Clinical Practice. Although not yet required by regulation in the United States, this guideline has been published in the Federal Register, and represents current thinking of the FDA on good clinical practices. Many sponsor companies require their studies to follow the ICH Guideline as well as the FDA regulations.

ICH stands for the International Conference on Harmonisation of Technical Requirements for Registration of Pharmaceuticals for Human Use. The ICH was organized to provide opportunities for standardized regulatory initiatives to be developed with input from both governmental bodies and industry representatives. There are three regions involved in the ICH: the European Union, Japan and the United States. The ICH guideline defines "Good Clinical Practice" and provides a unified standard for designing, conducting, recording and reporting on clinical trials involving human subjects. Compliance with good clinical practice ensures that the rights, well-being and confidentiality of human subjects are protected and that trial data are credible.[1]

---

1. ICH Guideline for Good Clinical Practice as published in the Federal Register May 9, 1997.

FDA Guidelines and Information Sheets

The FDA also publishes a number of guidelines and information sheets that are very useful in the conduct of clinical trials. These give further explanation to the regulations, including current interpretations and thinking of the FDA. They often include questions and answers for items that are of particular interest. Although the guidelines do not carry the weight of regulations, it is highly recommended that they be followed, as they are the FDA's expectations for the conduct of trials.

Links to specific guidelines can be found on the FDA web site. Some of the more useful guidelines are:

- FDA Information Sheets for IRBs and Investigators—1998 Update (www.fda.gov/oc/ohrt/irbs)
- Good Clinical Practice in FDA-Regulated Clinical Trials (www.fda.gov/oc/gcp/default.htm)
- Guidance: General Considerations for Clinical Trials (www.ich.org/ich5e.html, click on "E8, 9, 10: CT Design")
- Monitoring of Clinical Investigations (www.fda.gov/cder/guidance/index.htm, click on "Compliance," then click on "Monitoring of Clinical Investigations")
- Exception from Informed Consent Requirements for Emergency Research (www.fda.gov/ora/compliance_ref/bimo/err_guide.htm)
- Recruiting Study Subjects (www.fda.gov/oc/ohrt/irbs)
- Disqualified/Restricted/Assurance List for Clinical Investigators (www.fda.gov/ora/compliance_ref/bimo/dis_res_assur.htm)

CRCs should familiarize themselves with these guidelines as well as with the regulations. Especially useful for investigative site personnel is the first item, the FDA Information Sheets for IRBs and Investigators.

FDA Compliance Program Guidance Manuals

There is an FDA Compliance Program Guidance Manual (CPGM) that is helpful for a CRC and other site personnel. The CPGM manuals are used by FDA personnel when they do inspections of clinical investigators, sponsors or IRBs. Of particular interest to CRCs will be the CPGM for Clinical Investigators.[2] This manual will tell you exactly what the FDA will look at during inspections of clinical study sites.

---

2. http://www.fda.gov/oc/gcp/compliance.html

NIH Regulated Research

If your site is involved in doing trials under the auspices of the Department of Health and Human Services (HHS), you will want to be familiar with HHS regulations, which differ somewhat from the FDA regulations. For example, the HHS regulations contain specific sections on working with vulnerable subjects, such as pregnant women, children and prisoners, that are not found in the FDA regulations. There is an online document that compares the regulations for the two groups; it is called "Comparison of FDA and HHS Human Subject Protection Regulations."[3]

Exploring the FDA's web site is a wonderful way to find all kinds of information about conducting trials. Taking some time to look around and delve into different topics on the web will be time well spent for a CRC. The web site can be found at www.fda.gov. From this site, one can branch off into information about drugs, biologics and devices.

FDA Bioresearch Monitoring Program (BIMO)

The FDA requires that the biomedical research it regulates conform to GCP standards as found in the FDA regulations. To help ensure that GCP standards are followed, they inspect clinical trials. (Note that what the FDA calls "inspections" are commonly called audits by others.) The FDA's program of inspections/audits is called the Bioresearch Monitoring (BIMO) program and covers all of the parties involved in regulated clinical trials, including clinical investigators, IRBs, sponsors, monitors and contract research organizations (CROs). We will cover FDA audits in Chapter 11.

Good Clinical Practice (GCP)

Good Clinical Practice (GCP) is not a single document that can be referenced, printed or read. The phrase "Good Clinical Practice" was, in fact, coined by industry and is a standard for the design, conduct, performance, monitoring, recording, analysis and reporting of clinical trials. The purpose of GCPs is to protect human subjects in trials, as well as the general population who will use the products being tested once they are available on the market.

GCPs are made up of the FDA regulations and guidance documents, the ICH guidelines for good clinical practice, and codes of ethical conduct such as the Declaration of Helsinki and the Belmont Report. They are recognized as overall standard operating procedures for the conduct of clinical research

3. www.fda.gov/oc/gcp/comparison.html

and encompass the informed consent process, accurate collection of data, maintaining audit trails, reporting adverse events, and record retention. Compliance with GCPs ensures not only that the rights and safety of study subjects are not compromised, but that the integrity of the data collected is maintained.

Contacting the FDA

The FDA invites contacts from sponsors, investigators and IRBs with respect to questions about proper procedures or interpretation of the regulations. Appendix J of the Information Sheets for IRBs and Investigators[4] lists contact information for the FDA and is a useful document to have available for research compliance questions.

HIPAA

The Federal government implemented the Health Insurance Portability and Accountability Act (HIPAA) Privacy Rule in 2003 in an effort to protect individuals' rights to control access to and disclosure of private and confidential information, and to ensure continuity of coverage between health insurance plans. The HIPAA Privacy Rule has a far-reaching and significant impact on the clinical research process. It essentially pertains to all clinical research studies that utilize identifiable, personal health information. HIPAA regulations can be found in the Code of Federal Regulations (45 CFR Parts 160 and 164). All clinical investigators must comply with the Privacy Rule when any of their clinical trials involve medical treatments. Investigators must also comply with HIPAA if they request protected health information (PHI) from covered entities. Failure to comply with HIPAA can result in costly civil, or even criminal, sanctions against an institution or independent investigative site.

HIPAA Authorization

CRCs and other study site personnel must make reasonable efforts to use or disclose only the minimum necessary information on their study subjects. Although you may review a study subject's complete medical records and share this information freely with other clinicians involved with the subject's care, you must, in general, under HIPAA, obtain authorization from the sub-

4. www.fda.gov/oc/ohrt/irbs/phones.html

jects in order to use and disclose their identifiable and protected health information.

Since during a clinical research project, study subjects' medical records will be looked at, and perhaps even copied, by the sponsor and the FDA for scientific and regulatory purposes, study subjects must be provided with information related to their rights and recourse, and how their PHI may be used and disclosed. HIPAA authorization may be incorporated into the body of the informed consent form or it may be provided through the use of a separate authorization document.

Protected Health Information (PHI)

HIPAA regulations cover any subject information at your site that could be used to identify the person to whom the information pertains. This protected health information (PHI) includes, but is not limited to, the items shown below:

- Names
- Addresses (any geographic subdivisions smaller than a state)
- Employers' names or addresses
- Relatives' names or addresses
- All elements of dates related to a person except for year
- Telephone numbers
- Fax numbers
- Email addresses
- Social security numbers
- Medical record numbers
- Certificate numbers (including device serial numbers for implants)
- Member or account numbers
- Certification/license numbers
- Voiceprints
- Fingerprints
- Vehicle identifiers
- Device identifiers
- Biometric identifiers
- Full face photographs
- Any other unique identifying number, characteristic or code.

There is a difference between the terms "use" and "disclosure" of information (PHI). HIPAA regulations define these terms in the following way:

> "Use" happens within a health care organization and is under the direct control of the organization. Example: a CRC in a clinic "uses" protected health information when seeing a study subject.

"Disclosure" occurs when the information (PHI) is given to someone who is not part of the organization (not an employee). Example: allowing a sponsor monitor (CRA) to see a study subject's office chart/source document.

Recruitment of Study Subjects

PHI may be accessed for use in preparing a research protocol or to screen records for recruitment. It is acceptable to look through the records at your site to locate potential study subjects to contact about a trial. However, if an investigator is screening records that belong to another organization other than his or her own practice, then he or she is not allowed to contact the potential subjects associated with those records. Here are ways of recruiting subjects for trials that are allowable under HIPAA.

Patient Self-Identification

A physician may discuss a clinical trial with a patient during a regular patient visit. If the patient is interested in the trial, then the physician may refer the patient to the primary investigator or another source of information, such as a web site. This is the most conservative method, as the patient is the one who discloses his or her PHI. Also, the patient may sign a sheet that gives authorization to the physician to contact the patient about a clinical trial.

Reviewing Records to Identify Potential Research Subjects

The Office of Civil Rights (OCR) is responsible for HIPAA compliance. They have issued a guidance document saying that a researcher can look at PHI in medical records to identify potential study subjects, but that the information gathered cannot be taken outside the clinic or hospital (covered entity) and that the information cannot be used for anything other than research. Also, if the researcher is not an employee or in the workforce of the covered entity, he or she cannot contact the person unless the IRB has granted a waiver of authorization.

IRB Waiver

An investigator may use and disclose PHI for research without an authorization from each individual if the investigator has a waiver from an institutional review board (IRB). However, an IRB can only issue a waiver if all the following criteria are met:

- The use of the PHI involves no more than minimal risk to the individuals' privacy based on the following:

- There is a plan to protect the PHI from improper use and disclosure;
- There is an adequate plan to destroy the PHI as soon as possible after use; and
- There is adequate written assurance that the PHI will not be reused or redisclosed to any other person or entity (with a few exceptions).
- The research could not practicably be conducted without access to the PHI; and
- The research could not practicably be done without the waiver.

Research Databases and Repositories

It is acceptable for an investigator to keep information on potential study subjects for future use, but he or she should obtain a pre-research authorization from each potential subject. The investigator must also be careful not to use the PHI in this database for any purpose not covered in the pre-research authorization. Some investigators now routinely ask their patients to sign these authorization forms when they come in for an office visit.

Limited Data Sets

Researchers are allowed to keep data that are not fully de-identified. In this case, dates, geographic information (not actual addresses) and other unique identifying numbers, codes, etc., that are not expressly excluded (see list earlier in the chapter) may be retained. However, since the information in a limited data set does not include names, it probably will not be useful for recruitment.

Marketing with Authorization

It is acceptable to use protected health information to solicit authorizations from people, so it can be used to compose a mailing list of potential study subjects and writing to them to request authorization to use their PHI for recruitment. This means that the investigator can send a letter to his or her patients asking for written authorization to use their PHI for recruitment purposes; if you do this, you should include an authorization form in the letter.

Direct Communication

Under HIPAA, an investigator or a staff member, may communicate directly with patients without patient authorization to discuss the option of enrolling in a clinical trial. This means you can telephone or send letters directly to your patients to tell them about trials and their options for possible enrollment in them.

Obtaining Informed Consent under HIPAA

As was discussed earlier, under HIPAA an investigator must obtain permission from patients before using their PHI for most clinical research. Investigators may use a separate authorization for this, or it can be included in the informed consent document that will be used for the study.

In the authorization/consent, you must list all the health information that will be used or disclosed, including the standard PHI and the subject's medical history, physical findings and laboratory test results. If the investigator determines later that he or she needs to use information that was not included in the original authorization, a new authorization will probably need to be obtained. The items that need to be included in this authorization are:

- The specific information you intend to use.
- The people or organizations who may use or disclose the information (usually the investigator and the research team).
- The people or organizations who will receive the information (usually the sponsor, CRO, central laboratories, IRB, FDA, etc.).
- The purpose of the use or disclosure.
- The expiration date or event (such as 10 years after the end of the study).
- The right to refuse to sign the authorization.
- The right to revoke the authorization.

Subjects may, of course, withdraw from a study at any time. Under HIPAA, however, they must withdraw in writing to revoke the subsequent use or disclosure of their PHI. Even after a subject has revoked authorization to use his or her PHI, the investigator may still use enough of the PHI to inform the sponsor of the revocation. Also, if the investigator has already submitted the subject's data to the sponsor, those data do not need to be retrieved. In general, the investigator may not submit any additional data from a subject to the sponsor once a subject has revoked authorization to use his or her PHI. One thing an investigator may want to consider is having a study subject who withdraws from a trial sign a form that makes clear whether or not researchers may continue to use his or her PHI.

In summary, HIPAA rules and regulations are complicated, and they do have an impact on the way clinical trials must be conducted. The CRC should understand his or her site's standard operating procedures (SOPs) regarding HIPAA.

The Declaration of Helsinki (1964)

The World Health Organization spent more than ten years working on the statement of ethical principles that became known as the Declaration of Helsinki. This document defined rules for "therapeutic" and "non-therapeutic" research. It repeated the Nuremberg Code requirement for consent for non-therapeutic research but allowed for enrolling certain patients in therapeutic research without consent. The Declaration of Helsinki also allowed legal guardians to grant permission to enroll subjects in research, both therapeutic and non-therapeutic, and recommended written consent—an issue not addressed in the Nuremberg Code. In addition, the Declaration of Helsinki requires review and prior approval of a protocol by an IRB. Several revisions have been made to this document, including a Clarification, and it is still under revision today. The Declaration of Helsinki can be found in 21 CRF 312 (see Appendix D).

The Belmont Report (1979)

The National Research Act, passed by Congress in 1974, created the National Commission for the Protection of Human Subjects of Biomedical and Behavioral Research. This commission wrote a document entitled Ethical Principles and Guidelines for the Protection of Human Subjects of Research, which became known as the Belmont Report when it was published in 1979. The three basic principles of the Belmont Report are respect for persons, beneficence and justice.

1. Respect for persons is manifested by the informed consent process, as well as in safeguards for vulnerable populations, such as children, pregnant women, mentally disabled adults and prisoners. Other important concerns of respect for persons are privacy and confidentiality.
2. Beneficence has two general characteristics: do no harm, and maximize benefit while minimizing risk. Beneficence is manifested in the use of good research design, competent investigators, and a favorable risk/benefit ratio.
3. Justice implies fairness, and is manifested in the equitable selection of subjects for research, ensuring that no group of people is "selected in" or "selected out" unfairly based on factors unrelated to the research. This means that there must be appropriate inclusion/exclusion criteria and a fair system of recruitment.

The Belmont Report forms the cornerstone for the ethical treatment of human subjects of research.

Key Things to Remember

- The FDA regulations pertaining to clinical trials are found in 21 CFR parts 50, 54, 56, 312, and 314.
- The ICH Guidelines for Good Clinical Practice should be followed in clinical trials.
- The FDA publishes many guidelines and information sheets pertaining to the appropriate conduct of clinical trials.
- Good clinical practices are the ethical and clinical standard for designing, conducting, analyzing, monitoring and reporting on clinical trials.
- There are differences between FDA and HHS rules for doing research in human subjects.
- CRCs should read and be familiar with the regulations that pertain to clinical trials and the ICH guidelines.
- HIPAA was enacted in an effort to protect individuals' rights to control access to and disclosure of private and confidential information and to ensure continuity of coverage between health insurance plans.
- In general, authorization must be obtained before using a subject's protected health information (PHI) for research.
- The HIPAA Privacy Rule has a large impact on recruitment for clinical trials.
- The Declaration of Helsinki and the Belmont Report are critical documents for the protection of human subjects in research.
- The three main principles of the Belmont Report are respect for persons, beneficence and justice.

CHAPTER 5

An Overview of Research

Introduction

In this chapter we will present an overview of the research process for new pharmaceutical compounds, looking at both pre-clinical work and clinical development. We will also briefly discuss the two main documents that must be filed with the FDA. One of these is the Investigational New Drug application (IND), which is filed before studies can begin in humans. The other is the New Drug Application (NDA), which is the formal request for permission to market a new product.

It is important that CRCs comprehend the entire drug development process, even though they will not be involved in every step. This will help you understand why things happen as they do, and to participate knowledgeably in the process.

Pre-Clinical Research

In this section, we will look at drug discovery and the pre-clinical work that must be done before phase I studies in humans can begin. "Pre-clinical" refers to studies that do not involve human subjects. Clinical studies are studies done with human subjects. Sometimes people refer to "pre-clinical" research as "non-clinical" research, even though some of the non-human work can continue after clinical studies have begun. The two terms, non-clinical and pre-clinical, are used interchangeably.

The purpose of pre-clinical studies is to provide information on safety and, if possible, efficacy, in order to begin clinical studies in humans. The information received from pre-clinical studies provides the pharmaceutical company, the FDA and the IRB with enough evidence to make reasonable decisions about the compound. The information from pre-clinical studies includes: data on acute toxicity, the kinetics and metabolism of the drug, organ sensitivity and, most importantly, a starting dose with an acceptable margin of safety so that there is minimal chance of endangerment to human study subjects.

Drug Discovery

The discovery of new substances, which subsequently become marketed drugs or biologics, occurs in a number of ways. There is direct research, where medicinal chemists create compounds with structures likely to evoke the kind of physiological effect for which they are looking. Another approach is to change the molecular structure of known compounds in hopes of improving safety or efficacy, while creating a new chemical entity that is sufficiently different from the parent compound to allow for the filing of a new patent.

In addition to classical chemistry, there are many new laboratory tools for developing viable drug substances. Computer technology provides many methods for molecular structuring. There are also computer-readable chemical libraries, which may contain several hundred thousands of molecular structures. Many pharmaceutical companies have contracts with firms that provide these libraries; the companies take these chemical structures from the database, then perform structure/function/activity computations and computer modeling to look for a hit on a potential compound. Companies can also perform high throughput screening and other computer-related inquiries to look for hits. Other methods include gene sequencing, gene vector delivery and recombinant DNA.

In addition to the laboratory synthesis of compounds, naturally occurring compounds are another source of potential pharmaceuticals. A number of drugs originated from soil samples (antibiotics), plants (digitalis) and other natural materials such as coral (prostaglandins).

Serendipity plays a role in any research program. Some very exciting compounds have been discovered by accident. Many drugs are marketed for an indication that was discovered by accident during studies for the primary indication. One example is Rogaine®. This compound, minoxidil, was originally developed as an antihypertensive (Loniten®). Its hair growing capability wasn't known until subjects enrolled in the hypertension studies began exhibiting accelerated hair growth—in all the wrong places. Women weren't thrilled with their new mustaches and bushy eyebrows that grew together in the middle. Based on this unwanted side effect, the company eventually developed a topical formulation of minoxidil as a hair growth product; this was approved by the FDA and is marketed as Rogaine®.

Pre-clinical Studies of Product Candidates

Once a compound appears to be a viable product candidate, it must be determined if a compound is reasonably safe for initial testing in humans, and if it exhibits pharmacological activity that might justify developing it commercially. This pre-clinical work focuses on collecting data and information to establish that humans will not be exposed to unreasonable risks in early phase clinical studies. This evidence will be presented to the FDA in an Investigational New Drug application (IND).

The first step is to determine the basic physical, chemical and biological characteristics of a new compound. Once a compound is characterized and satisfactory stability data are in hand, pre-clinical studies can be initiated. The type of studies and their design will vary depending on the intended use of the drug or biologic being developed. The purpose of pre-clinical studies is to characterize the toxic effects of the compound with respect to target organs, dose dependence and relationship to exposure. Many of the studies are in lab animals, sometimes in multiple species with variable durations of dosing.

The pre-clinical studies will establish a number of different things, including:

- The highest dose of the compound that can be tolerated as well as a dose that evokes no overt toxicity, in order to determine initial dosing in humans and to characterize potential organ-specific adverse events.
- Proposed dose, route of administration and duration of treatment for phase I studies.
- Whether any adverse effects that are seen are reversible.
- Genotoxicity, teratology and reproductive toxicology.

The IND (Investigational New Drug Application)

The FDA becomes involved in a drug development program at the point when the sponsor has completed enough pre-clinical work with the compound to determine it is reasonable to start working with it in humans. This is when the molecule changes in legal status under the Federal Food, Drug, and Cosmetic Act. It becomes a "new drug" and is subject to specific regulatory requirements.[1] In order to do this, the sponsor must file an IND with the FDA.

INDs are not actively approved by the FDA, but may be disapproved. If a company has not heard to the contrary, clinical testing of a new compound may begin thirty days after the FDA has received the IND. This allows the

1. www.fda.gov/cder/regulatory/applications/ind-page-1.htm

FDA time to review the IND for any safety concerns. Even though it is not required, most companies will contact the FDA if they have not heard from them within the thirty days, just to verify that the FDA is in agreement about starting studies.

The IND contains information in the following areas:[2]

1. Animal pharmacology and toxicology studies. These make up the pre-clinical data that allow the FDA to make an assessment about whether the product is reasonably safe for initial testing in humans.
2. Any previous experience with the drug in humans. This might be from foreign studies, especially if the compound is marketed in other countries.
3. Manufacturing information.
4. Clinical protocols and investigator information. This will include detailed protocols so that the FDA can assess whether the initial-phase trials will expose subjects to unnecessary risks, as well as information about the qualifications of clinical investigators.

The IND must be updated on an annual basis. In the update, the sponsor includes any new information about the drug, as well as the results of any studies ongoing or completed during the year. This information includes current enrollment numbers, adverse event information and the overall study status. The update also includes the clinical plan for the next year. This information keeps the FDA abreast of what is happening with the compound over time.

Amendments to the IND may be filed at any time. Amendments are filed for any changes in protocols, medicine strength, investigators, or other changes in the development program. The regulations pertaining to INDs are found in 21 CFR 312.

A CRC will not have any involvement with the IND. However, when it is time for the annual update, sites working with the compound may be contacted for current information needed for the update. When this happens, there are often critical timelines involved, so the CRA will work with you to collect the information in a timely manner.

Clinical Trials

In this section we will discuss the clinical development of a compound. The term "clinical" implies human studies, as opposed to animal studies. Clinical studies are not started until a reasonable amount of pre-clinical work has been completed and there is evidence that the compound is potentially safe for use in humans.

---

2. 21 CFR 312.23.

Clinical trials are divided into phases: I, II, III and IV. Many companies also use the designation of phase IIIB, which will also be defined in this chapter. (Note that you may also see the phases numbered using Arabic numerals 1, 2, 3, 3B and 4.) The phases simply serve as markers or milestones in the drug development process and are not necessarily distinct, consecutive periods; for example, in some cases phases II and III can be combined, and phase II may start before phase I is complete. However, each phase does have distinct characteristics and purposes, and each is important to the development program.

Phase I Clinical Trials

During phase I, the investigational drug or biologic is given to humans for the first time.

Phase I studies, frequently referred to as safety studies, enroll a small number of subjects. The total number of subjects in phase I is usually between 20 and 100. Subjects are usually healthy volunteers, although in some cases, patients with the target disease are studied. The type of subject depends on the nature of the disease and the expected toxicity of the investigational drug. It would not be ethical, for example, to give healthy subjects a toxic new drug meant to treat one of the cancers.

The purpose of phase I studies is to determine the metabolic and pharmacologic action of the drug in humans, assess the adverse effects associated with different doses, and to perhaps get an indication of whether or not there is any evidence of efficacy. Because this is the first time humans are exposed to the drug, these studies are very closely monitored by medical personnel. Phase I studies are often done in special testing facilities designed for this work.

Essentially, phase I should provide the researcher with sufficient information about the drug's pharmacokinetics and pharmacological effects (safe dose range and adverse effects), to permit designing safe, well-controlled, scientifically sound phase II studies. The primary concern of phase I is subject safety.

Phase II Clinical Trials

When the appropriate phase I studies have been completed and sufficient safety data are in hand, phase II studies are initiated. Phase II studies are rigid, well-controlled studies in a relatively small patient population, usually no more than a few hundred subjects in total. These subjects have the target disease, but no other illnesses. Phase II usually consists of double-blind studies using a placebo or comparator drug, or both. Their purpose is to determine whether or not the investigational drug demonstrates efficacy for the proposed indication within the safe dose range established in phase I. Short term adverse effects and risks are also assessed. While the focus of phase II studies is primarily efficacy, they also assess safety, as this is always of primary concern. Dose range finding, e.g., establishing a minimum and maximum effective dose, and pharmacokinetic (PK) data correlating blood levels of the drug with pharmacological effect are also studied during phase II.

Phase III Clinical Trials

Phase III studies are only initiated if the data generated in phases I and II show a satisfactory safety profile and there is sufficient evidence of efficacy. The purpose of phase III studies is to demonstrate the long-term safety and efficacy needed to assess the risk/benefit relationship of the drug and to provide adequate data for the product package insert.

Phase III studies are expanded, controlled studies in large patient populations (often thousands of patients) that represent the types of patients the compound is intended to treat after it is marketed. They may extend over several years. The development plan for the compound usually includes many different studies, including more than one multicenter study using the same or similar protocols. Multicenter studies are those in which multiple investigative sites all follow the same protocol, and in which the data are intended for analysis together in one group.

The FDA requirement for registration of a drug is two "adequate and well-controlled" (primary efficacy) studies. However, under the FDAMA legislation of 1997, the FDA may allow one study instead of two for a product where it is determined (by FDA) that "data from one adequate and well-controlled clinical investigation and confirmatory evidence (obtained prior to or after such investigation) are sufficient to establish effectiveness." A fast track product is intended for the treatment of serious or life-threatening conditions and demonstrates the potential to address unmet medical needs for the condition. The decision to do one, rather than two, adequate and well-controlled studies is not one that a sponsor will make on its own; this decision will be made after consultation with and the support of the FDA.

The NDA (New Drug Application)

The NDA is a formal request to be allowed to market a drug. The sponsor submits the NDA to the FDA at the time that the primary efficacy studies (phase III) are complete. The company is essentially telling the FDA that it has completed the necessary safety and efficacy requirements needed for approval. This signals the end of phase III, although there are likely to be some studies still in progress.

In the NDA, as in the IND, the sponsor informs the FDA of everything that is known about the drug to date. This includes copies of all protocols and case report forms from studies. (These applications are enormous.) The regulations for NDAs are found in 21 CFR 314. They are very detailed, and delineate the particular information that must be included.

Again, CRCs are not involved in putting together the NDA, although there may be a last-minute push to retrieve and/or clean up data that are needed for the NDA; it seems that there are always some outstanding data that need to be collected and entered into the database very quickly in order to process material for the NDA. CRCs may also be asked to re-verify information from their sites when questions arise during the NDA writing process.

Part of the NDA is the proposed package insert that the sponsor would like to use with the drug. This is the information that goes with the drug that tells physicians about the drug and how it should be used. The package insert negotiations between the sponsor and the FDA can be significant.

There is an active approval process for an NDA, as opposed to the passive 30-day wait for an IND. The sponsor must receive a formal approval letter from the FDA before marketing of the drug can begin.

Phase IIIB Clinical Studies

A sponsor will frequently have some studies that are still ongoing at the time it files the NDA for a new compound. There are also studies that may be initiated and conducted while the NDA is pending approval. These studies are known as phase IIIB studies. The purpose of these studies may be to gather additional safety data, or to gather information on additional indications for the drug, or to assess its use in special patient populations such as pediatric or geriatric patients.

Phase IV Clinical Studies

Phase IV studies are those done after the approval of the NDA, often to determine additional information about the safety or efficacy profile of the compound. They consist of:

- Studies required as a condition of approval by the FDA, or
- Long-term safety studies required by the FDA, or
- Studies conducted to look at the compound in comparison with other marketed products, or
- Studies designed to familiarize physicians with the compound.

If the sponsor was allowed to file the NDA with one, rather than two, adequate and well-controlled studies, the FDA may require that one or more additional confirmatory studies be completed within a certain time period of the approval. This is a condition of the approval; if it is not met, the approval may be withdrawn.

The FDA may also require that a sponsor do a long-term safety study as a condition of approval. These studies are often referred to as epidemiologic or post-marketing surveillance studies. These may be required because the FDA has seen problems with similar compounds, or because the compound is novel and the FDA thinks additional safety information will be beneficial.

During the development time for the compound, other drugs may have been approved by the FDA and become the new standard of care for the disease or condition. In this case, the sponsor may want to do additional studies comparing their drug to these new compounds. The sponsor may also wish to look at different formulations, dosages, durations of treatments, or medical interactions with other compounds commonly used by people with the disease targeted by the drug. Note that if the sponsor wants to evaluate the compound for a new (additional) indication, then these studies will be considered as phase II studies; a new NDA will need to be filed for the new indication(s).

Studies designed to familiarize physicians with the new drug are sometimes referred to as marketing studies. Physicians may be given a relatively small amount of the new drug to use in an open label manner with appropriate patients, and will be required to collect some data, usually only safety data, as they use the drug. The goal of the sponsor of these studies is to have the physician like the product and begin to use it regularly.

Notes on Studies in Women and Children

Many compounds do not work the same in women or children as they do in men. Consequently, the FDA has determined that studies should include women and children if the compounds would be used to treat them after marketing. The rationale is that it is preferable to determine the effects of the compound under the controlled conditions in clinical trials as opposed to uncontrolled use of the drug after marketing.

Table 1: Timeline of Pediatric Testing Regulations

1997	**FDA Modernization Act—Pediatric Exclusivity Provision** Grants six month patent extension for pediatric testing of drugs already approved for adult treatments
1998	**Pediatric Rule** Requires pediatric testing of all new drugs used by children
2001	**Clinical Investigation of Medicinal Products in Pediatric Populations** Sets standards by which IRBs determine if a pediatric trial can be safely and ethically conducted; included requirement that children give their assent to participate
2002	**Best Pharmaceuticals for Children Act** Grants patent extensions to sponsors conducting pediatric trials or offers funding to third parties if sponsors choose not to
2003	**Pediatric Research Equity Act** Amends the Food, Drug and Cosmetic Act to authorize the Food and Drug Administration to require research in drugs used in pediatric patients

Source: CenterWatch, 2004.

The pediatric clinical trials market, which saw a flurry of activity in the late 1990s, has fallen flat during the early 2000s as the number of patent extensions granted under the U.S. Food and Drug Administration's pediatric exclusivity provision dwindled. During that time, many sponsor companies held back pediatric studies on new drugs after FDA's Pediatric Rule, which required pediatric testing of all new drugs used by children, was struck down by a federal court judge.[3]

Yet now that the Pediatric Research Equity Act (PREA) has become law, re-instating the provisions of the Pediatric Rule, sponsors must consider pediatric assessment as a routine part of drug development. The industry already has seen an increase in protocols for new pediatric studies since the legislation was signed in December 2003.[4]

And while industry experts don't expect a big jump in the demand for pediatric studies, such as was seen when patent extensions to encourage pediatric testing of drugs were first offered under the FDA Modernization Act (FDAMA), most predict PREA will prompt a slow, steady increase in the number of pediatric clinical trials conducted in the future. As a result, the legislation will help maintain the pediatric infrastructure built under FDAMA's pediatric exclusivity provision.[5]

Renee Simar, Ph.D., vice president of INC Pediatrics, said the transition from having a pediatric rule to a federal law implies an important shift in opinion regarding the need for well-controlled studies in the pediatric population. "The notion of conducting a pediatric trial is going to be less and less a phenomenon. It's going to be part and parcel of what we do. Now with the re-enactment of the Pediatric Rule, sponsors will be expected to have conversations with FDA at the end of their phase II meetings, so early in development they're going to be thinking about doing pediatric data for their compound," Simar said.[6]

As PREA places renewed pressure on pharmaceutical companies to conduct pediatric clinical trials, the Institute of Medicine issued a report in March 2004 called "Ethical Conduct of Clinical Research Involving Children" offering the industry concrete guidelines for addressing ethical and practical issues critical to the success of pediatric clinical trials such as the definition of minimal risk in children, the process of obtaining informed consent, evaluating whether children should be paid for participation in clinical trials, and the role of the institutional review board when reviewing research involving children. An abstract of the report can be found at www.iom.edu.[7]

---

3. Korieth, Karyn, "Pediatric Trials Come of Age," *The CenterWatch Monthly*, Vol. 11, Issue 4, April 2004.
4. Ibid.
5. Ibid.
6. Ibid.
7. Ibid.

In addition to children, women of childbearing potential are a major concern in clinical trials because of the possibility of unintentional exposure of an embryo or fetus before data are available relative to potential risk. Some teratology work (segments I and II) is usually done before entering women of childbearing potential in a clinical trial, although this is not essential.

Although the FDA recommended in 1993 that clinical studies include enough women to understand the unique ways in which their bodies respond to drugs, more than a decade later, women are still underrepresented in small, phase I safety trials. And when eligibility is restricted by age, older women are disproportionately excluded from studies of diseases that are more common in women at older ages. The possibility of becoming pregnant also excludes most women in their childbearing years.[8]

Generally a woman capable of conceiving a child won't be considered for a clinical trial unless she's not pregnant and agrees to use birth control. Many studies require that women of childbearing age use two forms of contraception during participation. Pharmaceutical companies don't want their drugs tested among women who are—or might get—pregnant, mostly because the risk of a lawsuit by the mother is too high. Many parents are quick to blame poor birth outcomes on drugs. Some doctors erroneously believe that certain drugs cause fetal abnormalities. But genes and chromosomes are the primary culprits, according to Marilynn C. Frederiksen, M.D., associate professor of obstetrics and gynecology at Northwestern University Medical School. All of this presents a major barrier to clinical trial participation by women who don't want, can't afford or are religiously opposed to contraception.[9]

As a direct result of the 1993 NIH Revitalization Act, NIH-sponsored clinical research now routinely includes sufficient numbers of non-pregnant women. Pharmaceutical companies following FDA guidelines, however, pay for most clinical trials. The FDA recommended back in 1977 that premenopausal women capable of becoming pregnant be excluded from early drug trials. In practice, the participation of women in all phases was affected. The FDA's current stance—that a "reasonable" number of women be included in all clinical trials—hasn't fully addressed participation inequities.[10]

In the U.S., women of childbearing potential may be included in early studies prior to completion of reproductive toxicology studies, provided that the studies are carefully monitored and all precautions are taken to minimize exposure *in utero*. This generally involves pregnancy testing and establishment of highly effective methods of birth control. Monitoring and testing should continue throughout the trial to ensure compliance with all measures intended to prevent pregnancy.

---

8. Anderson, D., *A Guide to Patient Recruitment and Retention*, Thomson CenterWatch, 2004.
9. Ibid.
10. Ibid.

If women of childbearing potential are used in a clinical trial prior to completion of the teratology studies, the informed consent process should clearly indicate the possible risk associated with taking the experimental drug since effects on the embryo or fetus are unknown.

If pregnant women are to be enrolled in clinical trials, all reproductive toxicity studies and genotoxicity tests must be completed. Data from any previous experience in humans will also be needed.

If children are to be included in clinical trials, repeated dose toxicity studies and all reproductive toxicity and genotoxicity studies should have been completed. In addition, safety data from previous studies in human adult populations should be available.

Summary

Table 2 shows the progression of activities in drug research, as well as some of the important milestones covered in this chapter. Drug discovery and development are long processes, and most compounds never make it all the way through. The time between a compound entering pre-clinical testing and the NDA approval averages about 10 years. The attrition rate is very high. For every 5,000 to 10,000 compounds screened, only 250 enter pre-clinical testing; of the 250, only five go into clinical testing, and only one makes it all the way to approval by the FDA.[11]

Table 2: The Research Process

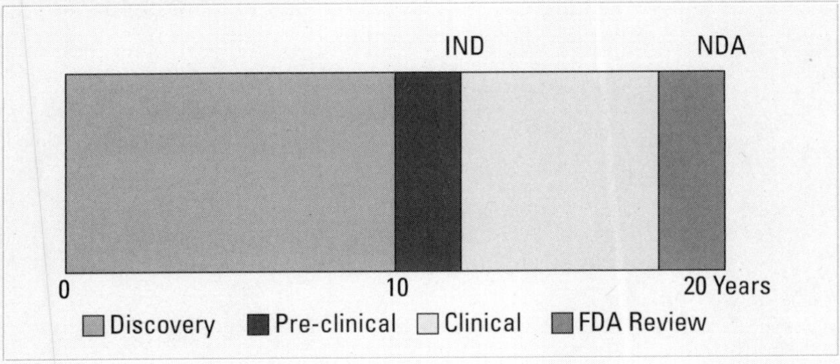

Source: FDA, Tufts Center for the Study of Drug Development.

11. Woodin, Karen, *The CRA's Guide to Monitoring Clinical Trials*, Thomson CenterWatch, 2003.

Key Things to Remember

- Pre-clinical trials do not involve human subjects.
- Clinical trials involve human subjects.
- Before clinical trials begin, the sponsor must file an IND with the FDA.
- The IND must include results from the pre-clinical studies.
- The IND is filed after significant pre-clinical testing has been done on a compound, and it appears to be reasonably safe for use in humans.
- There is no formal FDA approval for an IND. A sponsor must wait 30 days after filing the IND before starting studies in humans.
- INDs must be updated annually. The update contains what was learned about the compound during the year and the clinical plan for the following year.
- Phase 1 studies are small safety studies, usually done in healthy volunteers.
- Phase 2 studies are usually the first studies in patients with the disease or condition of interest.
- Phase 3 studies are large, comprehensive safety and efficacy studies.
- Phase 3B studies are those being done during the time the compound is in the FDA review cycle.
- Phase 4 studies are done after approval of the compound.
- The NDA is the sponsor's formal application to market a new drug.
- The NDA is filed when the primary safety and efficacy studies are complete.
- The FDA must formally approve a drug before it can be marketed.
- There is an increased emphasis on doing studies in women and children.

CHAPTER 6

Standard Operating Procedures (SOPs)

Performing clinical trials is a complicated business. It is bound by regulations and good clinical practice, with the overriding concern of protecting the safety and welfare of study subjects. Sites must follow each protocol exactly and meet other sponsor demands. One of the best ways to ensure that all these conditions are met is to formulate and follow standard operating procedures (SOPs). Standard operating procedures are just that: the "procedures" and processes that you use and "operate" under that have been "standardized" to ensure that you do them the same way each time. An SOP is nothing more than a clearly written description of how a particular task is to be performed. SOPs are critical tools in successful business operations for all those involved in doing clinical trials, including investigative sites, sponsors and IRBs. They are essential for standardizing processes, for ensuring that regulatory and organizational policy requirements are met, for training new personnel and for managing workload. This chapter will cover the importance and value of SOPs, as well as presenting an approach for the development of SOPs at your investigative site.

The regulations do not require that investigative sites have SOPs. However, the regulations do state that "A sponsor shall select only investigators qualified by training and experience..." (21 CFR 312.53) and that "[The investigator] will ensure that all [staff] are informed about their obligations..." (21CFR312.53). What does this mean? It means that investigators must be qualified to do trials, as well as qualified in the disease area. It also means that investigators must ensure that all others assisting in trials are knowledgeable about the obligations and responsibilities. One of the best ways to ensure this is to have SOPs that cover clinical trial procedures and responsibilities.

FAQ

If SOPs are not required by regulation, why should we bother with them?

Your site will be better prepared for doing studies well, your processes will be consistent, and you will look much more professional. Most sponsors (and the FDA) will expect a site that consistently does clinical trials to have SOPs.

SOPs have several purposes. They ensure that the site has consistent processes that meet or exceed regulatory and good clinical practice (GCP) standards and that all employees are familiar with the processes. They also ensure that processes are reviewed and updated on a regular basis. Having and adhering to good SOPs helps to ensure that audits by sponsors or by the FDA do not result in detrimental findings, and may also afford the site some legal protection.

Writing SOPs

Writing SOPs is not an easy process. It is very time-consuming and involves analysis of your processes. However, it pays big dividends when complete. There are many ways to approach the formulation of SOPs. One that has been used successfully by many organizations is described below.

Step 1. Map Your Process

Process mapping is a procedure of laying out all the steps in a currently used process and analyzing the process with the goal of making it more efficient and easier to follow. It involves taking each step in the process and "mapping" it into a process chart. All the people who are involved in doing the task should be involved in mapping it into a process chart, and there should be free and open discussion. It is often discovered during this process that all involved people do not do things the same way and have very different ideas about how the current process works and how it should be done in the future.

You will want to map the steps of your process into a flow diagram, with the primary and secondary steps shown. For example, if you were to map the process for making a cup of coffee, the primary steps might be:

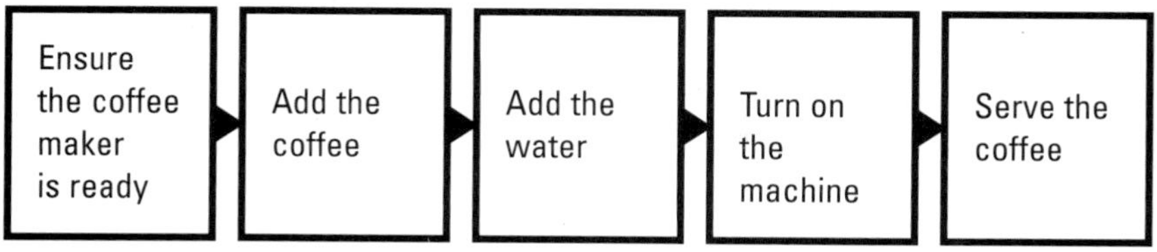

Adding the secondary steps to the flow chart might result in a process that looks like this:

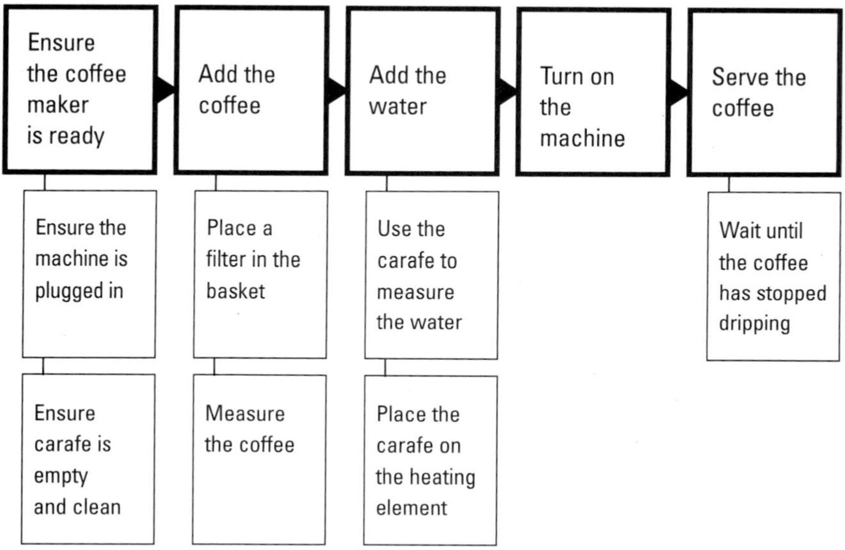

A convenient way to do mapping is to put a large, long sheet of paper on the wall (tablecloth paper) and write the steps on large (3" by 5") sticky notes. This allows you to move them around easily as you are mapping, which is very convenient.

Once you have the process mapped, you can add the people who are responsible for each step to your map. For this, it's easy to use the small sticky notes in several colors, with different colors representing the different person/position you need. For example, the investigator may be represented by green, the CRC by blue, the receptionist by yellow, etc.

When you have finished the mapping, convert your process map to an outline for ease of use. The outlines become the building blocks for your SOPs. The outline for the process we mapped above might look like this:

1. Ensure the coffee maker is ready.
   a. Plug in the machine.
   b. Be sure the carafe is clean and empty.

2. Add the coffee.
   a. Place a filter in the receptacle.
   b. Measure the coffee.
3. Add the water.
   a. Use the carafe to measure the water.
   b. Place the carafe on the heating element.
4. Turn on the machine.
5. Serve the coffee.
   a. Wait until the coffee has stopped dripping.

When a procedure has been mapped, it should be tested. Have the people who are involved try it out and see if it really works. Determine if there are any missing steps or redundant or unnecessary steps that can be eliminated. Does the process meet the requirements? Is it the best way to do the task? If not, make appropriate changes and retest it.

SOP: Making Coffee

SOP #000	Rev #000	Author:	Effective date:	Page X of X

Purpose

This SOP ensures that any company employee wanting to make coffee does so appropriately and according to company standards, thus ensuring a drinkable brew that satisfies and gives pleasure.

Scope

This SOP applies to all employees of the company and pertains only to use of the approved machine (name of machine) to make coffee. Coffee may be made only by employees who have been trained on the machine and are approved to make coffee (approved coffee makers).

Procedure

1. Ensure coffee maker is plugged in and the carafe is clean and empty.
2. Place a filter in the coffee receptacle and add the appropriate amount of coffee.
3. Fill the carafe with the desired level of water and pour into the water reservoir.
4. Place the carafe on the heating element and turn the machine on.

When the coffee has stopped dripping into the carafe, it is ready to serve.

A good approach to SOPs is to have a two-tiered system that includes both SOPs and guidelines. The SOPs give more of a bird's eye view of the process, and include all the main steps, while the guidelines are significantly more detailed. The guidelines should essentially allow someone to complete the process by following the steps in the guidelines. SOPs are usually approved at a higher level, and should not be able to be changed on a whim. One major advantage to a two-tiered system is that the SOPs will rarely need to be changed. The guidelines, on the other hand, may change much more frequently, due to changes in organizational structure, equipment or personnel functions. Guidelines are often formulated and updated at a departmental level, rather than a corporate level. There may be more than one guideline attached to an SOP, and some SOPs may not need guidelines.

SOPS often have the following sections: header, scope, purpose and procedure. An SOP might look like the example "SOP: Making Coffee."

Guidelines usually list the tasks necessary to complete the process, as well as the person or function responsible for completing each task. An example of a guideline for making coffee is shown below.

Guideline: Making Coffee

Date: February 4, 2004

Responsible person	**Activity**
Approved coffee maker	Ensure coffee maker is plugged in. ■ Plug is located at end of cord attached at back of machine ■ Outlet is on wall directly to the right of the machine ■ Insert plug into wall outlet, matching large side of plug to larger hole in outlet ■ Be sure plug is inserted firmly and completely
Approved coffee maker or custodial staff	Wash out coffee carafe if needed. ■ Dishwashing soap is located in the cupboard under the sink ■ Use hot water and a small amount of dishwashing soap ■ Brush with small brush located on hook under sink ■ Rinse thoroughly with hot water
Approved coffee maker	Pull out coffee receptacle. ■ Located in top half of machine

Guideline: Making Coffee (continued)

- Grasp handle flap firmly and gently pull toward you until receptacle is fully opened

Put a filter in the receptacle.
- Use a #4 cone filter
- Filters are located in the drawer directly under the coffee machine
- Be sure the filter is opened correctly
- Press the filter firmly against the sides and bottom of the receptacle

Prepare to fill the filter with coffee.
- Remove can of coffee from the cupboard just left of the coffee machine
- Remove the lid from the can
- Place the lid on the cupboard top

Measure and add the coffee to the filter in the pot.
- Use the red scoop found in the drawer next to the filters
- Measure the appropriate number of scoops of coffee and place the coffee in the filter
- For a full pot, use eight scoops
- For a half pot, use four scoops
- Rap the scoop gently on the rim of the filter receptacle to ensure it is completely empty after each scoop
- Rinse and dry the scoop and return to the drawer

Approved coffee maker

Put the lid back on the coffee and return the coffee to the shelf.

Push the filled coffee receptacle firmly back into the pot, ensuring that it is completely in place.

Fill the coffee carafe with water.
- Use cold water

Guideline: Making Coffee (continued)

- For a full pot of coffee, fill to the line near the top of the carafe
- For a half pot, fill to line midway up the carafe

Carefully pour the water from the carafe into the water reservoir at the back of the machine.

- The top of the machine opens up to allow access to the water reservoir
- If any water spills, clean it up with a paper towel (located in dispenser above sink)

Place the carafe on the heating unit at the foot of the machine.

- Be sure it is firmly in place
- Handle should be pointed toward the front of the pot

Turn the machine on by pushing the toggle switch on the left front to the "on" position.

- The red light next to the switch should be glowing
- Pot should start making gurgling noises

Wait until the machine has stopped making noise and coffee is no longer dripping into the carafe.

Pour into cup or mug.

Add cream and sugar to taste, if desired.

Enjoy.

Note that the guideline is much more detailed, and may need to be changed even if the SOP is still valid and appropriate. For example, if you changed the brand of coffee maker, you might need to change some of the steps in the guideline (type of filter, location of switch), but you would probably not need to change the SOP.

Approval, Training and Implementation

There should be an approval process for your SOPs and guidelines. In general, SOPs are subject to review by any groups or departments that are affected by them. This review (and re-review, if changes are made) will help to ensure that they are, in fact, processes that can and should be followed. The final sign off on SOPs should reside at a senior administrative level in the organization.

FAQ

We have SOPs, but most of our staff are not familiar with them. As long as we don't do anything wrong, does it matter?

Yes. When you are audited by a sponsor or by the FDA, you will be held to your SOPs. It is critical that everyone involved is trained on them and follows them. If an SOP cannot be followed, then it should be rewritten to reflect actual practice (assuming you are adhering to the regulations).

Once you have SOPs and guidelines, it is critical that all involved personnel are trained on them. SOPs are only functional if people know what they are and follow them. In general, SOPs should not be implemented until everyone is familiar with them. After they have been approved, training should take place, and then implementation should occur. Note that the approval date usually precedes the implementation date, in order to allow training to be done. Each employee should also have easy access to the SOPs and guidelines, either online, in hard copy, or both.

It is recommended that all SOPs and guidelines be reviewed at least annually to ensure they are still workable and being followed. If a process changes at any time, the appropriate SOPs and/or guidelines should be revised to reflect the change. There should also be someone who is charged with keeping the documents current and maintaining a history of the documents and any revisions. It is important to keep all previous versions of a changed SOP or guideline, with the dates during which it was in effect. This will enable the organization to know why things may have been done differently in the past and provides an audit trail for process changes.

SOPs for Investigative Sites

There are a number of SOPs that are useful for an investigative site to have. Following is a list of topics for which you will probably want to have SOPs and/or guidelines in effect at your site:

- Preparing, maintaining and training on SOPs
- Pre-study evaluation visits by potential sponsors
- Assessing protocol feasibility
- Study documents
- Preparation and maintenance of study files
- Investigator and site initiation meetings
- Informed consent process
- IRB submissions
- Various study startup activities
- Handling of case report forms (CRFs)
- Correcting CRF and source document errors
- Confidentiality of study materials
- Adverse event reporting
- Handling and storage of investigational materials, especially controlled/scheduled substances
- Investigational drug accountability
- Preparation and handling of lab samples
- Shipping of biological specimens
- Sponsor/CRO monitoring visits
- Study monitor visit logs
- Internal QA for study documents and case report forms
- Communications with sponsors/CROs
- Study closeout/termination
- Post-study critique
- Preparation for sponsor or FDA audits
- Retention and archiving of study documents
- Handling of subject/patient emergencies

Note that there are even SOPs on SOPs; these tell you what the process is for formulating, approving and training on these documents. Sometimes SOPs also have attachments, such as checklists or explanatory documents. To help you get started with SOPs, we are giving you an example of an actual SOP, guideline and attachment from a study site. This group of documents covers study closures.

SOP: Study Closure

Revision # 0 **Effective date:**

Purpose:

At the end of a study, it is important that all study materials are correctly taken care of and that all necessary documentation is appropriately filed.

SOP: Study Closure (continued)

Revision # 0 **Effective date:**

The purpose of this SOP is to ensure that proper study closeout is done for each clinical trial completed.

Scope:
This SOP applies to all clinical trials.

Responsibilities:
The investigator, clinical research coordinator, and other personnel, as appropriate, are responsible for ensuring that proper closeout activities are done.

Procedures:
1. A final report will be provided to the IRB and to the sponsor.
2. All study documentation will be verified and filed in the study file, including the Investigator Brochure.
3. Case report forms and supporting documentation will be filed.
4. All signed informed consent documents will be filed with the study documents.
5. All unused study materials, including drugs, case report forms, etc., will be disposed of or returned as directed by the sponsor.
6. Actions and problem resolutions will be documented in the study file, if not already done.
7. All materials will be filed together according to standard archiving procedures.
8. A post-study critique will be done.

Regulations and Guidances:
21 CFR 312.62 Investigator recordkeeping and record retention
21 CFR 312.64 Investigator reports
ICH Guideline for Good Clinical Practice, Section 4.9. Investigator Records and Reports
ICH Guideline for Good Clinical Practice, Section 4.10. Investigator Progress Reports

References:
SOP: Post-Study Critique
Guideline: Post-Study Critique
Guideline: Study Closeout

SOP: Study Closure (continued)

Revision # 0 **Effective date:**

Attachments:
Checklist: Study Closeout

Keywords:
Closeout, post-study critique, final report, archive

Approved by:______________________________ Date: ____________

Guideline: Study Closure

Revision # 0 **Effective date:**

At the completion of a study, all study documentation and materials must be properly filed or otherwise taken care of. It is important that proper study closeout procedures are done for each completed study.

Responsibility	**Action**
Investigator, Clinical Research Coordinator	Prepare a final report for the IRB and sponsor, including: ■ Number of subjects screened, enrolled, completed, dropped ■ Reasons for dropouts ■ Listing of all serious adverse events ■ Listing of any protocol deviations or violations ■ Other information as requested, or as appropriate Send the report to the IRB and the sponsor.
Clinical Research Coordinator	Prepare the study document file for archiving: ■ Ensure that all documents are present, including the final report (Refer to the Study Document Checklist.) ■ Include pertinent communications from the sponsor

Guideline: Study Closure (continued)

Revision # 0 **Effective date:**

Responsibility	**Action**
	■ Ensure that any problems occurring during the study (protocol violations, etc.) have been documented, including the resolution ■ Include documentation of the final return and/or disposal of unused study materials, including drug, case report forms, etc. ■ Include the Investigator Brochure in the file
Clinical Research Coordinator or other designated site personnel	Place all signed consent forms together within the file. ■ Verify that a signed consent is present for each subject
Clinical Research Coordinator or other designated site personnel	Ensure that all case report forms, including queries, etc., are present. ■ Ensure that any problems have been addressed and documented ■ Box these materials for storage
Study Coordinator or other designated site personnel	Return and/or dispose of unused study materials. ■ Contact the sponsor for directions
Designated site personnel	File all documents together according to standard archiving procedures. ■ Note in central files where these documents are stored
Investigator and/or Clinical Research Coordinator	Ensure that a post-study critique has been done.

Regulations and Guidances:

21 CFR 312.62 Investigator recordkeeping and record retention
21 CFR 312.64 Investigator reports

Guideline: Study Closure (continued)

Revision # 0 **Effective date:**

ICH Guideline for Good Clinical Practice, Section 4.9. Investigator Records and Reports
ICH Guideline for Good Clinical Practice, Section 4.10. Investigator Progress Reports

References:
SOP: Post-Study Critique
Guideline: Post-Study Critique
Guideline: Study Closeout

Attachments:
Checklist: Study Closeout
Checklist: Study Documents

Keywords:
Closeout, study documents, case report forms, informed consents, study materials, post-study critique, final report, archive

Approved by:_______________________________ Date: ____________

Study Closeout Checklist

Protocol: Sponsor:
Investigator: Date:

- ☐ Study documents file is complete (refer to Checklist: Study Documents).
- ☐ Final report has been made to the IRB and the sponsor.
- ☐ All case report forms (CRFs) are complete and have been submitted to the sponsor.
  - ☐ All CRF corrections/queries have been addressed.
  - ☐ Any patient diaries, etc., have been submitted as required.
- ☐ All source documentation is in order.
  - ☐ If not with study files, location of materials is noted in the document file.
- ☐ Study personnel form is complete.
- ☐ Subjects' signed informed consent forms are filed.
- ☐ Drug dispensing and disposition forms are complete.
- ☐ Study drug has been returned as per sponsor instructions.

Study Closeout Checklist

Protocol: ______________________ Sponsor: ______________________
Investigator: ______________________ Date: ______________________

- ☐ All other study materials (extra CRFs, etc.) have been returned to the sponsor.
- ☐ Investigator Brochure is filed with other study materials.
- ☐ All study materials are filed together as per archival procedures.
  - ☐ Location of materials is noted in records.
- ☐ Post-study critique has been held.

To sum up, SOPs are important for standardizing processes and procedures at the investigative site and for ensuring that all employees know the right way to perform their assigned tasks. They also help to ensure that regulations and good clinical practices are followed.

Key Things to Remember

- An SOP is a clearly written description of how a particular task is to be performed.
- SOPs are essential tools for standardizing processes, for ensuring that regulatory and organizational policy requirements are met, for training new personnel, and for managing workload.
- Two of the main keys to a successful research site are good, clearly written, functional SOPs and training on them.
- Process mapping is a procedure of laying out all the steps in a currently used process and analyzing the process with the goal of making it more efficient and easier to follow.
- One approach to SOPs is to have a two-tiered system that includes both SOPs and guidelines.
- There should be an approval process for SOPs and guidelines.
- It is critical that all involved personnel are trained on SOPs and guidelines.
- All SOPs and guidelines should be reviewed at least annually.
- All previous versions of SOPs and guidelines should be retained.

Note: There are two organizations that provide investigative site SOPs for purchase. They are the Center for Clinical Research Practice (www.ccrp.com) and JKK consulting (karenwoodin@mindspring.com).

CHAPTER 7

Protocols and Case Report Forms (CRFs)

Introduction

In this chapter, we will look at protocols and case report forms, the main "tools" of clinical trials. Although a CRC may never be involved in the writing of a protocol, he or she will use one for every study, so it is critical to understand what is in a protocol and what should be expected when a protocol is received from a sponsor. It may be that an investigator is also doing his or her own investigational research, in which case the CRC may be involved in helping to write a protocol. Case report forms (CRFs) are the data collection instruments for a trial; CRCs will be intimately involved in the use of these forms.

Protocols

The protocol is the plan for a study and describes how the study will be conducted. If the protocol is well written and the study design is sound, the study will be able to generate valid data that are acceptable to the scientific community, including the FDA. Even if CRCs are not involved in writing protocols, it is important for them to have an understanding of protocol basics. The protocol is the basic tool of clinical trials, and will be used in every study the CRC coordinates. Knowing the basics of a protocol makes the CRC more effective and the job easier.

A CRC should be able to read a protocol and determine whether or not it contains all the elements important to a trial, as well as the critical medical information. A CRC should be able to determine if a protocol is logistically feasible.

Contents of a Protocol

No two protocols are the same. Formats will vary from company to company and among different authors in the same company. The content will vary depending on the therapeutic area of investigation. Many sponsors have a pre-defined format for protocols that is dictated by their standard operating procedures (SOPs).

There are also differences in protocols because of the development phase of the compound. Phase I protocols are more flexible and less detailed than those for phases II and III because phase I studies are early in the development program and not much is known about how the investigational drug acts in humans. A phase I protocol is primarily an outline of the study and should include:[1]

- A description of the number of subjects to be studied
- A description of safety exclusions
- The dosing plan, including duration, dose or method being used to determine dose
- A detailed description of the safety procedures such as vital signs and laboratory evaluations

Phase II and III protocols are very detailed and describe all aspects of the investigations. The FDA defines some minimal requirements for these protocols,[2] which must contain at least:

- A description of the objectives and purpose
- The name, address and qualifications of each investigator
- The names of all sub-investigators working under the direction of the investigator
- The institution where the research will be done
- The name and address of the IRB
- The inclusion and exclusion criteria for study subjects
- The number of subjects to be evaluated
- The design of the study, including the type of control group being used, if applicable
- The methods employed to minimize bias (usually randomization and blinding)

---

1. 21 CFR 312.23 (6).
2. 21 CFR 312.23 (6).

- The method used to determine dose(s) used, the maximum dose and the duration of administration
- A description of the observations and measurements being used
- A description of the measures (laboratory evaluations, procedures, etc.) being used to monitor the effects of the investigational drug and to minimize risks to subjects

These are minimum requirements; almost all protocols will contain additional elements as well. The common elements of a protocol, in the order in which they usually appear, is discussed below.

Common Elements of a Protocol

1. **Title Page.** All protocols will have a title page. Essential information for the title page includes:

   - Title: The title should be specific enough to distinguish the protocol from those for similar studies. It should be a concise description of the study providing the reader with the drug, disease, design and study phase.

     Example: A randomized, double blind, phase III trial of (drug under study) in subjects with generalized anxiety disorder. A placebo-controlled, fixed-dose, parallel-group multicenter study of 12 weeks.

   - Protocol Number: This should be a unique number that identifies the protocol. Most sponsors have a specific procedure for determining this number that identifies the drug as well as the study.

     Example: 12AB345/0021, where 12AB345 is the drug identifier, and 0021 identifies the protocol within that drug development program.

   - IND Number: The IND number of the drug, for studies done under an IND.
   - Date: All protocols should be dated as part of their identifiers. This also allows various versions to be readily identified.
   - Sponsor Medical Monitor: The name and contact information for the sponsor's medical monitor.
   - Principal Investigator: The name and address of the investigator doing the study.
   - Some protocol cover pages include the statistician, CRA, sub-investigators, study coordinator and laboratory contact information, but these are optional.

2. **Protocol Summary.** The protocol summary should give a good overview of the study and is highly recommended. The sponsor may send your site the summary when it is interviewing potential investigators, even when the entire protocol is not yet complete. The summary will provide enough information for potential investigators to determine if they are interested in and have the capability to do the study.

   The summary is usually one to two pages long and typically includes:

- Protocol Title: Repeated from the title page.
- Study Objective: A statement of the main objectives and purpose of the study.

  Example: The primary objective is to show that (study drug) is more effective than placebo in the short-term (12 weeks) treatment of generalized anxiety disorder. The secondary objective is to gain information on the short-term safety of (study drug).

- Study Population: A brief description of the type of subjects to be included.

  Example: Study subjects will be male or female, 18 years or older, with diagnosed generalized anxiety disorder and no clinically relevant co-morbid psychiatric conditions.

- Study Design: A brief description of design, e.g., single dose, multiple dose, pilot, safety, efficacy, randomized or not, single or double blind, open label, parallel, crossover, etc.

  Example: The study is a randomized, double-blind, fixed-dose, placebo-controlled, phase III, multicenter trial.

- Study Medication, including the:
  - Generic name and trade name (if known) of the compound Example: alprazolam (Xanax®)
  - Dosage form. Example: 0.25 mg tablets
  - Route of administration. Example: Oral
  - Dose and regimen. Example: 0.25 mg three times a day

- Duration of Treatment: The time period during which the study medication will be administered to the subjects. If the treatment is not continuous, it should be described.

  Example: Subjects will be treated for 10 weeks, followed by a two-week single blind taper period.

- Methods and Materials: A general description of the procedures, tests, etc., required.
- Duration of Subject Participation: Total duration of subject involvement in the study, including screen and any follow-up.

  Example: Subjects who complete the study will have 12 weeks of study involvement.

- Anticipated Maximum Number of Subjects: Total number of subjects in all treatment groups.

  Example: There will be 440 subjects in each treatment group, for a total of 880 subjects.

  Number of Centers: If known.

3. **Abstract.** An abstract is optional. An abstract should be limited to one or two paragraphs describing the objective, design, population, sample size and major study activities.

4. **Table of Contents.** A detailed table of contents should be included in all protocols.

5. **Introduction.** The introduction should identify the reason for doing the study and place it in context with previous investigations and in the overall development plan. If the introduction is lengthy, subheadings should be used. Abbreviations and acronyms should be avoided when possible. If they are used, each abbreviation or acronym should be identified in full the first time it is used. Example: Hamilton Rating Scale for Anxiety (HAM-A). The introduction usually contains:

   - A brief discussion of the study medication, including the medical need and rationale for use.
   - A description of the design and major endpoints, including the rationale for use.
   - A description of how this protocol differs from other similar protocols for the same treatment.
   - An identification of the setting in which subjects will be studied (outpatient, hospital, etc.).
   - The rationale for the dose and regimen, citing supporting data.
   - A description of the study control (e.g., placebo) and/or comparator drug, plus the rationale for use.
   - A general description of procedures and length of the study.

6. **Study Objectives.** These should clearly state the primary and secondary objectives and identify the endpoints that will be used to satisfy

them. Primary endpoints are usually the key efficacy parameters to be studied. Secondary endpoints usually consist of efficacy variables that are of lower clinical significance and also the safety parameters of the trial. State whether the study is intended to show a difference or similarity between treatments (this could also be included under study design).

7. **Study Design.** This section should include a description of the study design, including:

   - Type of study (methodology, pilot, tolerance, efficacy, pharmacokinetics)
   - Controlled or uncontrolled
   - Single or multiple dose (fixed or variable)
   - Single site or multicenter
   - Open label or blinded
   - Randomization scheme
   - Design (parallel, crossover, matched pair, block, sequential)

8. **Randomization and Blinding.** This section should describe the randomization and blinding procedure, including any stratification. It should also contain instructions for breaking the blind, if it becomes necessary.

9. **Subject Selection.** This section will include a description of the study population, indicating the number of subjects to be enrolled. If appropriate, it will differentiate between the maximum number of subjects to be enrolled and the minimum number of subjects required to meet protocol objectives. The subject selection criteria (inclusion and exclusion criteria) should include:

   - A description of each requirement for subject eligibility. If there are any exceptions to a criterion, they should be stated.
   - Specific disease-related criteria.
   - Willingness to sign an informed consent form as an inclusion criterion.
   - Allowed and disallowed concomitant medications.
   - Criteria that will exclude subjects.
     - Subjects who are taking another investigational medication or who have recently taken an investigational medication within a specified time period (i.e., 30 days) are almost always excluded.

   This section should also include a description of when the entry criteria must be met, e.g., before or following a screening period, after a washout period, etc.

In some trials, subjects who meet basic study criteria are enrolled in a screening period. During this time, various tests are done (e.g., physical exam, laboratory tests) to determine if the subjects meet the additional criteria for entry into the entire trial. A washout period is a time when subjects are taken off their current (non-study) medications. When the carryover effect from these medications has had time to dissipate, subjects are entered into the main part of the trial.

10. **Subject Enrollment.** This section should identify the point at which a subject is considered enrolled. For randomized studies, this is usually at the time of randomization. Other possibilities might be after the informed consent form is signed or after successful completion of a screening period.

11. **Informed Consent.** The section about informed consent is sometimes located in the body of the protocol and sometimes in an appendix. The protocol section on informed consent should include:

    - A complete description of informed consent requirements, emphasizing the requirement for obtaining consent prior to a subject's involvement in any study-related activity.
    - The investigator's responsibility to obtain IRB approval of the consent.
    - Specific instructions if vulnerable populations, such as minors, will be included in the study.

12. **Screening Procedures.** This section should contain the following:

    - A description of all activities and tests related to the screening of subjects for study enrollment.
    - Specify timing relative to tests, meals or the start of treatment.
    - If results of any screening tests will be used as baseline for within-group comparisons, this should be stated.
    - Describe discontinuation of any concomitant medications, if required.

13. **Replacement of Subjects.** This section should specify whether subjects who drop out will be replaced and any conditions associated with replacement. If replacement is allowed, the protocol should specify how replacement subjects would be assigned to treatment groups.

14. **Treatment.** This section should provide the following information about the investigational medication and any comparator medication, including a placebo.

    - Generic, chemical and trade name (if known).

- Formulation of the placebo.
- Dosage forms and formulation, in general terms. If any medication contains excipients to which some subjects may be sensitive, such as lactose, this should be indicated.
- Packaging (e.g., bottles, blister packs).
- Special storage procedures and stability considerations. If the medication requires reconstitution, the stability in the reconstituted form should be specified.
- Route of administration; include any special instructions for reconstituting medication or preparing individual doses. If it is administered intravenously (IV), specify the infusion rate.
- The dosage regimen and time schedule for each dose. Clarify the duration of administration, including any medication-free periods or washout periods. As appropriate, specify the timing of dosing in relation to meals.
- Rationale for the dose and regimen.
- Procedures for dosage adjustments, if applicable.
- Compliance parameters, e.g., the number of allowable missed doses, etc.

15. **Concomitant Medication.** This section should include the policy on the use of concomitant medications, including over-the-counter (OTC) medications, herbals, and vitamin supplements. Indicate that all concomitant medication must be recorded. If concomitant medications are allowed, there should be information about how they may be used and why the use will not confound the treatment effect. Interaction data should be cited as appropriate.

    If the analyses will be stratified based on concomitant medication, this should be stated, with reference to the analysis plan.

    If smoking, alcohol, caffeine or illicit drugs are prohibited or restricted, this should be mentioned in this section.

16. **Study Activities and Observations.** This section will give all the activities that are to be done at each study visit. It should also include an overall activity schedule that shows at a glance each event, procedure, observation and evaluation that will be done for each visit. An example of a protocol activity schedule is shown below. Other considerations to keep in mind for this section are:

    - Each time period should be clearly defined.
    - All study activities, observations and evaluations to be made during each period should be listed and defined.
    - If any non-study medications are to be discontinued during a period (usually a screening period), the procedure should be described.

- The acceptable leeway or "treatment window" for each visit should be specified.
- If there is a tapered discontinuation of the investigational medication, the exact procedures, including the specific dose adjustments and time schedule to be followed should be described.

Clinical assessments also need to be described in this section, including:

- Specific criteria (as appropriate) for the various observations and assessments at each study period.
- The rationale for the selection of specific endpoints or assessment tools, unless discussed elsewhere.
- Any special conditions under which assessments are to be made or specific equipment that should be used.
- The rules or criteria for changing the management of the subject if there is either marked improvement or worsening of the subject's condition.

17. **Adverse Events.** There should be a very explicit section covering adverse events and adverse event reporting.

18. **Data Recording Instructions.** This section should:

- Indicate how data will be collected. If detailed instructions have been prepared, specify their location (e.g., study manual, appendix, etc.).
- Discuss the use and management of source documents.
- Discuss the procedure for correcting errors.

19. **Data Quality Assurance.** This section should:

- Describe procedures for assessing subject compliance.
- Describe any special training or other measures for site personnel to ensure valid data.
- Discuss source document review.
- Provide Good Clinical Practice (GCP) references.

20. **Analysis Plan.** Items that may be included are:

- Discussion of the general study design issues.
- A statement of the planned sample size, reasons for choosing it, and power calculations.
- Classification of study variables (e.g., primary versus secondary).
- Identification of statistical model(s) to be used.
- Description of specific analyses, including any subgroup analyses.

- Information about the timing and purpose of any planned interim analyses.
- Handling of missing or non-evaluable data.

21. **Risks and Benefits.** This section should briefly summarize the risks and potential benefits associated with the use of the test compound or procedure. This section should be consistent with the consent form.

22. **References.** All references for the protocol should be in this section.

23. **Appendices.** Appendices may be used to detail information that might be confusing if placed in the body of the protocol.

A very extensive guide for writing protocols can be found at: http://www.cc.nih.gov/ccc/protomechanics

After the protocol is written, case report forms can be developed.

Case Report Forms (CRFs)

Case report forms (CRFs) are used during a clinical trial to record the protocol-required data for each study subject. CRFs standardize the collection of study data and help to ensure that the medical, statistical, regulatory and data management needs of the study are met. It is the "deliverable" of the study and forms the basis for all analysis of the drug/device. Working with CRFs is a significant part of the CRC workload and is a major factor in the performance of a clinical trial.

Case Report Form Completion

When completing the case report forms for a subject, the CRC must keep a number of things in mind. You must be sure that the data entered on the forms are accurate, complete and legible. The CRC should ensure that each item has been completed and each blank filled in. Check that the answers are within range, the form is signed, if appropriate, and by the correct person, and the header is complete and correct. (The header is the top part of each form that lists the subject and study identifiers.)

Next, check all the pages for a single visit. Check for completeness, correct dates and that the visit was within the allowed window. Check to be sure that the timing of procedures was appropriate. If, for example, there was to be a blood draw, followed by another activity, then the blood draw should have been done first, and the times should reflect this. Any time there is a specific ordering to be followed for activities, that ordering must be followed.

The CRC should ensure that there is consistency across forms. If the subject is getting better according to various ratings, then the overall rating should reflect an improvement. If a form says there was a concomitant medication administered for an adverse event, then the medication should be listed on the concomitant medication form and the adverse event entered on the adverse event CRF. In addition, the CRC should think about what appears in the forms, and whether or not it makes sense, given the subject's condition and the study activities. Sometimes it's easy to see each tree, but miss the view of the overall forest.

The CRC should also check the current visit with previous visits. Are the data consistent from visit to visit? Was the timing of procedures appropriate? Do the data match where necessary? Are the visit windows correct over time? Usually each visit window is calculated by going back to the starting or baseline date, not from the previous visit. The reason for this is if a subject is always two days late, and if the window is always calculated from the last visit, you are adding two days and two more days and two more days...and so forth. After a while, there is not enough study drug for the subject to finish all the visits specified by the protocol.

Lastly, be sure you have correctly identified the same subject at each visit, with the same initials, numbers and other identifiers. It is always better to straighten out any problems you may find before the CRA comes to review CRFs at your site. Remember that monitors are on the same team with the same objective—clean accurate data.

Source Document Review

Source document review, sometimes called source document verification, involves checking the data recorded in the case report forms against data found in available source documents, including the patient chart, laboratory reports and other supporting documents. A source document is any document where the data are first recorded.

FAQ

One sponsor insists that we have a source document for every entry on the case report form. Is this in the regulations?

No. However, the sponsor may not agree to let you do the study if you cannot meet their internal requirement.

The purpose of source documentation is twofold: first, to verify that the subjects exist and, second, to verify that data in the CRF are consistent with the information found in the source documents, which verifies the integrity of the data.

For example, one would expect to see basic demographic information in an office chart for a patient, including name, address, phone number, insurance information and a social security number. When monitoring, the CRA is not interested in the particulars of this information, but only that it exists. The usual office chart will also contain lab reports or reports of other tests. The name and identifying information should match the other information in the chart. This information is indicative that the person entered in the trial actually exists.

When the data in the case report forms are in agreement with data contained in source documents, it is an indicator of the quality and veracity of the information being gathered for the study. It is not necessary for every entry in a CRF to have a matching entry in a source document, but where the data do appear in both, they should agree. Neither ICH GCPs nor FDA regulations require that source documents be kept for all entries on case report forms. Under 21 CFR 312.62(b), "An investigator is required to prepare and maintain adequate and accurate case histories that record all observations and other data pertinent to the investigation...Case histories include the case report forms and supporting data including, for example, signed and dated consent forms, progress notes of the physician,...hospital chart(s) and nurse's notes."[3]

ICH GCPs say only that the study monitor shall verify that "the data required by the protocol are reported accurately on the CRFs and are consistent with the source data/documents."[4] Despite the lack of any regulatory requirement, many companies are currently insisting on a matching source document for every case report form entry, in which case they may provide the site with source document templates to use, or the CRC may be charged with developing source documents to use during the trial. Whether or not this is the case, the CRA will verify that where matching data do exist in source records, they are consistent with the CRFs.

Upon occasion, the original collection of data may be done directly on the case report forms; in effect, the case report forms become source documents. This is frequently seen in rating scales, such as the Hamilton Depression Rating Scale, because it is easier to collect the information directly on the CRF as opposed to transcribing it later. It is not wrong to do this, but a note should be made to the investigator's study file saying that this is being done. The sponsor may request/require this to be done.

If a discrepancy is found between the case report form and the source document during monitoring, the CRA should always ask the investigator or coordinator to determine which one is correct, and to make the appropriate corrections. Usually the source document takes precedence. If the source document is corrected, the CRC should sign and date the document, including an explanation, as appropriate. Sponsor CRAs should not make changes on either the source documents or the case report forms; this is the responsibility of the CRC or other site personnel. The CRC must remember, however, that even one change on a CRF or in a source document can have

---

3. 21 CFR 312.62 (b).
4. ICH Guideline for Good Clinical Practice 5.18.4(m).

an impact on other data. Be sure to check this, both within the visit and across visits.

There are significant differences among sponsors with respect to the amount of source document review that a CRA must do, and there are no guidelines in the regulations. Some companies require "100% source document review," but the definitions of 100% source document review also vary, from the expectation of a source document for every data point for every subject, to 100% verification of the data insofar as it exists in source documents. Other sponsors have sampling schemes, and these also vary considerably. Whatever the scheme, however, all subjects' case report forms are normally reviewed for critical information, such as the inclusion and exclusion criteria, a signed informed consent form, adverse events and critical study-specific parameters.

Errors, Queries and Corrections

Some of the most critical errors made during a clinical trial are those that result in protocol violations. These include such things as a subject not meeting the inclusion and exclusion criteria, a wrong diagnosis, a subject taking disallowed medications, problems with visit windows and others. Often these are found during source document review by the CRA. Other errors found during source document review run the gamut from incorrectly transcribed data to things that are just plain wrong. There are also case report form errors, such as missing data or out-of-range values.

Fixing errors is easier if your CRA has an effective procedure for dealing with them when they are found. Many sponsors have an Error Query/Correction form that is specific to their CRFs. Some CRAs rely heavily on sticky notes. Although they are good reminders, and mark CRFs nicely, they can fall off and get lost, and they do not generate an audit trail. A written correction form/log is more effective overall.

FAQ

We have a new CRA, and she wants us to fill in the CRFs differently than the previous CRA said—plus, she wants us to go back and change all the previous entries for this variable. Do we have to do this? It's an enormous amount of work.

This can be a real problem. Your best bet is to contact the sponsor medical monitor, explain the problem, and ask for advice. Chances are that the difference can be resolved internally, not at the site. If you do need to go back and change all previous entries, you might ask for some additional financial compensation to pay for this "unbudgeted" time.

When potential errors are found during a monitoring visit, the CRA should note them in the corrections/questions log and discuss them with the CRC. When they are resolved, the CRC should make the necessary corrections to the case report forms; CRAs do not make the corrections. Corrections are made by drawing a line through the incorrect entry, making the correct entry, and dating and initialing it. If the reason for the change is not clear, a reason should also be added to the form. It is never acceptable to use whiteout or to erase a wrong entry before correcting it; anyone reviewing the forms must be able to see what was changed, when and why. Write-overs are also unacceptable. See the example below for a correctly done change.

Date 01/16/~~01~~ 02 JAK 2/5/02

It is in the CRC's best interest to correct errors at the site before sending the case report forms to the sponsor. However, despite everyone's best efforts, additional errors are often found when the CRFs go to data entry at the sponsor's. Computer-generated errors will be sent back to the site and/or to the CRA. These are usually called queries. Different sponsors have different methods of doing queries, but usually there is a query form that is sent to the site; it lists the errors, where the errors are located on the CRF, and asks for a correction or explanation to be made and sent in. Sometimes the CRA is involved in the correction process; sometimes it is solely between the site and data management.

Whether errors are found by the CRA or come in the form of queries, the CRC should think of them as training tools. If it is not clear, ask your CRA to explain why each one is an error and how it can be avoided in the future. It is important to have your CRA review and submit the forms for the first few subjects as early as possible, in order to give you timely feedback so that you can eliminate similar errors in the future. This is especially important in the case of consistent errors, which are usually due to misunderstanding.

Error rates should decrease as the study progresses, due to feedback and training by the CRA and data management, as well as to experience on the part of the CRC and other site personnel.

Errors are very costly, both in terms of money and people hours to correct. Although most of the cost is borne by the sponsor, about one-third of the cost of correcting errors is borne by the site.

Electronic Data Capture (EDC)

The advantages of electronic data capture (EDC) applications over paper-based clinical trials are numerous. First, as data are entered (for example, into a case report form or medical record), automated data edit checks alert the investigative site to possible errors in data entry. The site can check while the source document is readily available, rather than months later in a typical paper-based process. This immediate feedback can not only help the site in correcting the initial issue but can also help educate the site to avoid similar errors in the future. Since there is no delay as is typical in the paper process, costly errors can be avoided much earlier in the process.

A common type of EDC comes in the form of an "e-diary." Study subjects enter their personal and confidential data into an electronic diary device, for example, a cell phone or personal digital assistant (PDA), similar to the way they complete a paper diary. The study subject provides observations about side effects, symptoms and the perceived effectiveness of a medical treatment. Numerous e-diary data collection approaches have been validated. Screens may display an outline of the human body where, using a stylus, the patient can indicate where pain is occurring and its severity. Patients can enter the exact time a medication was taken. And subjects can respond to a number of different quality-of-life measures. Once collected, electronic diary data are transmitted back to study personnel through a wireless or landline modem.[5]

Impressed with improvements in volunteer compliance from e-diaries, the FDA has expressed interest in developing specific e-diary guidelines to ease adoption. Industry is finding that e-diaries can be a flexible and lower-cost technology solution that can be integrated relatively easily and quickly into research projects and existing processes. Given that more than 75% of all clinical trials now include a patient reporting component, investigative sites can anticipate that e-diary adoption will continue to progress at a much faster rate relative to other eClinical technologies.[6] There are many reasons why EDC has not been implemented as quickly as many people had hoped. The problems encountered include such things as: system crashes, training on multiple systems, set up/maintenance woes, time to enter data via keyboard and cumbersome data corrections. Over time, solutions will probably be found for many of these difficulties.

CRCs should remain vigilant to changes in the industry, and be prepared to adapt as new technologies come along. There is no question that sites and CRCs will see and be involved more and more with EDC in the future.

Good, High Quality Data

We talk a lot in this business about "good, high quality data," but this term isn't usually defined. By asking a number of people how they would define good, high quality data, the following list of characteristics was generated.

---

5. Zisson, Stephen, "Break-Away Adoption of e-Diaries," *CenterWatch*, Vol. 10, Issue 11, November 2003.
6. Ibid.

The general characteristics for good data are:

- They can be evaluated and analyzed.
- They allow valid conclusions to be drawn.
- They are complete and accurate.
- They do not need to be queried.
- They are consistent across subjects and sites.

More specific characteristics are:

- Subjects meet the entry criteria.
- All fields are complete.
- Entries are legible and understandable.
- Values are within range.
- Entries make logical sense.
- The units (for measurements) are correct.
- There are no extraneous comments.

If these characteristics are met, the data should lead to valid conclusions and results that are reproducible. This is the goal for clinical studies. If your site can provide high quality data in a timely manner, you should have many opportunities to do studies.

There are a number of things that sponsors can do to help sites eliminate errors and generate good, usable data. First of all, the sponsor should develop good case report forms that are readable, easy for sites to use and have clear directions. Clear, detailed instructions and good training are also instrumental in minimizing errors. Most errors are due to misunderstandings, and these misunderstandings can be eliminated with training. Asking your CRA to come and monitor soon after the first few subjects are enrolled is a big help in clearing up misunderstandings. Fast turnaround on edits and queries will eliminate repeat errors, as well as cross-form edits of which the site was not aware. All of these items will help the site achieve lower error rates, with big cost savings in terms of both time and money for both the site and the sponsor.

As a CRC, do not hesitate to ask questions and have items clarified. It will pay large dividends in the future and save you and the CRA unnecessary time and effort on making corrections.

Internal Quality Assurance

Sites that are dedicated to doing clinical studies often have their own plan for quality assurance (QA). They may have a person dedicated to this function, if the site is large, or they may manage it with part-time work by someone at the site. QA usually consists of checking the case report forms and doing source document review on all or part of them before the CRA comes to monitor them. The person carrying out this responsibility should be someone other than the person who completed the forms initially; often CRCs at a site act as the QA person for each other's studies. When doing QA, the person acts in the same capacity as the site monitor or CRA. He or she should check the case report forms, perform source document review, and tag any errors or questionable entries for CRC review. Doing internal QA prepares a site to present case report forms to the sponsor that are clean and ready to submit without needing additional work during the monitoring visit. This will help your site achieve a reputation for excellent work.

Like all QA, this is "error confirmation" after the fact. It is much better to ensure first-time quality by use of such tools as careful construction of source documents, lists of all visit day procedures, randomizations, checklists, etc. It is always better to do it right the first time.

Key Things to Remember

- The protocol is the plan for a study. It contains all the information necessary to do the study correctly and well.
- Protocols for phase I studies are relatively flexible, while those for phases II and III are more rigid and detailed.
- Certain information is required by regulation to be in protocols.
- Case report forms have a significant impact on data quality.
- The purpose of source document review is to verify subjects' existence and the integrity of the data.
- Quick feedback and explanation of errors and queries will help reduce the number of corrections needed in the future.
- Corrections or modifications to source documents or case report forms can only be done by site personnel, not by sponsor monitors.
- Correcting errors before CRA review and submission to the sponsor saves the site time and money.
- Internal quality assurance will help to ensure that the case report forms have minimal errors when reviewed by the study monitor.

CHAPTER 8

Preparing for a Study

Introduction

In this chapter we will discuss a number of activities that happen before a site is selected, as well as activities that must be completed before a study site can start enrolling subjects. Topics included are: site assessments, assessing protocol feasibility, budgeting, preparing the site for a study, study initiation documents, financial disclosure and investigator meetings. CRCs are usually involved in all these activities and need to have a thorough understanding of each of them.

Site Assessments (Site Evaluations)

The site evaluation is a critical step for both the sponsor and the site. For the site, these visits determine whether or not they will be selected to participate in the research, while for the sponsor, they are the primary method of determining the best sites to conduct their studies.

When a sponsor or contract research organization (CRO) is looking for investigative sites for a protocol, the first contact is usually by telephone. If it appears that there is a high level of interest in the protocol on the part of the potential investigator, and if the sponsor feels there is good potential for placing a study at the site, it will arrange a time to visit the site in person. This will enable the sponsor to better evaluate the investigator's capability to do the project. Many companies require a signed confidentiality agreement before sharing a protocol summary; in this case, they will fax or mail a confidentiality agreement to the site and have it completed and returned before sending the materials. Note that some sponsors and CROs send a preliminary questionnaire to sites to assess their suitability for a particular clinical trial. It is a point in the site's favor to return the signed confidentiality agreement and any questionnaires to the sponsor/CRO quickly.

When a sponsor representative, usually the CRA, makes an evaluation visit to a potential investigative site, he or she will be evaluating the investigator's experience, expertise and interest in the trial, as well as the staff, facility and potential patient population available. The sponsor may have a specific checklist that will guide the CRA in making an assessment. There is an example of such a checklist in Appendix D.

The main attributes assessed in an evaluation visit are the investigator's experience, expertise and interest. The sponsor will want a copy of the investigator's curriculum vitae (CV) in order to make a general assessment of the investigator's experience and expertise. Conversing with the investigator in person will allow the sponsor to determine his or her research activity, especially in the therapeutic area of interest. The sponsor will also want to know if the investigator has conducted trials similar to the one being proposed, or has worked with similar compounds. The investigator and CRC should read any materials (protocol synopsis) before the evaluation meeting so that they are prepared for the discussion.

The sponsor will also evaluate whether the site has sufficient staff and an appropriate facility to do the study. Many sponsors will not place a study at an investigative site that does not have a clinical research coordinator (CRC). During the evaluation visit, the CRA will want to meet and spend some time interviewing the CRC. Not only must there be appropriate people available for a study, but they must have sufficient time to do the necessary work. The CRA will also assess the general atmosphere at the site to determine if the people in the office are pleasant and friendly and how, if you were a study subject, you would feel about interacting with them.

During an evaluation visit, you should offer to show the CRA your facilities. The CRA will want to see that there are appropriate drug and study supply storage areas, equipment necessary for performing the study and a place for the CRA to work during monitoring visits.

The CRA will thoroughly assess the enrollment potential of the site, including whether subjects will come from the investigator's current patient population or if they will be drawn from elsewhere. Note that it is usually easier to assess enrollment potential for chronic disease studies than it is for acute disease studies. For chronic diseases, such as arthritis or diabetes, the investigator should already have appropriate patients among his or her current patient base. It does not necessarily follow that these patients will qualify for or want to participate in the research study, but it gives a base from which to start. For acute studies, one must rely on past statistics. For example, if a pneumonia study is being discussed, the CRA will want to know how many patients with pneumonia the investigator saw over the past year. In either case, the more thorough the records are concerning the patient population, the better the enrollment estimates will be.

FAQ

What are the most important factors in a sponsor's determination of which sites to pick for a study?

Past experience and current capability are probably the most important, but all the factors mentioned in this section will be taken into account. And—many sponsors won't even consider using an investigator who does not have a CRC.

There are several other items a CRA will want to discuss during an evaluation visit. One is whether or not the site is doing, or is planning to do within the same time period, any competing studies. A competing study is usually one in which similar subjects are to be enrolled. In order to meet the enrollment targets, it's important that a study does not have to compete for subjects with another sponsor's study. In assessing competing studies, it is not enough to assess only those studies being done at the investigator's site, but those being done in the same community. Those studies will also be in competition for subjects, and can have a great impact on the ability to meet enrollment targets.

Another factor is the timing for the study. If the site has too many active studies at the same time, a study may not get the attention it needs to be done well.

The CRA will want to check on the laboratory and pharmacy, if either will be used for the study, to ensure that laboratory accreditations are current and the facilities are adequate to perform the necessary study activities. If a pharmacy will be involved in drug dispensing, the CRA may wish to meet with the pharmacist.

The importance of the site evaluation visit cannot be overstated. It is this visit, more than any other factor, that determines whether or not your site will be selected to participate in the research. Consequently, the investigator and CRC should be well prepared for the visit and ready to show their site at its best.

Protocol Feasibility

The sponsor is not the only entity that needs to determine if a study should be done at a site. It is equally important for the site personnel to make an assessment of whether or not a proposed study is a good fit for their capabilities. It is always better to turn down a study that is not a good fit for your site than to accept it and fail.

Just as sponsors have checklists and specific items they need to assess at a site, the site should have specific things to assess before accepting a study. The CRC, the investigator, and any other people who will be involved in the study should read the protocol and supporting materials before making an assessment. Following is a list of some of the questions they should ask before agreeing to participate:

1. Have we worked with this sponsor before and was it a successful partnership?
2. Are the number of subjects to be enrolled and the timeline realistic?
3. Will our patients benefit from this study?
4. Do we have the necessary resources to do the study within the given time period?
5. Are we interested in the study?
6. Do we have access to the right kind of patients for this study?
7. How difficult will the protocol be to execute?
8. Is the budget reasonable?

FAQ

We've been offered a study, but we don't think we can really do it very well (enrollment will probably be difficult). We're worried that if we say no to it, the sponsor won't come back.

You will almost always be better off telling a sponsor you cannot do a study when you don't think you can do it well. Most sponsors will come to you again if they have a more suitable protocol. However, if you accept a study and fail, the sponsor can't afford to try your site again.

It is recommended that the site use a checklist when evaluating a potential study. There is a sample checklist provided in Appendix D. After each involved person has made his or her assessment, a group discussion is valuable in reaching a decision. Again, it is much better for a site to pass on a protocol than to take on a project and fail at it. Most sponsors will respect a decision not to participate when it is based on a thorough analysis, and will come back to the site with other studies that may be a better fit. However, once a site has failed at a study, most sponsors will not want to use the site again. Consequently, study feasibility is one of the most important pre-study tasks to be performed.

Grants, Budgeting and Contracts

Protocols have become more complex, calling for more procedures, on average. This means that sites must be careful about whether or not they can actually afford to do a study, without losing money, and that they will need to be very selective about the projects they decide to take on. There are many hidden costs that the investigative site has to beware of. Investigative sites are typically taking on clinical projects that require an estimated $4,000 to $6,000 in hidden costs per study that are not being reimbursed by sponsors and CROs.

Most sponsors operate on a fee-for-service basis. This means that they will pay for actual work performed, i.e., subjects enrolled and subject visits. Most grants are formulated on a per-subject amount and prorated for the number of visits a subject actually completes. The amount per visit will often vary, as some visits are more labor- and time-intensive than others. Sponsors feel that they are buying a service from the investigator and do not expect to pay if the work (subjects and data) is not delivered.

There are different ways in which sponsor grant figures are determined. Many of the larger companies subscribe to a service called PICAS from DataEdge. PICAS is a computer program that is used to calculate grant figures. Briefly, all the subscribers put their grant information into the system (blinded) by the type of study, the procedures involved, site locations and amounts. The data from all the companies form a huge informational database. When starting a new protocol, the subscriber can enter all the protocol procedures into PICAS and get back subject costs, including ranges, averages and deciles, overall and regionally. This gives the sponsor a very realistic grant range to work from when determining how much they wish to pay for per-patient grants. PICAS is probably the best method available for determining realistic grants based on actual data.

Some sponsors will determine a range or a single per-subject grant figure that they will pay and will not budge from this figure. Investigators either accept it or will not be able to do the study. Other sponsors will allow more flexibility, depending on experience with an investigator or geographic location. Costs do differ in different parts of the country, so it makes sense to allow some flexibility.

CRCs often help investigators when it comes to figuring a budget and determining an appropriate grant amount for a study. A good way to come up with a grant figure is to look at each study activity, attach a cost to it, add an additional amount for overhead and other required activities, and total it up. The charge for each item should also include the cost of the time of the

Table 1: Examples of Top Uncompensated PI Costs

Principal Investigator Activities	*Uncompensated costs for an 18-week, 10-subject trial*
Study Supervision	$1,733
Investigator Meeting Attendance	$1,541
Case Report Form Review	$963
Initiation Visit Attendance	$578
Adverse Event Management	$482
CRA Meetings and Interactions	$433

Source: RapidTrials, 2003.

Table 2: Distribution of Investigative Site Operating Income

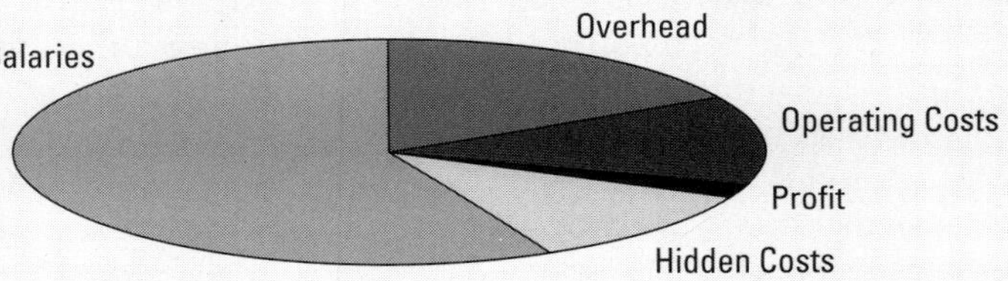

Source: CenterWatch, 2003.

person performing it. An example of a grant worksheet for a hypothetical study is shown in Table 3.

For this hypothetical study there are eight visits. One common way to determine a prorating schedule is to look at the visits and the amount of work to be done at each visit. If some visits demand considerably more work than others, count them as two visits; generally speaking, the baseline visit and the final visit are the most demanding.

In the example shown in Table 4, there are three visits that are more labor-intensive, (Visits 1, 5 and 8) the three that involve physical exams and stress testing. To determine the prorating dollar amount, each of these visits should count as two and the other five visits should each count as one, for a total of eleven. If the cumulative amount of $5,152 is divided by 11, the cost per visit is $468.36. Based on this, the three more intensive visits should be prorated at $937, and the other five at $468 (with the extra dollar added to the cost of the last visit). Note that if a subject drops out after visit 3, the investigator would be paid $1,837. For a subject dropping out at Week 7, the payment would be $4,214, and so forth.

This is a simple way of calculating grants and prorating visit costs, but it is quite effective if the initial amounts for each procedure and activity are realistic. It is easy to explain and should help the investigator and the CRC in negotiating a grant amount that is fair to both the sponsor and the site.

Table 3: Budget Worksheet—Protocol XXX

Study activity	Number of visits	Charge	Expanded charge
Phone pre-screen	1	50	50
Medical history	1	50	50
Physical exam	3	150	450
Labs	8	150	1,200
EKG	3	200	600
Treadmill stress test	3	250	750
Office visit—general assessments	8	75	600
Phone assessments	2	50	100
Subtotal for procedures			**$3,800**
Coordinator time	8	50	400
Pharmacy charge	8	35	280
Subtotal			**$680**
Total			**$4,480**
Overhead—15%			672
Grand total per completed subject			**$5,152**

Table 4: Grant Amounts for One Subject

	Visit 1	Visit 2	Visit 3	Visit 4	Visit 5	Visit 6	Visit 7	Visit 8
Amount per visit	$937	$468	$468	$468	$937	$468	$468	$938
Cumulative amount	$937	$1,405	$1,837	$2,341	$3,278	$3,746	$4,214	$5,152

Some companies utilize their monitor (the CRA) in determining when grant monies should be paid, while others handle all grant payments in-house without the CRA's involvement. These companies usually pay either on a timed schedule, such as quarterly, or on the basis of case report forms received in-house. Whatever the scheme, the site will want to know what it is ahead of time, so it is prepared accordingly.

Note that many companies will pay a small amount of the grant up front (maybe two subjects' worth), but will then apply this amount to the work being done. This allows the investigator to set up study procedures, pay for initial labs and other tests, etc., without having to use site funds. If subjects are not enrolled for whatever reason, the upfront money may have to be returned. Watch the contract wording. Sometimes a non-refundable startup amount can be negotiated for all the work preparing up to the point of startup. The investigator and/or the CRC should keep track of the work done and payments made to be sure that everything balances as it should.

FAQ

We'd like to work with a particular sponsor, but the grant they are offering us for a study will not cover our costs. Should we do the study anyway, hoping for additional work with the sponsor in the future?

Your first task should be discussing the grant in detail with the sponsor. Show the sponsor your actual figures, and see if they can make an adjustment in your grant amount. If not, you have to decide how much money you are willing to lose in the hopes of another study. Just remember, their next grant may not be any better.

If the CRC is involved in grants, he or she must have a good understanding of both the process and the specifics for each protocol in order to be able to discuss the grant with the investigator and the sponsor, and to track the figures to ensure that all sums are paid as appropriate.

A contract between the sponsor and the investigator will be signed before the trial starts at a site. This document usually contains the responsibilities of the investigator, including the number of subjects the site is expecting to enroll, timelines for enrollment, grant amounts and the regulatory requirements for the investigator. It also contains the responsibilities of the sponsor, including when and how grants will be paid, monitoring of the study and sponsor regulatory requirements. The investigator should always ask for an indemnification clause from the sponsor. It will be signed by the appropriate company representative, and by the investigator. (Note that in large institutions contracts may be signed by someone in the contract office, rather than by the investigator.) Contracts are rarely written, negotiated or signed by the CRC, although he or she may have input into the contract when working on it with the investigator.

Investigative Site Study Files

Before the study starts, the CRC should set up study files at the site. Good study files will have a significant impact on the quality of a study and, subsequently, the validity and usability of the data.

By regulation (21CFR 312.62), the investigator must keep records relating to disposition of the study drug, including dates, quantity and use by study subjects, and case histories, including case report forms and all supporting documentation. Supporting documentation includes the signed and dated consent form, medical records, progress notes, hospital charts, nursing notes and any other source documents. It should also be documented that informed consent was obtained prior to the subject's participation.

This is the minimum by regulation. In reality, study files contain much more information. One recommendation is to have three major categories for study files: regulatory, administrative and clinical. Site study files organized under this system would look like this:

In the regulatory files, the following will be kept:

- Completed Form FDA 1572 (Statement of Investigator)
- Copies of the curriculum vitae (CV) for the investigator and sub-investigators
- IRB-approved consent form
- Written IRB approvals of the study protocol and consent form, and advertising and subject compensation, if applicable
- Signed copy of the protocol and any amendments
- Copies of the laboratory certification and normal ranges
- Investigator brochure
- Investigational New Drug application (IND) safety reports
- Other similar items

In the administrative section of the file, the following will be kept:

- Correspondence, telephone logs and emails including contacts with the sponsor, contract research organization, CRO (if involved), IRB and the institution (if applicable)
- Instructional material
  - Case report form (CRF) completion/correction
  - Guidelines for handling adverse events
  - Procedures for handling and storing laboratory specimens
  - Study drug information, including instructions for storing, dispensing and accounting
- Drug shipment, dispensing and return records
- Sponsor/CRO contact information
- Log of study subjects (Master Study Subject Roster)
- Records of meetings and contact with the sponsor and/or CRO
- Monitoring log (a record of CRA monitoring visits)
- Miscellaneous

Occasionally things happen during a clinical trial that are outside the normal procedure and merit a note to the file. For example, a patient lost one bottle of medication. The note may say:

> Mr. Smith lost one bottle of medication while on vacation. The sponsor was notified (Carl White, 6/8/04). Mr. Smith had an adequate sup-

ply, so he did not miss any doses. The sponsor will send a replacement bottle for Mr. Smith.

Cynthia Rodgers, CRC 6/8/04

Follow-up—6/10/04
New meds received 6/10/04 and will be placed in Mr. Smith's medication box, as per sponsor (Carl White).

Cynthia Rodgers, CRC 6/10/04

The site will also have a clinical file for each study subject, which will include:

- CRFs and supporting documents
- Signed consent form

There are two items not mentioned in the list above: the grant and any reports from sponsor quality assurance (QA) audits. This information is not routinely made available to FDA auditors and should not be kept in study files.

File retention is discussed in Chapter 11, Study Closure. However, investigators and CRCs must be aware from the start of the study that all study documents must be retained long after the study is over.

If you have not set up study files before, your CRA can be a valuable help in assisting you with setting up and maintaining files throughout the study. The CRA will also check the files regularly throughout the study and again at study closure. Being sure that the files are complete and in order periodically during the study will ensure that they are in good condition in the event of an audit of the site by the sponsor, the IRB or the FDA. Some companies also provide clearly marked containers for study files to help minimize loss after the study is completed.

During a study, you will want to have your study subject files kept where they are ready to be easily accessed for sponsor monitor visits. Some sites have a special file room or area where they keep patient files for active studies. Not only are the files easy to access for monitoring visits, but they are also easy to access during patient study visits. These files usually contain not only the patient chart, but also any other source documents and the case report forms for the patient as well. Although these files should be easily accessible during a monitoring visit, sponsor monitors should not have free access to them. Rather, the CRC should pull the appropriate files and take them to the monitor's workstation for use. This is because sites frequently do studies for different sponsors at the same time, and no monitor should have access to another sponsor's confidential information. In fact, during a site evaluation visit, many sponsors will check on how confidentiality of materials is maintained at a site.

When a study is complete, a subject's regular office chart may be replaced in the usual office filing system. However, it should be marked as a study patient file in case it needs to be pulled for any study-related activities, such as audits, at a later date. It is always necessary to keep these charts and materials.

Some sites use special marking systems to designate charts of study patients. One way is to have a stamp made and stamp the outside of the chart with "STUDY SUBJECT." Others have a more elaborate system with a stamp that allows the sponsor and protocol to be written in, which allows easy identification of the chart/patient in the future (see example below).

STUDY SUBJECT

Sponsor:
Protocol:
Start date:

Other sites have brightly colored stickers printed with similar information on them. The stickers may be affixed to the outside of the chart, or may even be designed to fold over the edge so they are easily visible when the chart is filed in an upright position.

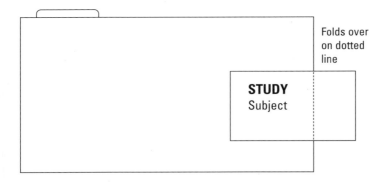

The keys to maintaining good files are to organize them at the start, to file things regularly throughout the trial and to file everything correctly. If you do this, your trial will run more smoothly, and you will be well prepared both for audits and for long-term storage of the documents.

Source Documents

A source document is any document where the data are first recorded. Your study monitor will check the source documents throughout the trial; this is known as source document review or source document verification. The purpose of source document verification is twofold: first, to verify that the subjects exist, and second, to verify that data in the CRF are consistent with the information found in the source documents, which verifies the integrity of the data.

The primary source document for a study subject is the regular office chart. One would expect to see basic demographic information in an office chart for each patient, including name, address and telephone number, insurance information, and a social security number. Your site monitor is not interested in the particulars of this information, but only that it exists. The usual office chart will also contain lab reports or reports of other tests. The name and identifying information should match the other information in the chart. This information is indicative that the person entered in the trial actually exists.

Other source documents include such things as laboratory reports and electrocardiogram (ECG) and other test readings and reports. Depending on the type of practice you are working in, and the types of studies that are conducted at your site, there may be other items that qualify as source documents. Upon occasion, the original collection of data may be done directly on the case report form or patient diaries; in effect, the case report form and/or diary becomes a source document in this case. This is often seen in rating scales, such as the Hamilton Depression Rating Scale, because it is easier to collect the information directly on the CRF as opposed to transcribing it later. When this is done, a note of explanation should be made in the investigator's study file.

Storage of Study Materials

Studies often necessitate the use of lots of materials. Not only is there the study drug or other test article to be stored, but there are the case report forms, laboratory kits and miscellaneous other materials. The CRC must be prepared to arrange appropriate storage space for these materials.

If your site is short of storage area—and many are—either for the drug or other study materials, discuss this with your sponsor representative before all the materials are sent. The sponsor may be able to send you smaller quantities at one time, and ship them more frequently. The downside for the CRC, however, is that you must remember to order more before you actually run out of the old supplies. Companies usually want at least two weeks to get new supplies to you, and you don't want to be left with the "perfect patient" ready to enroll and no drug for him or her.

It is critical to discuss the storage criteria for the study drug or other test article with the sponsor before the study starts. If, for example, you are required to have a -70° freezer, it is not acceptable to think you can use the -20° freezer that you have on site. Depending on your perceived value to the sponsor, they may even be willing to provide you with the -70° freezer, but only if it is discussed before the study commences. The CRC must also be prepared to keep such items as temperature logs to verify that the drug has been stored properly throughout the study.

Many studies use a central laboratory for all sites. These laboratories will send the site laboratory kits for the collection and shipping of samples for each study subject at each appropriate visit. These kits also take up a lot of space. Most laboratories are able to ship them to the sites in smaller quantities, but need to know ahead of time. (You can usually see the kits and find out how to handle shipments at the investigator meeting.)

Good planning and organization in advance of a study startup will help to ensure a study that runs smoothly and well throughout its course.

Study Documents

Before a trial can begin, a number of documents must be collected for each site. Most of these are required by FDA regulations, although some sponsors may require their own additional documents. Both the sponsor and the investigator must have copies of each of these documents; usually, the originals are kept at the investigator's site, while copies are sent to the sponsor. Most often the CRC is the one in charge of collecting and preparing these documents.

The documents listed below are the ones that a sponsor company must have from the site before the trial may start. Note that most sponsors will not ship the study drug before receiving all of the documents.

- Signed, IRB-approved protocol and any amendments
- IRB-approved informed consent, preferably containing an IRB-approved stamp
- IRB approval letter, verifying approval of both the protocol and consent document
- IRB approval of advertising and subject recruitment materials, including subject compensation, if applicable
- Signed, completed Form FDA 1572 (Statement of Investigator)
- Financial disclosure forms for the investigator and any other study personnel listed on the 1572
- Appropriate CVs for everyone listed on the 1572
- Current laboratory certification and laboratory normal ranges
- Signed contract or letter of agreement (not required by regulation, but required by most sponsors)

Some sponsor companies have specific people whose primary responsibility is to collect and maintain these documents, while in other companies the sponsor monitors (CRAs) gather the documents for their sites. Since the CRA is the person who visits the site, he or she will probably be involved in the collection and maintenance of documents even if another internal group has the primary responsibility.

The one document that generally takes the longest time to get is the IRB approval letter. This is the only document not under the direct control of the investigator. The IRB may have approved the study, but until the investigator receives written notification, it is not official. The CRC may need to keep contacting the IRB about the letter on a regular basis, as some IRBs are slow to issue their approval letters.

Most sponsors will not ship the study drug until all the documents have been received. Note that some companies do ship the case report forms and other non-drug supplies before receiving all the documents in an effort to speed the process, while others wait and ship everything only after documentation is complete.

Financial Disclosure

In February of 1998, the FDA published the final rule for financial disclosure. The requirement became effective a year later, and applies to any study of a drug, biologic or device that is used to support a marketing application. The regulation requires that sponsors certify the absence of certain financial interests of clinical investigators, disclose these financial interests, or certify that the information was impossible to obtain. If a sponsor does not do this, the FDA may refuse to file the application. A full description of the requirements is found in 21 CFR 54.

Disclosable financial arrangements, as taken from the FDA's "Guidance for Industry: Financial Disclosure for Investigators," are:

(a) Compensation affected by the outcome of clinical studies means compensation that could be higher for a favorable outcome than for an unfavorable outcome, such as compensation that is explicitly greater for a favorable result or compensation to the investigator in the form of an equity interest in the sponsor of a covered study or in the form of compensation tied to sales of the product, such as a royalty interest.

(b) Significant equity interest in the sponsor of a covered study means any ownership interest, stock options, or other financial interest whose value cannot be readily determined through reference to public prices (generally, interests in a nonpublicly traded corporation), or any equity interest in a publicly traded corporation that exceeds $50,000 during the time the clinical investigator is carrying out the study and for 1 year following completion of the study.

(c) Proprietary interest in the tested product means property or other financial interest in the product including, but not limited to, a patent, trademark, copyright or licensing agreement.

(f) Significant payments of other sorts means payments made by the sponsor of a covered study to the investigator or the institution to support activities of the investigator that have a monetary value of more than $25,000, exclusive of the costs of conducting the clinical study or other clinical studies, (e.g., a grant to fund ongoing research, compensation in the form of equipment or retainers for ongoing consultation or honoraria) during the time the clinical investigator is carrying out the study and for 1 year following the completion of the study.[1]

Financial disclosure became an issue with small biotech companies in their startup phases, as sometimes investigators and companies had closely tied financial interests, leading to conflict of interest in the testing of potential new products.

Having a financial interest in a company or product does not mean that an investigator cannot be involved in a trial; it simply means that all parties must be aware of the potential for conflict of interest. The sponsor will want to evaluate the potential for bias based on an investigator's financial interest before deciding whether or not to use that investigator. The FDA will do the same when reviewing an NDA.

FAQ

When accumulating the financial disclosure information for a sponsor, do I need to determine whether my mutual funds hold stock in the sponsor company, and how much might be included in my portfolio (in the mutual fund)?

No. It is not necessary to do this.

Financial disclosure applies to all the people listed on the Form FDA 1572 for a study, plus their spouses and dependent children. This is one good reason for not listing people unnecessarily on the 1572.

Financial disclosure information must be collected at study start. Any changes that result in exceeding the threshold(s) must be reported during the course of the study and for one year following its completion. There is no required form for the collection of this information from the investigator. Consequently, sponsors develop their own forms and ways of collecting and maintaining this information. Financial disclosure information must be reported to the FDA on Form FDA 3454 (certification of absence of financial interest) or Form FDA 3455 (disclosure of financial interest). These forms are submitted as a part of the NDA.

1. 21 CFR 54.2.

Although not popular with investigators or sponsors, financial disclosure information is required to be collected. CRCs may be involved in the collecting of that information, or, if they are listed on the 1572 for a study, will need to provide the information for themselves and their families. Because of their potential involvement, it is recommended that CRCs read the FDA's "Guidance for Industry, Financial Disclosure by Clinical Investigators," which is available on the FDA's web site (www.fda.gov).

Investigator Meetings

For multicenter trials (clinical trials involving several sites performing the same protocol) most sponsors hold an investigator meeting. Although not required by regulation, this meeting, which includes all investigators, their coordinators and appropriate sponsor representatives, is one of the most important activities pertaining to the conduct of a good trial. This meeting is often the first time the investigators and study coordinators meet the sponsor personnel; it creates an initial impression on both sides and sets the tone for the rest of the study.

Investigator meetings are scheduled and conducted by the sponsor, sometimes with the help of a contract research organization or a meeting planning company. The purpose of these meetings is to allow the participants to get to know each other, which facilitates communication throughout the study, and to review the entire study and its conduct. The major advantages of holding these meetings are that everyone hears the same thing at the same time and site and sponsor personnel become acquainted with each other; communications during the trial are easier when people have met in person.

Since these meetings are expensive, it is important that most sites are ready to start the study before the meeting. Sites that start the study more than a month or two after the investigator meeting will have forgotten much of the information by the time they actually start. Ideally, the study drug is shipped while the meeting is going on. CRCs should try very hard to collect and turn in all their study initiation paperwork before the meeting so that they are ready to immediately enroll the first patients upon their return to the site.

It is important for the investigator and CRC to thoroughly prepare for an investigator meeting. You should carefully read the protocol, the Investigator Brochure and any other materials provided by the sponsor before you arrive at the meeting. If you have any questions on these materials of study procedures, make note of them so you can clarify them at the meeting.

During the meeting, be sure that all your questions or clarifications are resolved. Be prepared to take careful notes, especially of any items that have changed or have an interpretation that differs from what was initially presented, so you have them to refer to during the study. It is also very important to become acquainted with sponsor personnel and personnel from the other study sites. It's easier to contact someone later by telephone if you have actually met him or her and know who they are. This facilitates problem solving throughout the trial. Also, be sure to attend all the sessions and be an active participant; not only will you learn more, but the meeting will be more enjoyable.

After the meeting, be sure that any necessary follow-up activities are done in a timely manner. After you have had time to review your notes and think about the meeting, if there are still items that are not clear, contact the appropriate person (whom you have now met) at the sponsor company for clarification. These meetings are very expensive for the sponsor to host and also cost sites in lost time, so it pays to benefit from them thoroughly.

Study Initiation Meetings

The study initiation visit, sometimes known as the startup visit, is held at the investigator's site just before the study begins. The CRA, and sometimes additional sponsor personnel, will meet with the investigator and the supporting staff. The purpose of the meeting is to review the study protocol, processes and procedures to ensure that all site personnel understand what is necessary to perform the study.

The study initiation should be held at the point when all regulatory paperwork is complete for the site and the study drug and other supplies have been shipped, but before any subjects have been enrolled. Many sponsors will not allow the site to begin enrollment until after this meeting is held. A good, thorough, informative initiation meeting may take half a day, or even longer for a very complicated study, so you may have to work with your sponsor to find a time when all your relevant staff are available for a meeting. Most sponsors are willing to work with sites to find an amenable time, even if it is in the evening or on a Saturday.

The CRA is almost always in charge of the initiation meeting, although the sponsor medical monitor and/or an in-house associate monitor may also be present. It is important that all site personnel who will be involved in the study attend the meeting, including ancillary personnel such as the subinvestigators, other coordinators, the pharmacist, dietician, lab person, etc.

If the investigator and coordinator attended an investigator meeting, the initiation visit will serve as a review and a more detailed discussion of the topics covered during that meeting. If there was no investigator meeting, or if it was held a month or more prior to initiating the study, then the entire protocol, processes and procedure should be discussed in detail. Since the investigator and study coordinator are usually the only site people who attend the investigator meeting, other site personnel will not be as familiar with the study. The initiation meeting provides an opportunity for everyone at the site to become familiar with the study and to understand everyone's study role.

The items to be covered at an initiation meeting usually include:

- Detailed discussion of the protocol, including:
  - Inclusion and exclusion criteria
  - Study procedures
  - Administration of the study drug
  - Randomization and blinding
  - Primary outcome measures
  - Other pertinent details
- Drug accountability
- Adverse event reporting
- Case report forms (going over each unique form in detail)
- Monitoring visits—how often, what should be ready, what will be covered
- Regulatory requirements
- Investigator responsibilities
- IRB interactions
- Any other study-specific or sponsor-specific items of importance
- Periodic reports of enrollment

If certain attendees are not able to stay for the entire meeting (investigator, pharmacist), the items critical to their participation should be covered while they are there. Other items, such as completing case report forms, can be covered with the coordinators and others who may be involved in a smaller group.

After the meeting, the CRA will complete a visit report detailing what was discussed and completed during the visit. Many companies have a special visit report for this meeting. ICH guidelines call for a trial initiation monitoring report that documents that trial procedures were covered with the investigator and his or her staff; this report is to be kept in both the sponsor and investigator study files.[2] The same purpose can be accomplished by the CRA sending the investigator a letter listing what was covered during the meeting.

If questions arose during the meeting that need further follow-up, the CRA should find out the information and relay it to the site. This meeting can go a long way in helping to ensure a successful study. It deserves the full attention of the CRC, the investigator and other involved staff.

Working with CRAs

For actual study conduct, the study coordinator or clinical research coordinator (CRC) is the most important person at the site and the CRA is the

2. ICH Guidelines for Good Clinical Practice 8.2.20.

most important sponsor representative. Since they will be spending a lot of time working on the study together, the CRC and the CRA must establish a good working relationship. Monitoring can be relatively easy and enjoyable or it can be a nightmare; the difference is often dependent upon the relationship between the CRC and the CRA.

It takes time to develop a rapport with the CRA and to develop a monitoring visit routine that works well for both of you. Each person needs to understand how the other works. The CRA should determine the best times and methods for routine communications with the CRC and let the CRC know the sponsor expectations.

Some CRCs, and some CRAs, simply have better interpersonal relationship skills than others do. It's amazing what a smile and good manners will do. Taking the CRA to lunch occasionally is a nice gesture. Remember, however, to always maintain a professional relationship. It's easy to develop a friendship over the course of a long study, but you still need to remember that it is a business relationship.

Other Sponsor Interactions

CRCs may need to interact with sponsor personnel other than the CRA upon occasion, such as a medical monitor, an in-house CRA or a data manager. The CRC should find out the appropriate people and best times to contact the sponsor with questions about the study. It is always easier if you have met these people at the investigator meeting, but if not, a friendly and professional demeanor will keep things running smoothly. Remember that you are on the same team—both the site and the sponsor have the best interests of the study subjects and the success of the study as top priorities.

Some sponsors will hire a contract research organization (CRO) to do the study monitoring for a project. The dynamics of the working relationships among the CRC, the CRA, the sponsor and the CRO can be complex. If not clearly defined during the investigator meeting, the study initiation meeting is a good time to clarify the communication channels for the study. The CRC may be required to communicate regularly with the CRO for some things, such as enrollment updates, and the sponsor for other things, such as serious adverse event reporting. Whatever the situation, being clear on the correct reporting and communication procedures will help the study progress smoothly.

A good relationship with the sponsor throughout a study is one of the major factors in obtaining more studies from the same sponsor. Being able to maintain a good relationship with the CRA, whether a sponsor or CRO person, and timely and correct communications about other issues is not only good for the study, but is good public relations for your site.

Shipping of Biological Samples

The packaging and shipping of biological samples is often the responsibility of the CRC. These activities are highly regulated, and there are significant fines for not complying with the regulations.

The following regulations apply to the packaging and shipment of biological materials:

- U.S. Department of Transportation, 49 CFR Parts 171-180 and amendments
- U.S. Public Health Service, 42 CFR Part 72, Interstate Shipment of Etiologic Agents
- U.S. Department of Labor, Occupational Safety and Health Administration, 29 CFR Part 1910.1030, Bloodborne Pathogens
- International Air Transport Association (IATA), Dangerous Goods Regulations
- U.S. Postal Service, 39 CFR Part 111, Mailability of Etiologic Agents, Mailability of Sharps and Other Medical Devices, and Publication 52, Acceptance of Hazardous, Restricted or Perishable Matter
- International Civil Aviation Organization, Technical Instructions for the Safe Transport of Dangerous Goods by Air
- United Nations, Recommendations of the Committee of Experts on the Transportation of Dangerous Goods

All North American airlines and FedEx, the largest shipper of infectious materials, use the IATA regulation (also referred to as the Dangerous Goods Regulation or DGR) as their standard. Meeting the conditions of this standard will ensure meeting the provisions of the other U.S. regulations.

Most clinics, hospitals, etc., are familiar with the regulations and procedures, but if you have responsibility for these tasks and are not familiar with them, you should read the regulations or get other training. One good source of information is a guide issued by Stanford University that can be found online at http://www.standford.edu/dept/EHS/prod/researchlab/bio/Shipping Guide.pdf. You may also find several references for this activity by doing a search on Google (www.google.com) using the terms "shipping biological samples." Many sponsor companies require evidence of training in this area when it is relevant for their trial.

Key Things to Remember

Site Assessments

- Sponsors make site assessment/evaluation visits to determine the expertise, experience and interest of the investigator, as well as the overall site ability to conduct a trial.
- It is critical for the investigator and CRC to be well prepared for a site evaluation visit.

Protocol Feasibility

- The investigator, CRC and site personnel should always assess the feasibility of doing each particular protocol before agreeing to participate.
- It is better to decline to do a study than to accept a study and not be able to do it well.

Grants, Budgeting and Contracts

- A CRC should be knowledgeable about grants and how they are calculated.
- The CRC must track the study progress to keep abreast of money owed.
- Most grants are prorated by visit for each subject.
- Contracts between the sponsor and the investigator are signed before the study starts at the site.

Investigative Site Study Files

- Investigators are required to keep study records and documents both during the trial and after the trial is closed.
- CRCs usually set up and organize these files and must check them regularly throughout the study.
- Maintaining files appropriately will ensure that they are in order for an audit.
- It is often simple to catch and correct problems with the files on an ongoing basis throughout the study. It may be impossible to correct the files when the study is over.

Study Documents

- There are a number of documents that are required before a study can begin at a site.
- Most sponsors will not ship the study drug until all required documents are collected.
- Copies of all documents must be kept in both the site's and the sponsor's study files.
- The CRC should keep track of the IRB approval process and letter, so the study is not unduly delayed.

Financial Disclosure

- The purpose of financial disclosure is to identify any potential conflict of interest that could bias a clinical trial.
- Financial disclosure information must be gathered for all people listed on the 1572, and their immediate family members.
- These data are collected for the time period of the study and one year following.
- Financial disclosure information is reported to the FDA when the NDA is filed.

Investigator Meetings

- All investigators and coordinators, as well as relevant sponsor personnel, should attend the meeting.
- The meeting should be held at the time when most sites are ready to enroll.
- The purpose of an investigator meeting is to ensure that all sites have the same understanding of all protocol and administrative procedures.
- CRCs and investigators should read all materials and be well prepared before attending the meeting.

Study Initiation Meetings

- The purpose of an initiation meeting is to ensure that everyone at the site has a clear and accurate understanding of how the study is to be done.
- This meeting should be held after a site has all the study supplies, including the study drug, but before study personnel enroll any subjects.
- All relevant site personnel should be present for the meeting.
- The meeting should be documented in both the investigator and sponsor study files.

Communications

- Good communications are critical for the success of the study and for repeat business from the same sponsor/CRO.

Shipping of Biological Samples

- The packaging and shipping of biological samples are highly regulated, and there are significant fines for not complying with the regulations.

CHAPTER 9

Working with Study Subjects

In this chapter, we will cover some of the most difficult aspects of conducting clinical trials: recruitment of subjects into the trial, scheduling of study subject visits, retention of subjects after they have been entered, and subject compliance with the protocol throughout the study.

Recruitment of Study Subjects

The majority (nearly 86%) of clinical trials conducted in the United States fail to enroll subjects within the contract period. This failure rate is up from 80% of trials in the late 1990s. Clearly these delays result in significant direct development costs for the study sponsor. Extended enrollment periods can also cause delays in new product introductions—a substantially higher cost that is due to missed market opportunity. Nearly two-thirds of investigative sites agree that the challenges of patient recruitment and retention are becoming more difficult.[1]

Government and industry sponsor more than 80,000 trials in the United States each year, representing as many as 5,000 to 6,000 protocols. The FDA alone reports that there are nearly 4,000 active investigational new drug

1. Anderson, Diana, *A Guide to Patient Recruitment and Retention*, Thomson CenterWatch, 2004.

applications in clinical trials at any one time. The largest numbers of subjects are needed for phase III programs.[2] It is necessary to attract a much higher number of patients through recruitment than are needed to finish the trial in order to yield the required number of subject completions.

Lasagna's Law

Knowing the patient population and being able to accurately estimate the number of subjects that can be enrolled are critical to completing a trial in the given time period. Before a study actually starts at an investigative site, there always seem to be more than enough potential subjects waiting in the wings. For some reason, however, it frequently happens that as soon as the trial starts, these potential subjects disappear. This is known as Lasagna's Law,[3] and can be shown visually as in Figure 1:

Figure 1: Lasagna's Law

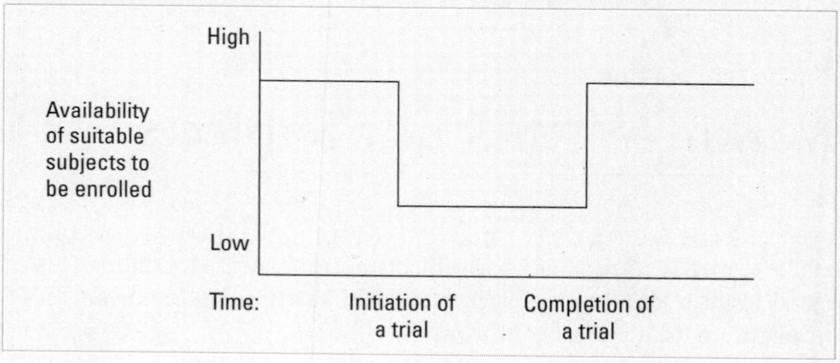

Lasagna's Law always seems like it should be a corollary to one of Murphy's laws, namely, "whatever can go wrong, will." In the case of Lasagna's Law, when the study is over, there seems, again, to be plenty of suitable subjects. Dr. Louis Lasagna was the Director of the Tufts Center for the Study of Drug Development for many years before his death in 2003.

Estimating Enrollment Potential at Sites

One of the most important pre-study activities a CRC performs is helping to accurately estimate the number of subjects that the site can reasonably expect to enroll in each trial. Investigators frequently overestimate the number of potential subjects they have. This is often due to the fact that they are looking only at the number of potential subjects who match the overall diagnosis, for example, depression. However, there are a number of other factors

2. Ibid.
3. Spilker. *Guide to Clinical Trials*, p. 87.

that must be weighed and taken into account, including the protocol and the subjects themselves.

Protocol considerations include the inclusion and exclusion criteria, activities and logistics. The largest constraints on enrollment are usually the inclusion and exclusion criteria for study entry. These criteria delineate the specific characteristics of the population to be enrolled. They will include demographic parameters, such as age and sex, disease and diagnostic criteria, and study-specific requirements. In a study of depression, for example, the following (simplified) inclusion/exclusion criteria might be found:

- Age 18 to 65 years.
- Men, and women who are post-menopausal, surgically sterile, or using acceptable birth control.
- Depression lasting at least six months, but no longer than one year.
- No previous depressive episodes.
- Not taking any other medications that might interfere with the study medication (list provided).
- Able to read and comprehend the informed consent document.
- Willing to sign the informed consent.
- Able to take pills.
- Able to make weekly visits to the clinic site for three months.

Let's look at how these criteria might affect the ability of a site to enroll subjects.

The upper age limit of 65 may limit enrollment from sites that treat a large geriatric population. Depression is a disease that tends to recur in people over time, so the criterion that disallows previous depressive episodes may be a problem. Willingness and ability to make weekly clinic visits is apt to interfere with a potential subject's life situation, especially when working. On top of these problems, many people are just not willing to participate in research, especially if the protocol requirements are burdensome and they do not see much potential value to themselves for participation.

How can these factors influence the ability to enroll? As a general rule, if you take the number of subjects in the practice who meet the diagnosis for the study (depression), then halve that number for each major inclusion/exclusion criterion, the number that remains is apt to be close to the number of subjects that will actually be enrolled. If we assume in our example that the site does not see many geriatric patients, then the three main criteria we need to be concerned with are: no previous episode, ability to make weekly visits and willingness to sign a consent form. Note that if most patients in the practice are under 65, then most of them probably work, so weekly visits to the clinic may be a problem. Let us also assume that the investigator says there are about 300 patients in the practice who suffer from depression. Take 300 and divide it in half for each of three major inclusion/exclusion criteria.

$$300 \rightarrow 150 \rightarrow 75 \rightarrow 37$$

It can be assumed that your site will probably be able to enroll about 37 subjects into the study, in total. This number may be acceptable, but the rate of enrollment needs to be factored in as well. (Note that if a site regularly does research similar to the protocol in question, they may be able to estimate enrollment much more exactly, based on their recent experience. In this case, there should be hard data about recent past trials, including the inclusion/exclusion criteria, numbers of subjects enrolled and rates of enrollment to back up the estimate.)

The CRC must help the investigator analyze the requirements for the rate of enrollment. The sponsor may expect, for example, two patients to be enrolled every week, for a total of 25. Two patients a week does not seem too onerous, but remember that we have a three-month study, and that subjects are seen on a weekly basis. Let's look at what happens as the site begins enrolling. At week one, the site enrolls two subjects. During the second week, it enrolls two more, for a total of four subjects on study. By week six, the site is up to twelve subjects, and by week ten, it has 20 subjects on study. Since this is a three-month study, all these subjects are still being seen on a weekly basis, and there are still five more to enroll. (We will assume no dropouts for the purpose of this example.) The site personnel must determine if they are able to see and manage that many study subjects within a given week. Assessments must be made that include the available staff and space, as well as the ancillary help needed for such things as scheduling visits and calling the subjects to remind them of their visits and other study responsibilities.

Table 1: Total Subjects Enrolled

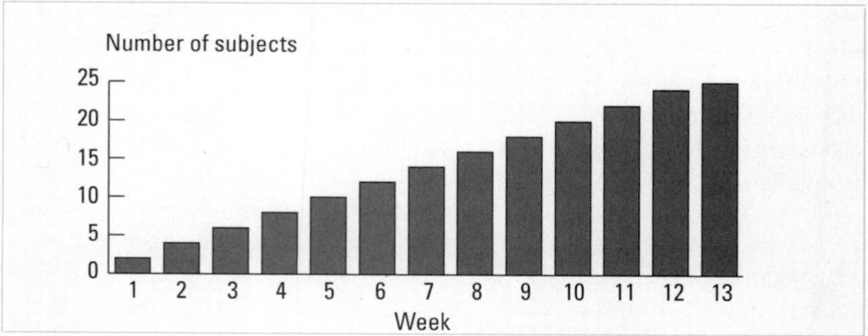

Unfortunately, most sponsors and investigators do not look at the cumulative workload as the study progresses. This is an area where a good CRC can make a significant difference in accurate assessments of enrollment and study load capacities. Before starting a study, the investigator and the CRC should feel confident that his or her site could manage the enrollment rate and numbers of subjects appropriately. Understanding what will be required in terms of time, staff and space throughout the trial will add to the overall chance of success.

Other Factors That Influence Enrollment

Another major factor influencing enrollment is that of competing studies. CRCs need to be aware of the enrollment problems that can result from having a competing study at the investigative site. Competing studies automatically reduce the resources available to each study, including the pool of available subjects. Even if the study is not competing for the same subject population, too many studies at a site can be a problem; study subjects will compete for other resources, including coordinator and investigator time, and space.

There can also be a significant impact from other studies within the same community. These studies may be trying to enroll the same type of subjects and will draw from the same community pool of potential subjects. For example, in the early 1990s, there were over 180 different AIDS study sites in San Francisco. The AIDS activists had a web site and an 800 number that listed all of the studies, plus the main inclusion/exclusion criteria for each, and contact names and numbers. The people interested in these studies were very well informed, and knew which ones had the most to offer in terms of potential benefit to subjects. Those studies with the newest and potentially best drug were meeting enrollment targets. Enrollment in the others languished. If a sponsor did not have an exciting compound, it was almost impossible to enroll sufficient numbers of subjects.

General interest in the trial, both on the part of the potential subjects and the investigator and staff, can have a major impact on enrollment. The more interesting the trial and the compound being studied, the faster enrollment will be. It is human nature to want to spend the most time on the most interesting projects; CRCs and investigators should carefully assess their interest in a trial before agreeing to participate. It is also important to thoroughly consider the available staff and space at a site, even if there are not any competing studies. If the CRC and other involved personnel do not have sufficient time to conduct study activities, or if there is not room to put study supplies and perform study activities, they will be more hesitant to enroll additional subjects.

Advertising for Study Subjects

Sometimes advertising for study subjects is planned right from the start of a study. In general, advertising planned from the start is used when it is expected that subjects will be difficult to find and enroll, when the timeline for enrollment is extremely ambitious, or when a site routinely advertises for all their studies. In other cases, it becomes necessary to advertise for study subjects when enrollment targets are not being met as the study progresses; i.e., there is already an enrollment problem. The goal of advertising—to find and enroll suitable subjects into a trial—is the same no matter when it begins.

The FDA has deemed that advertising for potential study subjects is not objectionable. In general, advertising is anything that is directed towards potential study subjects, with the goal of recruiting them into the study. It may consist of radio or television spots, newspaper ads, posters on bulletin boards, flyers, or any other items that are intended to directly reach prospective subjects. For example, one large general practice that does studies has multiple copies of a notebook in their waiting room. Each study they are doing has a brief explanatory page in the notebook that gives basic details about the study and whom to contact for further information. The explanatory pages in these notebooks count as advertising.

The FDA considers advertising for study subjects to be the start of the informed consent process.[4] Consequently, all advertising should be reviewed and approved by the IRB before use. Note that advertising may not be needed until later in the study, when it is apparent that enrollment goals are not being met. It does not matter that advertising materials were not submitted to the IRB when the study was first reviewed and approved; they simply must be approved before they may be used.

FAQ

Can we advertise our site as a study site—doing studies in many different areas—instead of advertising for only one specific study?

Yes. These are often referred to as "generic" ads. They still must be approved by an IRB.

There are some items that do not count as advertising under FDA rules. Not included as advertising are "(1) communications intended to be seen or heard by health professionals, such as "dear doctor" letters and doctor-to-doctor letters (even when soliciting for study subjects), (2) news stories and (3) publicity intended for other audiences, such as financial page advertisements directed toward prospective investors."[5] However, some sponsors require that doctor-to-doctor letters have IRB approval.

Submitting all advertising to the IRB for review and approval is probably the best course, as this eliminates the doubt and the need to make the determination of what is and is not appropriate material for the general public. Most sponsors also require that you submit advertising for their approval before it goes to the IRB; some IRBs also want to see the approval from the sponsor when the advertising is submitted for review.

4. Guidance for IRBs and Clinical Investigators. FDA. Sept. 1998, p. 29.
5. Ibid.

Advertising is reviewed by the IRB to ensure that it is not coercive and that it does not make promises about a cure or favorable outcome, or promise things other than what appears in the protocol or the consent. This is especially important if the study involves subjects who are considered vulnerable according to the regulations—children, prisoners, and economically or educationally disadvantaged people.[6]

For written advertisements, such as those designed for use in newspapers, the IRB may want to see a finished copy so that they can evaluate the whole ad, including type size and any visual effects. For advertising with an audio component (radio, television), the IRB may review both the written text and the audio version. Most IRBs will advise the investigator to submit the text first to be sure it is acceptable before the actual audio- or videotaping is done.

Advertising must not make any explicit or implicit claims that the drug, biologic or device is safe and effective, or that it is equivalent or superior to any other product. Remember that the reason the clinical trial is being conducted is to determine these things; they are not yet known. The ads must be sure to explain that the test article is investigational (experimental). Using a term such as "new treatment" implies it is a proven and approved product, and is not appropriate.

Advertisements may say that subjects will be paid for participating in the study, but the payments should not be emphasized by big, bold type or other methods.

Here is an example of an unacceptable advertisement. Note that it says "new treatment," promises to cut the time of the cold in half, and emphasizes the overly high payment amount.

New Treatment For The Common Cold!!!

Cut your sniffle time in half!!!
Get paid $1,000 after only 7 days

Study subjects needed. Three shots a day for 4 days. Call Success Clinical at 1-800-999-9999

6. 21 CFR 56.111 (a)(3) and 21 CFR 56.111 (b).

A more appropriate advertisement might look like this:

> **Research Study**
>
> **Subjects needed for a study to investigate the effects of an investigational medicine on lessening the symptoms of the common cold.**
>
> Subjects must be seen by the second day of the cold and must be at least 18 years old.
>
> For details, contact Shirley Williams at Eastside Clinic. (222) 222-2000

What information should go into an advertisement? In general, the information should be limited to what prospective subjects need to know to determine whether or not they might be interested in and eligible for the study. These may include the following items, although the FDA does not require that they all be included:

1. Name and address of the investigator or research facility;
2. Condition under study and/or purpose of the research;
3. Brief summary of the primary criteria for study eligibility;
4. Brief list of benefits (e.g., no-cost health examination);
5. Time or other subject commitment; and
6. Contact information.[7]

CRCs should be familiar with the information about advertising in the FDA's Guidance for IRBs and Clinical Investigators, so that they may better assist investigators in the proper development and use of advertising materials.

Other Recruitment Methods

Although advertising comes immediately to mind when discussing recruitment for study subjects, there are several other methods of finding subjects. The starting place for most sites is their own records. Many sites have their patients in a computer database that allows them to search based on diagnostic criteria. After they have found patients with an appropriate diagnosis, they are able to contact them to ascertain their interest and suitability for the trial. In the case of studies in chronic diseases, such as diabetes or hypertension, most subjects will probably come from the investigator's own practice.

7. Guidance for IRBs and Clinical Investigators. FDA. Sept. 1998, p. 30.

In the case of acute diseases, such as pneumonia and other infectious diseases, searching the records from the investigative site may not be particularly useful.

Many potential subjects hear about a trial by word of mouth, perhaps from a friend who is in the trial. Sites that do a number of trials often have "free advertising" from current or past study subjects spreading the word. Subjects also find clinical trials by talking to people, contacting organizations, including disease-related groups and pharmaceutical companies, and doing web searches.

There are many web sites available to potential study subjects that list trials that are in process or about to start. Thomson CenterWatch, for example, has an online database listing of clinical trials that is easily accessible (www.centerwatch.com). There are other web sites, particularly through the NIH, that list active trials with information for potential subjects. For an example of one of these, sign on to www.cancer.gov/clinical_trials. The U.S. Food and Drug Administration Modernization Act (FDAMA) legislation of 1997 contains a provision requiring that information about clinical trials for serious or life-threatening diseases be accessible to potential subjects.[8]

Advocacy groups for various diseases, such as AIDS, are sources of information about trials; sites may receive interested subjects from these groups or from people who have been in contact with them.

Frequently other physicians or healthcare professionals will refer potential subjects to a trial. Investigators often contact other physicians in the community to inform them of the trial, and ask that it be mentioned to suitable subjects. The investigator may make these contacts by phone, or may send letters to other healthcare professionals in the community. CRCs often help make these contacts.

Usually finding subjects for a trial is accomplished by a combination of methods. The more difficult it is to enroll, the more variety there will be in the methods used to attract potential subjects. It is important for a CRC to monitor enrollment and enrollment rates right from the start of each study, and to think about ways to enhance enrollment before it becomes a major problem. It is usually much easier to make changes when things are just starting to look like there may be trouble, than to wait until there is no question that a major problem has occurred. For enrollment problems, the way to fix things is often by implementing several small ideas and suggestions; not everything works in each case, and one change is frequently not sufficient.

---

8. FDAMA, Section 113.

Information for Potential Study Subjects

Potential study subjects are often not very knowledgeable about clinical trials and the clinical trial process. They tend to think that receiving treatment in a clinical trial is the same as receiving treatment as a regular patient in a medical practice. This is not true. Clinical trials are designed to answer scientific questions, not to provide medical treatment. Anyone who is thinking about participating in a clinical trial needs to understand the difference between participating in a clinical trial and receiving treatment at a doctor's private practice. It is the responsibility of investigators and CRCs to help educate their potential subjects about the differences in these activities.

There are, of course, many benefits to participating in clinical trials. Many subjects receive treatment with new compounds that may be much more efficacious in treating their disease or condition than standard treatments. Individuals with severe and life-threatening illnesses may receive treatments that offer them hope. Some subjects receive treatment that they are unable to pay for otherwise, and some, especially in phase I trials with normal healthy volunteers, participate to earn extra money. People often participate from a desire to help others with similar afflictions. No matter what reason a person has to participate in a clinical trial, however, it is important to the person to know and understand that clinical trials are not a substitute for other regular medical care, but rather an enlargement of his or her regular care team and support.

If your potential subjects want more information on participating in clinical trials, you may wish to have a few brochures available to explain. Thomson CenterWatch offers two: "Understanding Informed Consent" and "Volunteering for a Clinical Trial."

Compensation to Research Subjects

It is quite common for subjects to be compensated for participating in clinical trials, especially in the early phases of development. When subjects are compensated, however, it is viewed by the FDA as a recruitment incentive, not as a study benefit. All compensation schedules must be approved by the IRB in advance of the study, or in advance of being used. The IRB will look at both the compensation amounts and the timing of the compensation, to be sure they are not coercive and would not present an undue influence on the subject's trial-related decisions.[9]

Subjects are usually compensated on a regular basis throughout the trial, based most commonly for each completed visit, although they do not have to be compensated at each visit. It is rarely appropriate to compensate subjects only if they complete the entire trial; this might encourage them to con-

9. Guidance for IRBs and Clinical Investigators. FDA. Sept. 1998, p. 31.

tinue with the trial even if they would have normally discontinued due to side effects or other reasons.

The amount of compensation to subjects varies with respect to the complexity of the study and the involvement of the subjects. Compensation is usually designed to cover any costs the subjects might incur by participating such as for transportation, parking, lunch and childcare. Compensation must not be so large as to be coercive; that is, the subjects should not be entering a trial only because of the compensation. Before approving subject compensation, the IRB will also take into account where the study is being conducted and the patient population. Compensation of $25 per visit may be no enticement at all to people in some neighborhoods, but may constitute a great deal of money and enticement to subjects in other areas.

Some sites routinely compensate subjects for participating in trials, while others never compensate study subjects at all. Either is acceptable. The important things to remember about compensation to study subjects are that it must not be coercive or present undue influence and that it must be pre-approved by the IRB.

Incentive Payments to Healthcare Professionals

There are two types of incentive payments, those paid by the investigator to other professionals to encourage them to find study subjects, and bonus payments by study sponsors to investigators and their staff to enhance enrollment.

Incentive payments to healthcare professionals by an investigator for the referral of study subjects are known as referral fees or finder's fees. Examples are payments made to a coordinator or nurse, resident or intern physicians, or other local physicians for each subject referred and entered into a study. These payments are usually not acceptable, and may compromise the integrity of a trial. They may also be in violation of regulations or institutional policies.

Some states have laws that prohibit referral fees. For example, the California Health and Safety Code § 445 clearly prohibits referral fees. It states:

> "No person, firm, partnership, association or corporation, or agent or employee thereof, shall for profit refer or recommend a person to a physician, hospital, health-related facility, or dispensary for any form of medical care or treatment of any ailment or medical condition."[10]

---

10. California Health and Safety Code § 445.

Also, the American Medical Association (AMA) has stated in its Code of Medical Ethics that referral fees for research studies are unethical. Section 6.03 of the code, Fee Splitting: Referrals to Health Care Facilities, states:

> "Offering or accepting payment for referring patients to research studies (finder's fees) are also unethical."[11]

Many IRBs have taken a firm stand on the issue of finder's fees, and will not permit them.

Incentive payments to healthcare professionals also include bonus payments by the study sponsor to investigators and CRCs for enhanced (faster or more) enrollment. True bonus payments are usually not acceptable because they may encourage the enrollment of "borderline" subjects, or the enrollment of subjects the investigator would not otherwise recruit. This creates a conflict of interest and should be avoided.

There is no problem, however, with a sponsor covering true extra costs for enrollment procedures. These payments might be for additional people to help with the screening of potential subjects, advertising costs or other direct costs borne by the investigative site. This is frequently decided upon before the study starts, even though not implemented unless necessary to increase enrollment or to speed the rate of enrollment. For example, a sponsor may be willing to pay a per-screen amount for the prescreening of study candidates. In this case, there is usually a limit on the number of screen failures that they will pay you for in relation to the number of subjects actually entered into the trial. This ensures that the site is actually looking for and pre-screening suitable candidates. If site personnel are not sure whether or not a payment plan is appropriate, they should contact their IRB for an opinion before implementation.

Summary: Recruitment

Timely and appropriate recruitment and enrollment of subjects into clinical trials is essential for a drug, biologic or device development program. CRCs must be aware of the regulations regarding recruitment, and have an understanding of the potential problems and solutions for enrollment. It is important to remember that at each step from initial recruitment to actual study enrollment, the number of potential subjects decreases. The following Venn diagram patterned after one developed by Burt Spilker[12] shows this in graphic form.

---

11. AMA Code of Medical Ethics § 6.03.
12. Spilker. *Guide to Clinical Trials*, p. 237.

Figure 2: Venn Diagram Showing Shrinking Pool for Enrollment for a Clinical Trial

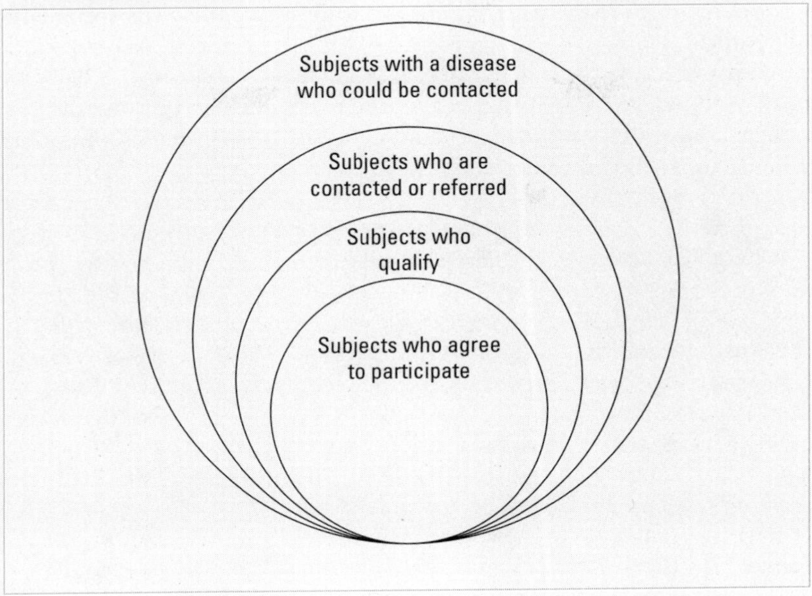

Scheduling Subjects

Scheduling subjects for their study visits is more difficult than scheduling normal office visits. This is because study visits must be in accordance with the protocol, and there is not much flexibility around the required visit dates. Since it is not always possible for subjects to come in for a study visit on the exact date, most protocols allow a few days prior or after the calendar date; this is known as the visit window. If a subject is not seen during the visit window, that visit is usually regarded as a missed visit; this is a problem for the analyses of the data, and some sponsors will not pay for these visits. You can, however, call the sponsor to discuss a specific case when it occurs; the sponsor may make an exemption on the visit window in certain circumstances.

For example, let's assume that a subject is to come in every week for a visit. If a subject starts on Tuesday, ideally he or she would come in every week on Tuesday. The visit window might be plus or minus one day, which means that it would be acceptable for the subject to come in on Monday, Tuesday or Wednesday for the visit. This allows some flexibility in case there is a reason that the subject can not come in on the usual Tuesday. Usually each visit window is calculated by going back to the starting or baseline date, rather than from the previous visit. The reason for this is that if a subject is always two days late, and if the window is calculated from the last visit, you are adding two more days and two more days and two more days…and so forth. Because the subject must take the drug every day, after a while, there is not enough study drug for the subject to finish all the visits specified by the protocol.

If your study sponsor does not give you a reference sheet with dates and study windows, you might find it useful to make one on your own, as it is a very valuable tool to use when scheduling subject visits. Here is an example of how a visit schedule sheet might look:

Table 2: Visit Schedule and Visit Windows

Patient Number	Baseline (+/- 1 day)	Week 1 Visit (+/- 1 day)	Week 2 Visit (+/- 1 day)	Week 4 Visit (Final visit) (+/- 1 day)
001	April 4 (Actual)	April 11 (April 10, 11, 12)	April 18 (April 17, 18, 19)	May 2 (May 1, 2, 3)
002	April 8 (Actual)	April 15 (April 14, 15, 16)	April 22 (April 21, 22, 23)	May 6 (May 5, 6, 7)

Notice that in this visit window schedule, the baseline dates are when the subjects actually came in for their baseline visits. At each other visit, the top date is the projected visit date, starting from baseline at each time period, and the bottom dates are the potential dates that the subject is allowed to come in based on the acceptable visit windows. Dates other than those in parentheses would be outside the window for each visit. There are other ways of making visit window schedules, but no matter which format is used, this is a useful tool for the CRC.

It also helps, in relatively short studies, to schedule all the subject visits when each subject comes in for the baseline visit. This allows everyone to plan ahead, and will help to eliminate scheduling problems. In longer term studies, the CRC should at least schedule the next few visits in advance. Scheduling in advance does not eliminate the need for visit reminders for study subjects. Some sites send post card visit reminders, and most sites find that telephone reminders a day ahead are very good aids in helping study subjects keep their appointments. Coming in on the appropriate days for study appointments is very important for study compliance, which will be discussed later in this chapter. A good CRC will do everything possible to maximize compliance with study visit dates.

Retention of Study Subjects

Once subjects are enrolled into a trial, it is important that they stay in the trial until it is complete, if at all possible. CRCs should be familiar both with the reasons that subjects drop out, and how retention can be enhanced. In this section, we will explore the reasons that subjects leave trials, and what can be done to increase retention.

Reasons That Investigators and/or Sponsors Discontinue Subjects

Before discussing reasons that subjects choose to discontinue their participation in clinical trials, it is important to differentiate between subjects who choose to drop out on their own and subjects who are discontinued by the investigator and/or the sponsor.

Investigators may discontinue a subject for a number of reasons. Some of these reasons are medical, some are based on the patient's compliance and cooperation, and some are trial-related. Some of the more common reasons for discontinuing a subject are listed below.

Medical reasons for potential discontinuation:

- Lack of efficacy of the drug
- Intolerable adverse events
- Serious adverse events (SAEs)
- Patient's condition deteriorates
- Patient develops an intercurrent illness (an illness other than the one under study, but which occurs during the course of the trial)
- Pregnancy
- Abnormal laboratory values
- Did not meet original entry criteria (discovered after study entry)
- Died

Patient compliance and cooperation reasons:

- Unacceptable compliance with protocol activities
- Unacceptable compliance in taking the study medication
- Not keeping appointments
- Not cooperating with study staff and/or study procedures
- Use of non-approved concomitant medications
- Moved out of the area

Trial-related reasons:

- Trial was terminated by the sponsor due to
  - Safety concerns

  - Benefit so great trial is no longer ethical because some subjects are not receiving active treatment
  - Business reasons
- Investigator no longer able to continue the trial (retired, died, moved)
- Investigator did not meet enrollment targets or did not comply with the protocol or the regulations

Since it was either the investigator or the sponsor who decided to discontinue patients for these reasons, we will not discuss them further. The main concern for CRCs is helping to retain subjects who would have decided to drop out of the study on their own.

FAQ

Our sponsor wants us to drop a subject from our study because he does not come in during the specified visit windows. He is a busy professional, and is often out of town during the visit times. Do we have to drop him?

Remember that compliance is ultimately a safety issue, as well as a statistical issue. You may discuss this with the sponsor, but the subject will probably need to be discontinued if he cannot adhere to the protocol requirements.

Other Reasons That Subjects Drop Out of Trials

There are many reasons that study subjects decide to stop participating in a trial. The most common are valid medical reasons such as intolerable adverse events or a lack of efficacy of the treatment. These cases are usually discussed with and agreed to by the investigator.

There are, however, other reasons that subjects drop out, which are not so compelling and could perhaps be avoided. This is where the CRC needs to understand what causes some of the problems, and how they might be prevented from occurring. The key for the CRC is catching problems, or patterns of problems, early so they can be fixed. After all, once subjects are lost from a study, they are lost forever. The CRC wants to ensure that losses do not become the standard and that they do not exceed what would normally be expected during a study. Some reasons subjects drop out are that:

- The subject does not understand the importance of remaining in the trial even when the disease condition has improved.
- The study requirements are too burdensome.
- The subject loses interest in the trial.

- The medication is unpleasant to take.
- The subject does not like some of the study staff.
- Unfriendly people at the site (could be anyone, including the receptionist).
- The subject has to spend too much time at the clinic.
- Difficulties with transportation, childcare or time off work.
- The subject is upset about some aspect of the trial.
- Friends or family are unhappy about the subject's participation.
- The subject has a change in his or her personal situation.

Many sponsors will want the site to keep a list of all subjects who drop out with the reasons categorized by general headings such as adverse events, lack of efficacy, lost to follow-up, withdrawal of consent, etc.

When a patient does not return for study visits, a diligent effort should be made to contact the patient and either have him or her return, or to find out why he or she is unwilling to return. Most sites will try to call the person at least three times, followed by a registered letter with a stamped return envelope included so the patient can easily reply. Proof of each contact should be kept in the patient's records. After several documented unsuccessful contact attempts, the patient can be classified as "lost to follow-up."

Maximizing Retention in Clinical Trials

The secret to subject retention in clinical trials is easy. It is not really a secret at all, but is just plain common sense (although sometimes sense is not so common). All site people have to do is be nice, treat subjects well, spend time with them, listen carefully to what they are saying and communicate openly and often.

Investigators and study coordinators are very busy people. They get rushed and behind on things, have good and bad days, and experience all the problems the rest of us do. Nevertheless, if a study is to go well, they must be able to set aside their concerns and problems when study subjects are in for their visits. Study subjects want to feel that their contribution is important, and they want to be the sole focus of attention during their time with the investigator and/or coordinator.

When a study subject comes in for a clinic visit, he or she wants to be able to discuss what has happened since the last visit, to have any study concerns allayed, to be praised for doing well, to have questions answered, and to be treated like an important partner in the study venture. In short, a study subject wants to be appreciated. After all, there are risks in becoming part of a study, there is no guaranteed outcome, and it is voluntary—no one has to participate at all. People who volunteer for studies are special people, and they should be treated as such.

Given the premise of wanting to be treated well, there are many things, frequently small things, that can make a subject decide that trial participation may not be worth the effort. Some of these things are:

- Having to wait when coming in for an appointment.
- Not being treated nicely and with respect.
- Not seeing the investigator or the coordinator, but being seen by a "substitute" that he or she doesn't know.
- Not seeing the same person at most visits (developing a one-to-one relationship).
- Being rushed and hurried through the appointment.
- Feeling that the investigator/coordinator doesn't really want to see him or her.
- Not being asked about how he or she feels and how the study is going for him or her.
- Not having the opportunity to ask questions.
- Being afraid to ask study-related questions.
- Being made to feel dumb or silly when asking questions.
- Being berated for doing something wrong.
- Having the investigator or coordinator disparage the study.

There are also situations where the subject does not return and is lost to follow-up, or where the subject drops out but refuses to give a reason, other than personal choice. These situations are difficult to combat, and the study site cannot do much about them. If there are many of these cases at a site, however, they should serve as a wake-up call. Chances are that the real reasons are in the list above, but the subject just doesn't want to say anything about them to site personnel.

These problems are all fixable, but first they need to be recognized and acknowledged. It's critical to catch them early. Some problems are easy to fix. For example, if a subject has a logistics problem, such as transportation to the site, one solution may be to pay for a taxi to transport the subject back and forth. If childcare is a problem, perhaps the visit time can be adjusted to an evening or weekend time so that the subject can come in when a spouse is home to stay with the children. Questioning the subject about problems and being willing to help with arrangements or adjustments may allow the subject to continue participating.

Some successful sites have very clever ways of making their study subjects feel happy, important and wanted. Some of the ideas and little things that have added to retention success for sites are:

- Reminder calls the day before each visit
- Giving each volunteer a special study T-shirt ("I'm a research volunteer," "Volunteer for XXXXX (study acronym)," big smiley face)
- Mugs, tote bags, gym bags for a study where there was exercise testing
- Separate waiting room with coffee, tea and doughnuts—and current magazines and newspapers
- Sending a cab to pick someone up if transportation was a problem
- Thank you notes from the coordinator after a few weeks on a study

- Thank you notes at the end of the subject's participation (leads to repeat volunteering)
- Balloons
- Birthday cards
- Bonus gift certificates

If you want to use these ideas, check with the sponsor and your IRB regarding the need for prior IRB approval; it's better to check than to assume it is OK without approval.

It helps if the CRC and the investigator plan out a strategy at the beginning of the trial to help retain subjects. Many sponsors are willing to foot the bill for little extras, such as mugs or T-shirts, that may encourage subjects to feel good about their participation and remain in the trial until completion.

Anytime there is a pattern of more than expected dropouts due to nonmedical issues, the sponsor monitor should meet with the investigator and coordinator to discuss the situation. Each case should be analyzed. Perhaps the reasons are clear cut and recognizable, or perhaps they are not. It may be time to reflect on the atmosphere at the site, and to take a hard look at how subjects are being treated. The site might even want to talk with subjects about their perceptions of how the study is going, how they feel when they come in for visits, and if they feel there are ways in which the site could improve the study process. Difficult as it is, site personnel must take an honest look at their interactions with study subjects. Sometimes it helps to think about how you would feel if you were in the study, or how you would feel about having one of your loved ones participating.

Summary: Retention

Retention of subjects in clinical trials is critical to the completion of an informative, sound clinical trial. Sites should help subjects understand that a successful trial is a partnership between the subjects and the investigative staff. Respect, courtesy, honesty and open communication on the part of both subjects and investigators will increase the chances of successfully completing a study.

Subject Compliance

Clinical trials are done in order to assess the safety and efficacy of a new drug. To be able to accurately assess safety and efficacy, study subjects must take the medication as it is prescribed. Unfortunately, subjects do not always do this. In this section, we will look at compliance, what can go wrong, and how to increase the probability of good compliance.

Undetected poor compliance can lead to invalid study results. Lack of compliance in one subject may have impact on only that particular subject; if several subjects are non-compliant, however, it can invalidate the entire study. Non-compliance can have the following results:

- An effective medication may look ineffective.
  This can mean that a medication that would be effective, and that would be of benefit to patients, never makes it to the marketplace. This is an unfortunate result for the company that has made the development investment in the drug, and even more unfortunate for those people who would have received benefit from it.
- An ineffective medication looks effective.
  This result is worse than the one above, because, once marketed, the medication will be relied on to effect a cure, and will not be effective in doing so.
- Failure to detect a drug-related safety issue.
- Inappropriate dosage recommendations.
  Depending on the type of noncompliance, the drug labeling could recommend either too high or too low a dose. This is not good in either direction—patients could be taking too little to be an effective treatment, or more than they need, which could lead to an excess of adverse reactions.

The effects of the drug in noncompliant subjects cannot be extrapolated to compliant subjects. It is very important that all study subjects are as compliant as possible during their involvement in clinical trials.

Negative Study Results

There are a number of reasons for negative study results. They may be due to the failure of the medication; that is, the drug just might not work. Remember that the reason clinical trials are done is to find out if the drug is safe and effective. Although it would be nice if every drug under development worked as expected, they do not always do so. Sometimes they are not safe, and sometimes they are not effective. In these cases, it is better if they are never marketed.

Negative results can also be due to poor subject compliance, although it usually takes more than just a few noncompliant subjects to affect the entire study. We will explore subject compliance in detail as we go along.

Reasons for Noncompliance

Sometimes study subjects are noncompliant for disease-related reasons. One reason is a lack of symptoms, or what can be called the "antibiotic effect." As many of us know from personal experience, it is hard to remember to take medications when you feel better and have very few or no remaining disease symptoms. A prime example of this is the standard 10-day course of treatment with many antibiotics. After five or six days, when the patient appears to be over the disease, it is very common to stop taking the pills. The subject has become noncompliant with the medication schedule; this happens in trials as well as in general practice.

There are also compliance problems with people suffering from terminal diseases. When people knows they are going to die soon anyway, they do not have the same incentive for taking a course of medications that they might have otherwise.

There are many other reasons subjects are not compliant when it comes to taking medication. Sometimes they just forget to take their pills. Sometimes there is a lack of belief in the treatment—"it isn't going to work anyway, so why bother..." If the medication is unpleasant to take, such as not tasting good, or pills that are so big they are hard to swallow, compliance may be poor.

Noncompliance can result from the way the drug is packaged. Think about using safety containers (childproof lids) in an arthritis study, for example. The subjects may not be able to open the containers without help, which will surely affect compliance. Sometimes study drug is packaged in large blister packs containing several days' worth of drug and with each day's drug clearly marked as to when it should be taken. At first glance, it appears this would help compliance, but think about it a bit more. What happens when a subject has to go to work? Most people do not want to carry a large blister pack to work with them, and have others asking about it. Consequently, subjects might take the day's drug out of the package and just carry it in a pocket, not knowing that the ordering of the pills for the day is important—they become non-compliant.

Sometimes subjects just do not understand the dosing scheme, especially if it is complicated. "Oh…it's two white ones and one pink one? I thought it was two pink ones and one white one. That's why I ran out of pink ones last week." Sometimes it is the regimen that is confusing, with too many pills, too many different times per day to take them, or confusion about the times and/or doses. It may also be the duration of the study, as subjects can lose interest over time.

Subjects may also become noncompliant because of adverse reactions. If a subject becomes nauseous after taking the medication, or thinks it is causing headaches, he or she may not take it as often as required, if at all. A subject may not take medication appropriately because of mistrust, either in the medication or in the physician. A subject may be influenced by family or friends in ways that affect compliance also; if people important to the subject do not want him or her to take the pills, or be in the study, this may impact compliance. "I'm not sure you should be taking anything not approved by the government, dear…."

Other ways in which subjects may be noncompliant that are related to the study medication are by not filling their prescriptions, by prematurely discontinuing the drug, or by sharing the drug with other people. Other examples of noncompliance include:

- Taking other medications at the same time, when the other medications are not allowed by the protocol.
- Using alcohol or other disallowed substances such as marijuana while in the study.
- Changes in their living situations that influence when and how the study drug is taken.
- Their mental conditions have a negative impact on their ability to follow protocol instructions.

There are also compliance issues in studies that are not related directly to the medication. Subjects may be noncompliant by missing visits, or not coming in for visits within the visit windows. They may not adhere to other study requirements such as special tests (eye exams, for example), dietary requirements or keeping diaries.

Sometimes compliance problems stem from investigator-related reasons. Subjects will be less compliant if it is difficult to schedule study visits, or if they are kept waiting when they come in for a visit. If study staff do not keep appointments, subjects are apt to do the same. Worst of all is a poor physician-patient relationship. In general, subjects want to please the physician and do things correctly, but if the relationship is poor, the subject is not as likely to care about complying with study requirements.

Unfortunately, there are many ways to be noncompliant, both on purpose and by mistake. The key is finding out about them and fixing the problem before it has a negative impact on the entire study.

Managing Compliance

Study protocols should be designed to enhance compliance as much as possible. They should also make it possible to monitor compliance.

CRCs and investigators must understand why compliance is important and how they can help to ensure compliance during the study. They need to work with their patients, both before and during the trial, in order to assure compliance. There are certain things that study patients must be aware of and do during the study. Just as clinical trials are different than clinical practice for investigators, they are different for study subjects. The investigator and CRC must ensure that potential study subjects are aware that if they are in the study, they must:

- Come in for all study visits on time and within the visit windows.
- Answer the questions truthfully, especially with respect to their medical histories and disease history.
- Cooperate fully with study procedures. This is one reason it is critical that the investigator fully explains the study to potential subjects.
- Allow tests to be done as appropriate, and on time.
- Take study medications as prescribed.
- Follow all study directions.

- Ask if something is not clear, and inform the site of any problems or snags.

The CRC should tell the study subjects how important it is to answer questions truthfully, especially about their compliance during the study. Subjects need to know that it is better to let the investigator and coordinator know that they missed some doses than to just not say anything at all, and that they will hurt the study if they are not forthcoming with this information. The CRC or the investigator must thoroughly question each subject about compliance at each visit. They should let subjects know that they should call if they are having any problems complying with study activities or are confused about what needs to be done.

There are a variety of ways of testing for compliance in studies. Every study will have some way of asking about and maintaining drug accountability. Usually a record is kept for each subject of the amounts and dates drug is dispensed, and the amounts and dates of drug returned. Subjects are told to bring back any unused medications at each visit. The returned drug is counted and recorded by the coordinator. This is a reasonable way to assess compliance, but, unless the subject admits a problem, there is no way of knowing about the pill that fell down the drain, or was swallowed by the dog. The person seeing the subject should also question him or her about whether or not all doses were taken.

Watching subjects take the pills in person would encourage good compliance, but studies are not usually set up in such a way that the subject is at the site each time a dose needs to be taken. This would work only if there is a single dose of medication being given, or if an IV drug is being administered, or if the drug is being given in an inpatient hospital setting, etc.

Subjects are sometimes asked to keep diaries and record when each medication dose was taken. This is probably valid with very compliant subjects, but for the others, it is as easy to forget writing in the diary as it is to forget to take the medication.

The "gold standard" for testing for compliance is to check blood levels. This is done in some studies, but mostly only the very early (phase I and II) studies. It is expensive, and not feasible to do most of the time.

What can site personnel do to maximize compliance? First, it helps to know the subjects enrolled. If an investigator and CRC have worked with a subject before, they should have an idea of whether or not the person will be compliant. They should question subjects before entering the study on their willingness to comply with study activities, if they can swallow the pills, if they can come in for visits, etc.

The investigator and coordinator must pay attention to the signs of potential non-compliance. Does the patient show up for visits? And on time? Did the subject complete any necessary pre-study activities? Is the person really interested in the study and aware of the requirements?

The CRC should ask the subject about anything that may interfere with completing the study. Does the subject have a vacation planned during the time of the study? Does he or she understand what is involved in participating? Does the patient's lifestyle allow for complying with the study rules and activities?

In short, if the CRC or the investigator knows or thinks that a subject will not be a good, compliant patient, he or she should not be enrolled in the study at all. This is a safety issue—if a subject is not compliant with the study protocol, he or she could be putting him- or herself at a greater than acceptable risk.

When Noncompliance Happens

If the CRC is aware that a subject has been non-compliant, either in taking the medication or other study activities, he or she should call and inform the sponsor of the noncompliance issue. Details of any noncompliance situations should be documented both in the site's source documents and in the case report form. The CRC or the investigator should discuss the situation with the subject, and do some retraining in study procedures. If the subject continues to be noncompliant, he or she may need to be dropped from the trial. Keeping subjects who are not compliant in a trial is not good for the subject (safety concerns) or the trial. When subjects are dropped from a study for noncompliance, the relevant information must be recorded both in the source documents and in the case report form.

By working closely with each potential subject before enrollment into a trial, and by working closely with the subjects throughout the trial, compliance can be maximized, and study results will be more reliable than if there had been major compliance problems.

Good study designs and protocols will anticipate non-compliance and give instructions for minimizing it and handling it if it occurs. If the CRC and the investigator do their jobs, both to minimize noncompliance and to detect and report it, the study should remain valid.

Key Things to Remember

Recruitment

- Timely enrollment of subjects is critical to a drug, biologic or device development program.
- It is important for investigative sites to accurately estimate the number of subjects they can expect to enroll in a study.
- Sites need to have the necessary personnel, time and space to handle the enrollment needed for each trial.
- Protocol requirements, especially the inclusion and exclusion criteria, are the primary limiting factors for enrollment.
- Assessment of the rate of enrollment is critical to managing a trial at the investigative site.

- Competing studies, both at the site and in the community, can have a significant impact on enrollment.
- The FDA allows advertising for study subjects, but it must not be coercive or exert undue influence on potential subjects.
- All advertising must be approved by the IRB before use.
- Study subjects often refer themselves to clinical trials.
- Payments to study subjects must be approved by the IRB and must not be coercive or exert undue influence on study subjects.
- Finder's fees or referral fees are usually not acceptable.
- Sponsors will usually pay true extra costs for enrollment procedures.

Scheduling

- Scheduling all (or many) subject visits at the initial visit aids in meeting protocol visit requirements.
- A visit window is the number of days allowed around a specific date that the patient may come in for each study visit.
- A visit window chart is a useful tool for scheduling appointments appropriately.
- Visit reminders are important for ensuring visit dates are appropriate.

Retention

- Investigators or sponsors may discontinue subjects from a trial for medical reasons, compliance or cooperation issues, or because the sponsor is stopping the trial.
- Subjects have many reasons for dropping out of a trial, including medical reasons and logistics problems.
- Determining problems as early as possible is the first step to retaining subjects in trials.
- Respect and open communication are the biggest factors in subject retention.
- CRCs can help by preparing their sites for good retention.

Compliance

- Good compliance is critical for valid conclusions from clinical trials.
- Subjects need to be aware of the importance of compliance.
- CRCs and investigators need to determine if potential study subjects are likely to be compliant, and not enroll subjects who probably will not be compliant.
- There are many different ways in which subjects may be non-compliant with study procedures.
- The CRC and investigator need to be alert to compliance problems throughout the study.
- If non-compliance occurs, the CRC should notify the sponsor.

CHAPTER 10

Study Closure

Introduction

When a study is over at an investigative site, it must be officially closed. Closing duties are usually shared by the CRC and the CRA. In this chapter we will look at the reasons studies are closed, and what must be done to close a study. We will also discuss a site post-study critique.

Reasons for Study Closure

The primary reason to close a study is that it is complete and finished: enrollment has stopped, all subjects have completed their study-related activities, and the data are complete and correct. This is the best and most desired outcome, and the most frequent.

There are also reasons for study discontinuation before they are complete. Studies may be terminated early for both favorable and unfavorable reasons. Some of the reasons are listed below.

Favorable or positive reasons for study termination:

- The treatment is so beneficial that it would not be ethical to have a trial where subjects might not be receiving the active treatment.

- Overall enrollment was met in the trial, so all sites are being closed even if they did not complete the site enrollment goal.

Unfavorable or negative reasons for ending a trial:

- The investigational product was found to be unsafe.
- The investigational product was not effective.
- It was not possible to find and enroll sufficient study subjects.
- The sponsor decided the potential product was not viable for marketing.
- Compliance or other problems at the site.

More studies are terminated early for negative reasons than for positive ones.

A trial may be discontinued at all sites at the same time or at individual sites at different times. Whatever the timing, the activity is essentially a single site activity, that is, it must be done at each site without regard to the activity at all other sites.

One cautionary note: if the study is stopped abruptly, while subjects are still taking the study medications, there should be an orderly plan for discontinuing each subject. This plan will be formulated by the sponsor and communicated to each investigator. The CRC should be prepared to explain the plan to the subjects. The site must also be prepared to notify subjects promptly, and assure them of appropriate therapy and follow-up outside of the trial.

Closing a study because it is finished and complete is the most common situation. It is also the easiest to handle. Everyone is usually pleased that it was finished and hopeful of a favorable outcome. If a study was closed for a negative reason, it may have been over all sites or just a particular site. No matter what the reason is for closing the study, the same procedures must be followed. In the rest of the chapter, we will discuss what needs to be done to close a study.

Closure Procedures

A CRA will visit the site to do a closure visit. The main items the CRA will address during a closure visit are: case report forms, drug accountability, the investigator's study file, and administrative items. The CRC should be prepared for this visit by having everything completed and ready before the CRA arrives.

Case Report Forms

If the case report forms have not already been reviewed, submitted and corrected, this must be done now. If the study has come to its natural end, this activity has probably been done. If the study has been stopped abruptly or early, this may not be complete. It is always better to have the case report forms submitted and reviewed, in case final corrections need to be made, before the closeout visit. The CRC should make sure that all the case report forms, as well as any corrections or query forms, are complete, in order, and ready for storage.

Drug Accountability

If there are still drug supplies at the site, the CRA will complete a final inventory at the closure visit. The drug should then be packaged for return to the sponsor, according to company policy. A copy of the drug inventory form should be placed in the investigator's study file.

Hopefully, drug reconciliation has been done throughout the study, rather than left to the end. In this case, it should be relatively easy for the CRA and the CRC to finish the reconciliation. Otherwise, drug accounting is apt to be the most time consuming study closure activity.

Investigator's Study File

The CRA will thoroughly check the investigator's study document file at this visit. The CRC should check it before the visit to ensure that nothing is overlooked. This is a good time to use a checklist (see Appendix D). All documents must be present, including appropriate re-approvals and correspondence from the IRB. If there were protocol amendments during the study, or amendments to the informed consent form, all versions should be in the file, including their dates of use.

Informed consent forms for each subject must be present. The CRA will double check to be sure they were all signed and dated appropriately. There should also be documentation for any protocol variations, whether they were previously approved or not. The investigator brochure should be available in or with the file.

If any documents are missing from this file, the CRA can help the site to obtain copies. When the file is complete and in order, it is ready for storage.

Investigator's Final Report to the Sponsor and the IRB

The investigator is required to make a final study report to the sponsor.[1] This report should include an enrollment summary, including the numbers of subjects entered, those who completed, and those who dropped, including

1. 21 CFR 312.64c.

the reasons for dropping. It will also include information about adverse events, and any other information relative to the trial at that site. The investigator will also make a final report to the IRB. It will contain the information above, plus any other information specifically requested by the IRB. Frequently the report done for the IRB is also sent as the final report to the sponsor. The investigator must notify the institution that the study is complete, if appropriate. Frequently it is the CRC who will draft these final reports for the investigator.

At the closing visit, the CRA will verify that these reports were done, collect copies for the sponsor, if appropriate, and ensure that the reports are in the investigator study file.

Administrative Issues

Since this is probably the last visit the CRA will make to the site for the trial, any outstanding business or issues should be resolved before the closure is complete. Any loose ends should be resolved and taken care of before the site is completely closed.

The investigator and/or CRC will want to verify that all appropriate grant monies have been paid or requested.

If there are unused study materials at the site (case report forms, unused laboratory kits, etc.), they should be returned or disposed of according to the sponsor's direction.

Any outstanding issues from previous visits, or issues that arose during sponsor review, should be resolved before the site is closed. If not documented elsewhere, a note detailing the resolution should be put in the investigator's study file.

Record Retention

The CRC should discuss record retention with the CRA. Not only do the records need to be stored and maintained, but also there must be a record of where they are stored; it is not easy to remember these things as the years go by. According to the regulations, records must be kept for two years after the NDA is approved for marketing, or, if an NDA is not filed or is disapproved, for two years after the investigation is discontinued and the FDA notified.[2] However, most sponsors expect the investigator to retain all study records until notified by the sponsor that they may be disposed of; this will usually be in the contract that the investigator signed before starting the study.

---

2. 21 CFR 312.62c.

Sites do not always keep study records as long as they should. Years go by, and things happen—they run short of storage space, or move to a new facility, or just don't think they need to "keep all that old stuff" around any longer. Unfortunately, these records may be needed years after the study is over. For example, the sponsor may decide to file a new application based in part on old studies. When the FDA visits investigative sites as part of the NDA review process, it will expect to see all the documents in place, even if the study was done many years previously. It will be an embarrassment to the investigator if he or she has thrown them away, and it may have a negative impact on the sponsor's NDA. The site may want to bill the sponsor an annual storage fee.

It is recommended that the boxes in which study information is filed be labeled on the outside "DO NOT DESTROY," with the names of both the investigator and the sponsor as contacts for questions about them. If there is some reason that a site can no longer maintain the records, the site should contact the sponsor. In most cases, the sponsor will arrange storage for these materials so that they are not destroyed.

FAQ

We have some boxes of old study papers that have been sitting in our storage room for years. Can we get rid of them? We need the space.

Contact the sponsor first. You should not dispose of study records without the concurrence of the sponsor; this is usually in the written contract. If you no longer have room for the materials and the sponsor does not want them destroyed, the sponsor may assist by arranging for off-site storage.

When everything is complete and accounted for, the site may be officially closed.

Post-Study Critique

After a clinical trial has been completed at your site, it is very beneficial to perform a post-study critique. During the critique, the study will be critically evaluated in terms of enrollment, procedures, successful completion and financial viability.

Before the critique, the investigator and/or the CRC should compile a summary of pertinent data from the study. The summary should include:

- Number of subjects
  - Screened
  - Enrolled
  - Completing
- Time frame for enrollment, completion
- Serious adverse events
- Summary of problems encountered, protocol violation, changes to the research, etc.
- Any other pertinent information

A copy of this summary, plus the pre-study assessment sheets, should be sent to all the people on the site's study team, including the investigator, subinvestigator, CRC(s), and other involved personnel. Everyone should review the material before meeting for the actual post-study evaluation and critique.

The investigator will also want to review the grant and costs associated with the study to determine if it was actually economically practicable to do the project. If not, perhaps budget assumptions will need to be adjusted for future work.

During the meeting, the group should discuss and determine what went well during the study and what did not. They should also check the validity of the initial assessments that were made before agreeing to do the study (from the Protocol Feasibility Assessment Checklist in Appendix D). Finally, the group will want to determine where consistent improvements can be made in the future. The Post-Study Critique Worksheet found in Appendix D is a useful tool for this review. Once it is completed, it can be filed for future reference.

By the end of the post-study critique session, the group should have a good handle on how the study went, whether or not it was a good fit for the site, if it was beneficial for the subjects involved, if the workload was manageable and appropriate, and if the study was financially beneficial. The last determinations to be made should be:

- Was the overall study experience favorable?
- Would we like to work with this sponsor again?

By completing a post-study evaluation after each clinical trial, you will be more adept at picking those projects that are best suited to do in the future. This evaluation will also show you where you need to make changes or adjustments in site procedures for increased efficiencies in your clinical trials.

Key Things to Remember

- Studies can be stopped because they are complete, or for a variety of other reasons.
- The CRA is the sponsor representative who will do a study closeout at a site.
- All study documents, including case report forms, informed consent forms, drug accountability and study regulatory documents must be complete and filed at the end of the study.
- All study drug and other supplies must be returned to the sponsor or otherwise disposed of at the end of the study.
- The investigator must prepare a final study report to the sponsor and to the IRB at the end of the study.
- The investigator must be aware of record retention requirements at the end of the study.
- The CRA will verify in a final visit report that the study was properly closed.
- A post-study critique should be done at the completion of each study done by a site.

CHAPTER 11

Adverse Events and Safety Monitoring

In this chapter, we will discuss adverse events and safety monitoring. It is critical that adverse events are monitored during clinical trials, for the protection of the subjects enrolled in the trial as well as for protection of the patients and proper use of the drug once it is marketed.

Reporting on safety during a clinical trial is one of the most important tasks the investigator and the CRC perform. At the same time, safety reporting is one of the most difficult things for a study site to do correctly. There are often misunderstandings about what is necessary for reporting on safety issues in trials, stemming at least in part because of the differences in clinical studies as compared to clinical practice. Also, although the regulations charge the investigator with protecting the rights, safety and well-being of subjects in trials, they don't give much information about actual safety reporting. We will look at the regulations in detail.

Regulations

21 CFR 312.64 (Investigator reports) requires investigators to report adverse events during clinical trials. It states:

> *Safety reports. An investigator shall promptly report to the sponsor any adverse effect that may be reasonably regarded as caused by, or proba-*

bly caused by, the drug. If the adverse effect is alarming, the investigator shall report the adverse effect immediately.

By signing the 1572, the investigator also commits to reporting adverse events to the sponsor that occur during the course of a trial, in accordance with 21 CFR 312.64.

The ICH Guidelines for Good Clinical Practice have somewhat more information. In the glossary both adverse events and adverse drug reactions are defined as follows:

Adverse Event (AE)
An AE is any untoward medical occurrence in a patient or clinical investigation subject administered a pharmaceutical product. It does not necessarily have a causal relationship with this treatment. An AE can therefore be any unfavorable and unintended sign (including an abnormal laboratory finding), symptom, or disease temporally associated with the use of a medicinal (investigational) product.

Adverse Drug Reaction (ADR)
In the preapproval clinical experience with a new medicinal product or its new usages, particularly as the therapeutic dose(s) may not be established, all noxious and unintended responses to a medicinal product related to any dose should be considered adverse drug reactions. The phrase "responses to a medicinal product" means that a causal relationship between a medicinal product and an adverse event is at least a reasonable possibility, i.e., the relationship cannot be ruled out.

Regarding marketed medicinal products: A response to a drug that is noxious and unintended and that occurs at doses normally used in man for prophylaxis, diagnosis, or therapy of diseases or for modification of physiological function.[1]

The ICH GCPs also contain a section (4.11) on safety reporting. In this section, it states that:

All serious adverse events (SAEs) should be reported immediately to the sponsor except for those that are designated in the protocol or investigator brochure as not needing to be reported immediately. The initial report should be followed by a detailed written report.

The investigator should comply with regulatory requirements for reporting unexpected SAEs to regulatory authorities and the IRB.[2]

---

1. ICH Guideline for Good Clinical Practice, as published in the Federal Register May 9, 1997. Part I. Glossary.
2. ICH Guideline for Good Clinical Practice, as published in the Federal Register May 9, 1997. Section 4.11.

In clinical studies, sponsors are required to report serious, unexpected, related events that are fatal or life threatening to the U.S. Food and Drug Administration (FDA) by telephone and/or facsimile within seven calendar days of the date the sponsor first becomes aware of the event. The reporting clock starts when the first person in the sponsor company hears of the event. If the sponsor company is using a CRO, the CRO becomes, in effect, the sponsor company; in this case, the reporting clock starts even if a person in the CRO is the first to become aware of the event. Note that the first person may be a secretary or any other person who happens to answer the telephone or receive the fax—it doesn't have to be someone involved in managing the study.

A written report detailing all the information the sponsor has about the event is sent to the FDA within a fifteen-day time period. This is a total of fifteen calendar days from the initial report of the AE, eight days after the seven-day telephone or facsimile report. The sponsor must also send out IND Safety Reports, which will be covered later in this chapter.

Adverse events that are serious, unexpected and related to the investigational drug but not fatal or life threatening, must be reported to the FDA by the sponsor in writing within fifteen calendar days of the date that anyone in the employ of the sponsor first becomes aware of the event. Anyone in the employ of the sponsor is defined exactly as described above for seven-day reporting.

Definitions

There are a number of definitions related to adverse event reporting that are important to know and understand. These are regulatory definitions, not clinical definitions, which is an important distinction to understand when working with investigative sites. These definitions are:

- Adverse event. An adverse event is any untoward medical occurrence in a subject administered a drug (biologic, device). It does not necessarily have a causal relationship with the treatment/usage.
- Serious adverse event. Serious adverse events are those that result in death, are life threatening (immediately as it occurred, not had it become worse at some time in the future), require hospitalization (or a prolongation of hospitalization in already hospitalized patients), result in a persistent or significant disability or incapacity, are congenital anomalies or birth defects. For clinical studies, these serious adverse events also include any other event that the investigator or the sponsor company judges to be serious, or is defined as serious by the regulatory agency in the country where the event occurred.

It is important to distinguish between the terms "serious" and "severe." The term "serious" is used with the definition above and categorizes events (i.e., they either meet the definition for serious or they don't). The term "severe" refers to the intensity of the event and can be used with any event, without regard to whether or not it meets the criteria for being classified as "serious." For example, a subject can have a severe headache, but it is not a serious event.

- Related to or associated with the drug. This is defined to mean that there is a reasonable possibility that the event could have been caused by the investigational product (drug, biologic, device).
- Expected/unexpected. An expected event is one where the specificity and severity of the event are consistent with the information in the investigator brochure or labeling for the product. Unexpected events are all the others.
- Life-threatening. A life-threatening event is one where the patient is in immediate danger of death unless intervention is done. It does not mean that the patient may die at some time in the future from the event or may have died if the event had been more serious or specific.
- Significant disability. A significant disability is one that causes substantial disruption to the person's normal life and activity.

Adverse Events (AEs) on Marketed Products

Companies must collect safety information on each of their products throughout the entire life cycle of the product—from the first time it is used in people during clinical trials to the time the last dose of marketed drug is sold and used.

Events collected after a product is marketed are called spontaneous adverse events. They are called spontaneous adverse events because medical professionals, patients or others report them spontaneously or voluntarily to the sponsor, as opposed to being collected systematically during clinical trials. Since these events are reported voluntarily, they are all classified as "related" to the drug for reporting purposes. The reasoning behind this classification is that if someone feels there is enough of a relationship to report the event, it makes sense to assume it is related in some way. Remember, however, that an adverse event must meet all three criteria to need expedited reporting to the FDA; it must be serious, related and unexpected.

The bulk of spontaneous adverse event reports come to a pharmaceutical company from health professionals. Health professionals often call a pharmaceutical company to report unusual things they have seen in patients who are taking the drug; frequently these are calls asking for further information about the compound. Reports may also come in from patients, other consumers, or from the FDA or other regulatory agencies.

The requirement for reporting adverse events on marketed products stems from the fact that clinical trials are never sufficient to provide a full adverse event profile for a drug. Some of the differences between clinical trials and marketed use of a drug are shown in Table 1.

Table 1: Differences Between Clinical Trials and Marketed Use of a Product

Clinical Trials	Marketed Use
■ Relatively small number of patients	■ Millions of patients
■ Tight control	■ No control
■ Extra care	■ Standard care
■ Highly trained physicians	■ Any physicians
■ Narrow patient population	■ Anyone prescribed the drug

All these differences can have an impact on the adverse event profile of the drug. As an example, assume there is an adverse reaction to a drug that occurs only about once in every 50,000 people who take it. Chances are that this adverse reaction will never be seen during the clinical trial program, which usually consists only of several thousand patients. Even if the clinical program enrolled 20,000 subjects, an event occurring only once in 50,000 probably will not show up more than once, if at all. When the drug is marketed, however, and is available for use by millions of people, these events will become apparent. The purpose of the FDA's safety surveillance program is to ensure that there is a mechanism to report, and learn about, these events.

Adverse Events (AEs) in Clinical Trials

The adverse events that CRCs will be most involved with are those that are collected during clinical trials of drugs that are usually not yet marketed, but are still in the development process. All adverse events that occur during studies are collected. They are further classified by the definitions for serious, related and unexpected, as given above.

Most of the adverse events seen during clinical trials will not be serious, as defined in the regulations. In general, these non-serious adverse events will be recorded regularly on case report forms and will be reviewed and collected by the CRA during regular monitoring visits. Remember that non-serious events can be severe in intensity but still not meet the definition of serious.

Most sponsors want all serious adverse events that occur during a trial to be reported to them by the investigator as soon as he or she becomes aware of them. This is for two reasons: first, to ensure the continued safety of subjects in the trial; and second, to meet the reporting requirements for the FDA. The FDA reporting rules for serious adverse events occurring during clinical trials are similar to those for spontaneous adverse events, although there are some differences.

Sponsors must still report (in writing) all AEs that are serious, related and unexpected to the FDA within fifteen calendar days, and those that are also serious and alarming (death, immediately life-threatening) must be reported by fax or phone within seven days, with a written report within the next eight days.

Safety Reporting Sections in Protocols

Every protocol for a clinical trial should contain a detailed plan for the collection and reporting of all adverse events, both serious and non-serious. There are several key items that should be included.

Definitions

The protocol should include the regulatory definitions for an adverse event and a serious adverse event, as well as the definitions for related/associated and for expected/unexpected events.

Sources of AEs

In general, the standard sources of all adverse events will be the investigator reporting of:

- All directly observed events. [I see you have a rash on your arm…]
- Events elicited from the subject by means of a general non-directive question. [Have you had any problems with your health since you were here the last time?] The use of a specific question allows the sponsor to standardize procedures across all sites. A non-directive question does not prompt a subject to answer in a specific way. Asking subjects about specific events [Have you had any headaches?], although appropriate in some studies, will lead to a higher reporting rate for the specific event than a non-directive question.
- Events spontaneously volunteered by the study subject. [You know, Doc, ever since I started taking these pills, I have had an upset stomach.]
- Laboratory, EKG or other test results that meet protocol requirements for classification as adverse events. [Example: laboratory values more than 10% outside the normal range.

Event Collection Periods

The study periods during which adverse events will be collected should be specified. Some protocols require adverse events to be collected during a pre-treatment period as baseline data, while others only require collection during active treatment. It is also quite common to collect AEs during a post-treatment follow-up period. Adverse events are always collected during the entire period that a subject is on, or could be on (in the case of blinded trials), the investigational product or study drug.

Diaries and Other Data Collection Instruments

Whenever data collection instruments are used that may elicit information about adverse events (e.g., quality of life questionnaires, patient diaries), the methods for handling these events should be specified in the protocol. Although they certainly have a place in data collection, instruments such as diaries can complicate the orderly collection of adverse events. The problem is that subjects may write comments in diaries that refer to potential adverse events, and there is often no orderly way to officially collect the pertinent information. There is an example of a patient diary with a written comment about a potential event in Table 2.

Table 2: Example: Patient Diary

ACMEPHARMA STUDY 1234 — Patient Diary—Week 4

Name: Betsy Smith

Each day, please enter the time you took your study medication. Remember, you should always take one pill just before breakfast (about 8:00 am) and two pills before dinner (about 6:00 pm).

Sunday	Date: 2/2/98		
	Morning dose time	______ am	
	Evening dose time	______ pm	
Monday	Date: ______		
	Morning dose time	______ am	
	Evening dose time	______ pm	
Tuesday	Date: ______		
	Morning dose time	8 am	
	Evening dose time	6 pm	migraine - felt dizzy

Notice that this patient was filling in the times she took her investigational medication, but she also added some additional information—the migraine headache. Certainly, the study site personnel would want to know about the migraine, but this is not the place for it to be recorded. The CRC will need to ensure that this event is recorded on the appropriate adverse event case report forms, and not missed.

Unresolved Adverse Events

Sometimes adverse events that occur during a study are unresolved at the time the subject's study participation ends. The protocol should state what is to be done in this case. Usually serious AEs are followed to resolution, that is, until they resolve, disappear or become stable.

There is often a time period during which any events that are ongoing at the end of the study are followed. Thirty days is a frequently used time period, but it varies depending on the compound, its half-life, the amount of time the subject was in the trial and the complexity of the diagnosis and protocol.

Exposure *in Utero*

If women of childbearing potential are allowed entry into the trial, then the protocol should include instructions for reporting exposure *in utero* and the subsequent outcome of the pregnancy. In general, the investigator will be required to follow up on any cases of pregnancy that occur during the study until the child is born or the pregnancy is terminated. There is usually no requirement for interim visits throughout the pregnancy, just an assurance that the subject will be contacted periodically to determine the outcome.

Timely Notification

The sponsor will want to be notified of serious events by the investigator in a timely manner, usually within 24 hours. It is extremely important that the investigator notify the sponsor of each serious adverse event as soon as possible, even if all the details are not yet available. Additional details can be reported as they become available; the initial report should never be delayed while awaiting more information.

An investigator may not know about an event for some time after it has occurred, especially if he or she is not the subject's primary physician. The study site may not know about the event until the subject comes in for his or her next appointment, or fails to show up for the appointment because of the event. However, the investigator should inform the sponsor of the event as soon as he or she becomes aware of it.

Non-serious adverse events are also reported to the sponsor. This reporting is done by way of the case report form and regular data collection process. Final reporting is done within a reasonable time following completion of the study (usually within three months). There are no FDA requirements for expedited reporting of non-serious events.

Investigator Reporting Responsibilities

Investigators are required to collect, assess and report all the adverse events that occur during a trial. The following information is usually gathered for each event: onset (date/time), duration, severity (mild, moderate, severe), relationship to the study drug, and whether or not it is serious. All events are to be recorded on the CRF. In addition, if an event is serious, the investigator is usually expected to report it to the sponsor very quickly (e.g., within 24 hours).

Not only must the investigator report adverse events to the sponsor, but he or she also has a requirement for reporting these events to the institutional review board (IRB), in the manner in which the IRB has requested. As with sponsors, some IRBs will want notification of all serious events, while others will want to hear only about events that are serious and related, or only those that are serious, related and unexpected. The IRB will let the investigator know what is expected, and what the report timing and mechanisms are. It is important that the investigator notify the IRB according to the rules the IRB has established.

It is a regulatory requirement that the investigator notify both the sponsor and the IRB of adverse events.[3]

The investigator may receive IND Safety Reports (discussed in the next section) from the sponsor. Whenever one is received, the investigator must forward the information to the IRB.

Sponsor Responsibilities

Sponsors are required to review safety data throughout a trial. This is so appropriate adjustments can be made if there are any relevant safety issues. For example, the protocol might be amended, or, if there are serious safety concerns, the trial might be stopped. Remember that the sponsor is the only entity that has access to all the safety data for a drug; investigators and IRBs only see safety data from the site or sites with which they are involved. Therefore, the burden is on the sponsor for prompt and thorough review of safety information as it is generated.

Sponsors have the responsibility of reporting adverse events that are serious, related and unexpected to the FDA within the expedited reporting time frames, as was discussed earlier.

Sponsors have an additional reporting requirement for serious adverse events in clinical trials; they must also inform all investigators who are currently working with the drug of any serious, related, unexpected adverse event. The investigators need to receive the same information as that sent to the FDA and within the same fifteen-day time period. These reports are

3. 3. 21 CFR 312.64, 66.

called IND Safety Reports. Note that IND Safety Reports are sent to all investigators working with the compound, not just those doing the same protocol. The requirements for IND Safety Reports are found in 21 CFR 312.32.6.

There may be rare instances where an adverse finding or a series of adverse events indicate that the drug has a safety issue that is so serious that the continued use of it in clinical trials is unacceptable. If this occurs, the sponsor must notify the FDA and all investigators who ever participated in a clinical trial with the drug immediately of that decision. This includes all investigators who ever studied the drug, not just those with currently active clinical trials. The investigators of open trials must then, in turn, immediately notify their IRBs of the trials' discontinuation for reasons of safety.

Differences Between Clinical Studies and Clinical Practice

One reason that adverse event reporting is fraught with problems stems from the fact that clinical practice and clinical research are not the same thing, and it is easy to get the two confused when it comes to safety reporting. It is often confusing for investigators and CRCs to realize that the definitions used for adverse event reporting in trials are regulatory definitions, not clinical definitions. A good CRC understands the definitions and reporting requirements, and takes the time to thoroughly train other staff members on the requirements before subjects are enrolled.

In studies, the investigator has a dual role as a physician and an investigator. It is a physician's duty to act in the best interest of the patient, while at the same time, it is the duty of the investigator to perform good research. These duties are not necessarily in conflict, but there are differences in the roles that must be understood.

Some examples of these differences are the following:

- Concomitant medications that might normally be prescribed for a patient may not be allowed under the protocol.
- Treatment periods may be longer or shorter under the protocol than are usual in general practice.
- Adverse events that are "normal" for the disease must usually be reported under study rules.

A worsening or progression of the disease may or may not be reported as an adverse event. For example, a worsening of anxiety in an anxiety trial would usually require reporting, while a progression of Alzheimer's disease in an Alzheimer's trial might not be reported, as this is a progressive disease.

Occasionally investigators do not understand the importance of reporting adverse events if they do not seem to be connected with the trial or the study medication, or if they are commonly seen with the disease under study. An investigator may say something on the order of "we see that all the time in this disease..." or "it's not connected to the trial..." or "that isn't of any importance...." These remarks signify a misunderstanding of the differences between clinical practice and research. The investigator, the CRC and other site staff must remember that the study is being done to find out about the investigational drug, including safety as well as efficacy. That is why studies are done—we never really know what we will learn about a drug or device when it is under investigation.

The investigator must remember his or her regulatory responsibilities with respect to doing trials, which include proper reporting of adverse events. He or she is also bound by the contract with the sponsor, and most contracts require the investigator to report adverse events as mandated by the regulations.

Assessing the Relationship of an AE to the Study Drug

Investigators are usually asked to assess the relationship between an adverse event and the investigational product by picking the term that best characterizes the relationship of the adverse event to the investigational product. The choices are commonly on the order of: not related, probably not related, possibly related, probably related, definitely related. Because not much is known about the product, investigators are often uneasy about making this decision. Here are some aids that investigators and CRCs might use when making these decisions.

Temporal Relationship

Does the timing of taking the investigational drug make sense in relationship to the timing of the event? For example, assume that the subject takes the drug, comes in two days later and is diagnosed with cancer. The cancer is probably not related, because it occurred too soon after taking the study drug. Or, assume that a subject has been taking the study drug without a problem but develops an adverse event just after the dose was titrated upward; in this case, the event might well be related to the drug.

Known Patterns of Reaction

Assume that the study drug causes a distinctive rash, and a study subject develops that type of rash. Chances are good that the rash is related to the study drug.

Other Potential Causes

Is there something else that would explain the occurrence of the event? For example, assume that the subject is allergic to chocolate, but couldn't resist that piece of devil's food chocolate birthday cake last night. He ate some and ended up with hives. The hives are probably not related to the study drug, but to the chocolate.

Does it Make Sense?

Assume that a study subject suffers from regular migraines, takes the study drug and has a migraine. It's probably not related. However, assume that the subject usually has one or two migraines a month, but ever since starting the study drug, she has them every two or three days. They are probably related to the study drug. This might, in fact, be reported as an exacerbation of a previously existing medical condition, e.g., a change in severity.

Dechallenge/Rechallenge

In this scenario, the subject has an adverse event. The study drug is stopped (the dechallenge), and the event stops. The study drug is restarted (rechallenge), and the event occurs again. It is probably related to the drug under study. This is a very definitive test, but may not be done unless allowed in the protocol. Although an investigator may stop a study drug (dechallenge) at any time it is deemed appropriate, he or she may not restart it (rechallenge) unless allowed by the protocol or after discussion with and agreement by the sponsor.

Common Reporting Problems

There are a number of common misunderstandings that result in incorrect adverse event reporting. Many of these errors can be avoided if the sponsor takes time to clarify them to site personnel in advance. One of these misunderstandings involves symptoms vs. a syndrome. Usually sponsors want a syndrome reported rather than the individual symptoms, for example, flu vs. cough, sniffles and sore throat all reported separately.

Another common error is the reporting of a procedure, as opposed to reporting the disease/condition that resulted in the procedure. An example of this is reporting a coronary bypass as the event, instead of reporting the heart condition that necessitated the bypass.

Changes in severity are frequently reported incorrectly, or not at all. The general convention is that if an event worsens in severity, it is reported as a new event, even if the event is in the pre-study history for the subject. Some protocols also require the reporting of changes in events when the change is for the better.

Although it was mentioned earlier in this chapter, it is critical for the investigator and CRC to understand the distinction between the terms "serious" and "severe" where the "severe" refers to the intensity of an event, without regard to whether or not it meets the criteria for being classified as "serious."

In case of exposure *in utero*, it is a good idea for the CRC to make a note to follow up with the subject in any case of pregnancy. It is easy to forget to do this when the subject is not being seen on a regular basis.

Key Things to Remember

- Subject safety is paramount in clinical trials.
- There are differences between clinical practice and clinical trials when it comes to reporting adverse events.
- The definitions used in adverse event reporting are regulatory definitions, not clinical definitions.
- Adverse events that are serious and related and unexpected require expedited reporting to the FDA.
- All investigators working with an investigational drug must be informed of any event with the drug that is serious, related and unexpected. The sponsor sends an IND Safety Report to each investigator for any adverse event meeting these criteria.
- The investigator must inform his or her IRB of any IND Safety Report received from a sponsor.
- Serious adverse events must be reported to the sponsor of the study within a very short time period (usually 24 or 48 hours).
- Protocols should contain explicit directions for collecting, assessing and reporting adverse events.

CHAPTER 12

Audits

During the clinical development process, the FDA may conduct audits (also called inspections) of investigative sites. Sponsors and IRBs may also conduct their own audits of investigative sites. In this chapter we will discuss these different types of audits, as well as the CRC role in audits. We will start with audits conducted by sponsors and IRBs, but will concentrate primarily on those audits done by the FDA, as they are the most critical to the investigative site and to the drug approval process.

Sponsor Audits of Investigative Sites

There are two main purposes for a sponsor to audit a study site. The most common reason is to ensure that a site is complying with the regulations and protocol when doing a study, and that everything is in order in case of an FDA audit. These are referred to as routine audits. The second reason is because there is evidence that the site is out of compliance, and the sponsor wants to either verify the problem or be reassured that no problem exists. These are called for-cause audits.

A sponsor's right to audit a site is based on both the regulations and (usually) on the contract between the investigator and the sponsor. Most contracts will state that the investigator agrees that the sponsor may conduct audits of the site. The regulations under which sponsor audits are loosely covered is found in 21 CFR 312.56(a)(b), which state:

> "(a) The sponsor shall monitor the progress of all clinical investigations being conducted under its IND," and "(b) A sponsor who discovers that an investigator is not complying with the signed agreement (Form FDA 1572), the general investigational plan, or the requirements of this part or other applicable parts shall promptly either secure compliance or discontinue shipments of the investigational new drug to the investigator and end the investigator's participation in the investigation."[1]

Routine Audits

If the sponsor knows or suspects that a site will be audited by the FDA, a routine audit may be done, either while the study is in process, or after it has been completed and during the NDA review period. The sponsor knows that the FDA will inspect some sites during its review of the NDA, so the sponsor will focus on the sites that are logical for the FDA to pick: those where enrollment was the highest or where multiple studies contributed to the NDA. If your site contributed a significant number of subjects for a primary registration study, your chances of an audit by the FDA are relatively high.

For a routine audit the sponsor will send in an audit team, who will follow the same inspection plan used by the FDA. This inspection plan can be found in the FDA Compliance Program Guidance Manual for Clinical Investigators (Program 7348.811) or can be found on the Internet at www.fda.gov/oc/gcp/compliance.html.

A written report of sponsor audit results is not often given to the investigator. This is because FDA inspectors do not have routine access to sponsor audit reports, and sponsors do not want to have these reports freely circulating, either at the site or internally. If a written report is sent to an investigator, the sponsor will usually ask that it be destroyed after corrective action is taken.

If any problems are found during the audit, the investigator will be asked to remedy them, with the goal of ensuring that the site is ready for an FDA audit.

For-Cause Audits

For-cause audits of investigator sites by a sponsor may be handled somewhat differently. These are audits done because of suspected noncompliance at a site, either with the regulations or with the protocol. They have the potential for being much more serious, both for the sponsor and ultimately for the investigator. The sponsor is unlikely to tell the investigator it is a for-cause audit. The audit team will look at most of the things they would inspect for any audit but will pay particular attention to the area(s) of sus-

1. 21 CFR 312.56(a)(b).

pected noncompliance. Depending on the results of the audit, a number of things could happen:

- If everything appears to be in compliance, the results will be handled as for any routine audit.
- If the problem was not found but is still suspected another group may be sent to look, or the sponsor might inform the FDA and ask them to inspect the site.
- If problems were found, they will either be rectified, or enrollment may be put on hold pending further investigation, or the study may be stopped at the site. In this case the FDA will be informed, if appropriate.

IRB Audits of Investigative Sites

IRBs also visit or audit sites upon occasion. A central or independent IRB may visit sites simply because they are not located nearby, and they want to be assured that the site is managing studies correctly. These are routine audits.

An IRB may also make for-cause visits if there is reason to think that the site has ethics or compliance violations. IRBs are required to report to the FDA any instances of unanticipated problems involving risks to human subjects, serious or continuing non-compliance with the regulations or IRB requirements, or any suspension or termination of IRB approval.[2]

FDA Audits of Investigative Sites

The FDA conducts three types of inspections at investigative sites: study-related, investigator-related and bioequivalence study. Bioequivalence study inspections are done when one study is the sole basis for a drug's approval; we will not discuss these further here. The other two types are important for a CRC to be aware of. For either study- or investigator-related audits, the purpose is threefold:

1. To determine the validity and integrity of the data
2. To assess adherence to regulations and guidelines
3. To determine that the rights and safety of the human subjects were properly protected

We will take a detailed look at both study-related and investigator-related audits.

2. 21 CFR 56.108(b).

Study-Related Audits

Study-related audits/inspections are almost always done on the studies that are important to an NDA or product license application that has been submitted to the agency. These studies are the primary efficacy studies on which a sponsor relies for showing that the product works and should be approved for marketing.

The sites selected for auditing are usually those that contributed the most data to the application, either by high enrollment or by doing multiple studies. Because of this, sponsors usually have a reasonable idea of which sites have a high probability of being audited. The sponsor also knows that studies will be inspected during the NDA review time, which is now six months or less for a fast track product, and one year or less for all others, from the date the FDA receives the application. The primary efficacy studies are closed at this point, as the trials are complete and analyzed before being submitted in the NDA; in fact, they may have been closed for quite some time.

FAQ

What are our chances of being audited by the FDA?

Not very high, as they audit only a few hundred sites each year. However, if your study is a primary efficacy study for an NDA, and you were among the top enrolling sites, your chances are much higher. They are also higher if there is a suspicion of regulatory noncompliance or other major problems at your site. Remember—if you do everything correctly during a study and follow all the regulations, you do not have to worry about an audit.

The sponsor will usually alert those sites that are most likely to be audited to this possibility. Often, CRAs are sent to the sites with high probability of being audited in order to ensure that all the study materials are available and organized for FDA review. Also, a site should inform the sponsor when they are contacted by the FDA to schedule an audit, in which case the sponsor may send the CRA in to help the site prepare. If missing documents or other problems are found during this review, the situation may be able to be remedied before an FDA audit occurs.

Investigator-Related Inspections

Investigator-related inspections are initiated for a variety of reasons, many of which are listed below:

- Investigators have done a large number of studies, or have done work outside their specialty areas.
- An investigator has done a pivotal study that is critical to a new product application and it merits extra attention.

- The safety or efficacy findings of an investigator are inconsistent with the results from other investigators working with the same test product.
- The sponsor or IRB has notified the FDA about serious problems or concerns at the site.
- A subject has complained about the protocol or subject rights violations at the site.
- There were an unexpected number of subjects with the diagnosis under study, given the location of the study.
- Enrollment at the site was much more rapid than expected.
- The study and investigator were highly publicized in the media.
- Any other reason that piques the curiosity of the agency.

Site Preparation

The best preparation for an audit is for the site to have done things correctly to begin with, in which case an audit will reveal no problems. However, once an audit is scheduled, the site should prepare by amassing all the study documents in one easy-to-get-to place, and by reviewing them to be sure everything is accounted for, complete and well organized. The study documents that should be available for review include all informed consent forms, patient charts, case report forms and the study regulatory file. When an inspector asks to see a document, the site should be able to retrieve it easily and quickly. Sometimes, although this is seen most often when the FDA audits non-U.S. sites, the FDA may ask the site to send them a letter of availability of records; this letter certifies that all study records will be available for FDA review upon their arrival.

The Audit Process

The first thing that happens with an audit is the notification to the site. The inspector usually contacts the site by telephone to arrange a mutually acceptable time for the audit visit. Sites are usually given one or two weeks' notice; it is acceptable to negotiate a delay in the visit date, as long as the investigator has a good reason and the time is not lengthened too much. If the audit is investigator-related, and if the FDA has concerns about subject safety or compliance, the time between the notification and the visit will probably be very short and delays will not be acceptable. If there are serious concerns, the FDA could just appear at the site without advance notice. Most sponsors ask and expect their investigators to let them know immediately of an impending audit.

The role of the investigator and the CRC in the audit is to be present, to provide the inspector with a quiet, comfortable place to work and to assemble the necessary documents. You should be polite, courteous, cooperative and reasonable when interacting with the FDA inspector; antagonism is inappropriate and will undoubtedly be regretted later. The investigator should provide all the materials/documents the FDA inspector requests, but should never give the inspector free access to the files. All questions should be answered, but extra information should not be volunteered. The inspector knows what he or she is asking for, and will continue to question until the needed information is detected. Although the responsibility for the audit remains with the investigator, it is usually the CRC who prepares the materials for the audit. Both the investigator and the CRC will usually interact with the inspector.

FAQ

Can FDA auditors ask to see anything they want to see?

Yes. But only give the auditor what he or she requests. Do not give the auditor free rein to look at any and all of your files.

Site personnel should not offer the inspector anything beyond a cup of coffee, such as a meal; the offer may be misconstrued. At this time, the FDA is not privy to grant information or to sponsor audit results, so if the inspector asks for this information, the investigator should nicely refuse to answer. If the inspector is treated politely, the audit will be more pleasant for everyone.

When inspectors arrive at sites, they will present their credentials (a photo ID) and a Notice of Inspections form (482) to the clinical investigator. If the inspector does not present these credentials, the investigator should ask for them. The investigator should check the date on the inspector's credentials to be sure they are still valid.

During the inspection, the inspector will meet with the investigator, the CRC, and any other appropriate study staff, and will review study documents. If people who played substantial roles in the study are no longer at the site, the investigator should be able to contact them, if at all possible, during the audit if the inspector wishes to talk with them. There are two main aspects of the study that will be looked at during the inspection, study conduct and study data. According to the FDA Guidance for IRBs and Investigators, the conduct of the study will be considered by reviewing the following items:

- who did what,
- the degree of delegation of authority,
- where specific aspects of the study were performed,
- how and where data were recorded,
- how test article accountability was maintained,
- how the monitor communicated with the clinical investigator, and
- how the monitor evaluated the study's progress"[3]

3. FDA Guidance for IRBs and Investigators, FDA inspections of clinical investigators, p. 75.

Notice that the monitor (CRA) is mentioned in two of these items. At the very least, you should have the monitor sign a study visit log at each monitoring visit to verify that the site was actually visited. There is an example of a study visit log in Appendix D.

When the inspector audits the study data, he or she will compare the data that were submitted to the agency with the site records that support the data, i.e., investigator copies of the case report forms and all the available source documents, including patient charts, laboratory reports, other test reports and so forth. Sometimes the inspector will also have copies of the case report forms from the sponsor, and will compare all three versions. The inspector will pay close attention to:

- the diagnosis,
- whether the patients were properly diagnosed based on their past history,
- whether or not the subjects met the protocol inclusion/exclusion criteria,
- concomitant medications, especially those that were not allowed, and
- appropriate follow-up of adverse events.

The inspector may look at data for only a sampling of subjects, or, if there appear to be problems, he or she may look at the data from all subjects. All informed consents are usually reviewed.

An FDA audit usually takes one to two weeks, although it depends on the amount of data to review, the findings and the amount of time the inspector has available for the audit. The days may not be consecutive for the entire period, but rather a day or two at the site at one time until the review is complete.

FAQ

If an FDA auditor is at our site for several days, are we expected to provide lunches and/or dinners?

No. In fact, you should not offer an FDA auditor anything beyond a cup of coffee, etc. An offer of anything beyond this could be misconstrued.

At the end of the inspection, the inspector will meet with the investigator to review the audit findings. During this meeting, the investigator may ask questions about anything that is not understood, and may clarify things that the inspector has interpreted incorrectly. Sometimes a misunderstanding or negative finding of the inspector can be explained satisfactorily at this point. If there are significant findings, the inspector may issue a Form FDA-

483 (Notice of Observations) to the investigator. This form will detail the findings from the audit that may constitute compliance violations.

Most sponsors ask that an investigator call them after the inspector leaves and let them know the results of the audit. If the investigator has received a 483 form, the sponsor will usually offer to help the investigator formulate his or her reply (a reply is mandatory).

After the Audit

After the audit is completed, the FDA inspector prepares an Establishment Inspection Report (EIR). This report goes through FDA compliance channels, and a classification is assigned to it. The investigator will receive a copy of the report a few months after the audit. The report is also available through the Freedom of Information Act, and most sponsors will request copies for their files.

The EIR classifications are:

- No action indicated (NAI). This is the best outcome, and means that no significant deviations from the regulations were found. The clinical investigator is not required to respond to this report.
- Voluntary action indicated (VAI). This report will provide information about findings of deviations from the regulations and good clinical practice. The letter may or may not require a response from the investigator. If a response is required, the letter will specify what is necessary. A contact person will also be listed for any questions.
- Official action indicated (OAI). This is the worst result to receive. This report identifies serious deviations from the regulations that require prompt action from the investigator. For OAIs, the FDA may also inform the sponsor and the IRB. The FDA may also inform the sponsor that the Agency believes that monitoring of the study was deficient. In addition to issuing the warning letter, the FDA may take other action, such as regulatory and/or administrative sanctions against the investigator. All in all, this is a very unpleasant process and should be avoided at all cost.

Consequences

The consequences of problems found during audits can be significant, especially when they impact a large amount of the data for a pivotal trial. The study at a particular site may be invalidated, especially if sufficient source documents were not available, if there were significant unreported concomitant therapies, or if there was a failure to follow the protocol. If the site was a high enroller and generated a significant amount of data in support of the sponsor's NDA, these problems could delay the NDA or result in a disapproved application. A sponsor may even have to repeat a study, which could add years to the drug development cycle.

There are also significant consequences for the investigator in these cases. An investigator may be disqualified or restricted from conducting clinical trials. This puts him or her on the infamous "black list," known more formally as the List of Disqualified and Restricted Investigators. Investigators can be added to the list through a court hearing or through a consent agreement; they can be totally disqualified from ever doing clinical studies, or may have other restrictions placed on them, such as only doing studies as a sub-investigator, or not doing more than one study every two years, etc. Once on the list, an investigator stays on the list forever, even if corrective action has been taken. It does not happen often, but in the worst cases an investigator can be fined and/or sentenced to prison.

Starting in 2000, the number of complaints to the FDA dramatically increased (about 15 to 20 complaints per year prior to 2000; over 100 per year since).

Because of the increase in the number of inspections, the compliance system is stretched. We can expect to see more audits, tighter controls and more training requirements for all clinical researchers in the future.

Remember that doing everything correctly throughout the study will ensure a successful audit. CRCs can help by educating themselves and ensuring that their site is compliant and performs research according to good clinical practices. A conscientious, knowledgeable CRC is a key to a good, valid study and favorable audit results.

Key Things to Remember

- Sponsors audit clinical investigator sites for studies that make a high contribution to their development programs. They also audit sites where it appears that there may be compliance problems.
- IRBs can also audit sites, especially if they suspect ethics violations.
- The FDA performs both study-related and investigator-related audits.
- The best preparation for an audit is to do the study correctly.
- CRCs should understand the audit process and how to prepare for audits.
- There are three classes of Establishment Inspection Reports that result from an inspection, NAI, VAI and OAI.
- The consequences of noncompliance are great, and can result in delays in an NDA, or in disqualification and other penalties for investigators.
- There has been an increase in compliance problems during the past few years.

AFTERWORD

This book covers a great deal of information, and I hope you will find it useful and helpful as a CRC. Remember that it's the little things that often make a big difference, both in how your job goes and in the success of clinical trials at your site. There is no doubt about it—the job of the CRC is not for the faint-hearted. It carries a lot of responsibility and an enormous amount of work. It requires multiple skills and the ability to keep organized under pressure. It's also fun and challenging, with constant opportunities for learning new things and meeting new people. I hope you enjoy both the job and the chance to make a difference in the lives of everyone who benefits from new drugs and devices after they are marketed. I'll leave you with a few last thoughts that will help you as a CRC.

- The safety and well-being of your study subjects always comes first.
- Establish a good, collegial working relationship with your investigator.
- Know your protocols and case report forms thoroughly.
- Keep organized.
- Read the regulations.
- Think of your sponsor monitors (CRAs) as the other half of the team.
- Don't be afraid to admit you don't know something—find out.
- Don't burn bridges. It's a small world.
- Don't be afraid to admit mistakes.

- Remember that you are making a difference in people's lives.
- Be nice.
- Smile.

Appendix A

Acronyms

ACRP	Association of Clinical Research Professionals
ADR	Adverse drug reaction
AE	Adverse event
AMA	American Medical Association
BIMO	Bioresearch Monitoring Program
CCI	Certified Clinical Investigator
CCRC	Certified Clinical Research Coordinator
CCRI	Certified Clinical Research Investigator
CDER	Center for Drug Evaluation and Research
CFR	Code of Federal Regulations
CI	Clinical Investigator
CPGM	Compliance Program Guidance Manual
CRA	Clinical Research Associate
CRC	Clinical Research Coordinator
CRF	Case Report Form
CRO	Contract Research Organization
CV	Curriculum vitae
DHHS	Department of Health and Human Services
DIA	Drug Information Association
DGR	Dangerous Goods Regulation
ECG	Electrocardiogram
EDC	Electronic Data Capture
EIR	Establishment Inspection Report

FDA	Food and Drug Administration
FDAMA	FDA Modernization Act
GCP	Good Clinical Practice
GLP	Good Laboratory Practices
GMP	Good Manufacturing Practices
HAM-A	Hamilton Rating Scale for Anxiety
HIPAA	Health Insurance Portability and Accountability Act
HHS	Health and Human Services
IATA	International Air Transport Association
IC	Informed Consent
ICH	International Conference on Harmonization
IEC	Independent Ethics Committee
IND	Investigational New Drug application
IRB	Institutional Review Board, Independent Review Board
IV	Intravenously
NAI	No Action Indicated
NDA	New Drug Application
NIH	National Institutes of Health
OAI	Official Action Indicated
OCR	Office of Civil Rights
OTC	Over-the-counter
PA	Physician Assistant
PDUFA	Prescription Drug User Fee Act
PhRMA	Pharmaceutical Research and Manufacturers of America
PHI	Protected Health Information
PI	Principal Investigator
PM	Project Manager
PMS	Post Marketing Surveillance
QA	Quality Assurance
RDE	Remote Data Entry
SAE	Serious adverse event
SC	Study Coordinator
SI	Sub-investigator
SMO	Site Management Organization
SoCRA	Society for Clinical Research Associates
SOP	Standard Operating Procedure
Sub-I	Sub-investigator
VAI	Voluntary Action Indicated

APPENDIX b

Glossary

Adverse Drug Reaction
An unintended reaction to a drug taken at normal doses.

Adverse Event (AE)
Any untoward medical occurrence in a study subject administered a pharmaceutical product; it does not necessarily have to have a causal relationship with this treatment.

Beneficence
Doing no harm. Maximizing benefits while minimizing risks.

Biologic
A virus, vaccine, toxin, antitoxin, blood product, therapeutic serum or similar material for the prevention, treatment or cure of disease or injury in humans.

Biotechnology
Any technique that uses living organisms or substances from living organisms, biological systems or processes to make or modify a product or process, to change plants or animals, or to develop microorganisms for specific uses.

Blinding
The process through which study subjects, the investigator and/or other involved parties in a clinical trial are kept unaware of the treatment assignments of study subjects.

Case Report Form (CRF)
A record of pertinent information collected on each subject during a clinical trial, based on the protocol.

Certified Clinical Investigator (CCI)
A clinical investigator who meets required experience and educational levels and has earned certification by passing an exam.

Certified Clinical Research Coordinator (CCRC)
CRC with more than two years experience and certification earned by passing an exam.

Clinical Trial (clinical study, clinical investigation)
Any experiment that involves a test article (drug, device, biologic) and one or more human subjects.

Clinical Research Associate (CRA)
The sponsor monitor who visits sites periodically during a study to monitor the data and assess progress.

Clinical Research Coordinator (CRC) (Study coordinator)
The person at an investigational site who manages the daily operations of a clinical investigation and who is responsible to the investigator.

Clinical Research Organization (CRO)
A person or entity that assumes, as an independent contractor with the sponsor, one or more of the obligations of the sponsor.

Contract Research Organization (CRO)

Control Group
A group of subjects who are not treated with the investigational product. This group is used as a comparison to the treatment group.

Data Management
The process of handling the data generated and collected during a clinical trial, usually including data entry and database management.

Demographic Data
The characteristics of study subjects, including age, sex, medical history and other information relevant to the study.

Device
An instrument, apparatus, implement, machine, contrivance, implant, *in vitro* reagent or other similar or related article, including any component, part or accessory, which is intended for use in the diagnosis, cure, treatment or prevention of disease. A device does not achieve its intended purpose through chemical action in the body and is not dependent upon being metabolized to achieve its purpose.

Double-Blind
The design of a study in which neither the investigator nor the subject knows which treatment the subject is receiving.

Drug
An article (other than food) intended for use in the diagnosis, cure, mitigation, treatment or prevention of disease in man or other animals.

Efficacy
A test product's ability to produce a beneficial effect on the duration or course of a disease.

FDA
The United States Food and Drug Administration.

Generic Drug
A medicinal product with the same active ingredient(s) as a brand name drug. Generic products may only be marketed after the original drug's patent has expired.

Good Clinical Practice (GCP)
The regulations and guidelines that specify the responsibilities of sponsors, investigators, monitors and IRBs involved in clinical trials. They are meant to protect the safety, rights and welfare of the subjects in addition to ensuring the accuracy of the data collected during the trial.

Human Subject
An individual who participates in research, either as a recipient of the test article or as a control. A subject may be either a healthy subject or a patient.

Inclusion and Exclusion Criteria
The characteristics that must be present (inclusion) or absent (exclusion) in order for a subject to qualify for a clinical trial, as per the protocol for the trial.

Informed Consent
The process by which a subject voluntarily confirms his or her willingness to participate in a clinical trial.

Institutional Review Board (IRB)
Any board, committee, or group formally designated to review biomedical research involving humans as subjects, to approve the initiation of and conduct periodic review of such research.

Investigator (Clinical Investigator [CI], Principal Investigator [PI])
An individual who actually conducts a clinical investigation, i.e., under whose immediate direction the test article is dispensed, or, in the case of an investigation conducted by a team of individuals, is the responsible leader of that team.

Investigator Brochure
A compilation of all information known to date about the test product, including chemistry and formulation information and preclinical and clinical data. It is updated at least annually. Once the product is marketed, it is replaced by the labeling (package insert) for the product.

Investigational New Drug
A new drug or biologic that is used in a clinical investigation.

Investigational New Drug Application (IND)
The application to start clinical testing of a new drug, biologic or device in humans.

***In Vitro* Testing**
Non-clinical testing conducted in an artificial environment such as a test tube or culture medium.

***In Vivo* Testing**
Testing conducted in living animal and human systems.

IRB Approval
The determination of the IRB that the clinical investigation has been reviewed and may be conducted within the constraints set by the IRB and applicable regulations.

Legally Authorized Representative
An individual or judicial or other body authorized under applicable law to consent on behalf of a potential subject to the subject's participation in research.

Medical Monitor (Sponsor Medical Monitor)
The physician at the sponsor who is responsible for the clinical investigation of a test product.

Minimal Risk
The probability and magnitude of harm or discomfort anticipated in the research are not greater than those ordinarily encountered in daily life or in the performance of routine physical or psychological examinations or tests.

New Drug Application (NDA)
The marketing application for a new drug submitted to the FDA. The NDA contains all the nonclinical, clinical, pharmacological, pharmacokinetic and stability data required by the FDA.

Open Label Study
A study in which the subjects and the investigator are aware of the drug that is being administered.

Placebo
An inactive substance designed to resemble the drug being tested.

Preclinical Testing
Studies conducted on animals to determine that the drug is safe to use in studies on humans.

Protocol
The formal plan for carrying out a clinical investigation.

Quality Assurance
Systems and procedures designed to ensure that a study is being performed in accordance with Good Clinical Practice (GCP) guidelines and that the data being generated are accurate.

Randomization
A method in which study subjects are randomly assigned to treatment groups. It helps to reduce bias in a trial by ensuring that there is no pattern in the way subjects are assigned to treatment groups.

Serious Adverse Event (SAE)
Any untoward medical occurrence at any dose that results in death, is life-threatening, requires hospitalization (or a prolongation of hospitalization in a patient who is already hospitalized), results in persistent or significant disability or incapacity, or is a congenital anomaly/birth defect.

Site Management Organization (SMO)
A group of investigational sites that have banded together and organized centrally to do studies.

Sponsor
The person or entity who initiates a clinical investigation, but who does not actually conduct the investigation.

Standard Operating Procedures (SOPs)
Official written instructions for the management and conduct of clinical trial processes. SOPs ensure that processes are carried out in a consistent and efficient manner.

Study Coordinator (Clinical Research Coordinator)
The person at an investigational site who manages the daily operations of a clinical investigation and who is responsible to the investigator.

Sub-Investigator
Any member of an investigational team other than the investigator.

Test Article
Any drug, biologic, or device being tested for use in humans.

Unanticipated Event
Problem involving risks to human subjects or others participating in a clinical research study, e.g., breach of confidentiality, incarceration of subject, suicide attempt, incorrect labeling of study drug. These, too, need to be collected and reported.

APPENDIX C

Resources

Books and Videotapes

Acres of Skin: Human Experiments at Holmesburg Prison—A True Story of Abuse and Exploitation in the Name of Medical Science
Allen M. Hornblum, 1998

Bad Blood—The Tuskegee Syphilis Experiment
James H. Jones, 1981

Code of Medical Ethics
American Medical Association, 150th Anniversary Edition, 1997

Factories of Death—Japanese Biological Warfare, 1932-45, and the American Cover-up
Sheldon H. Harris, 1994

Guide to Clinical Trials
Bert Spilker, Lippincott-Raven, 1996.

Human Radiation Experiments—(The) Final Report of the President's Advisory Committee
Advisory Committee, 1996

Nazi Doctors—(The) Medical Killing and the Psychology of Genocide
Robert Jay Lifton, 2000 (reprint)

(The) Placebo Effect
Edited by Anne Harrington, 1997

(The) Plutonium Files—America's Secret Medical Experiments in the Cold War
Eileen Welcome, 1999

Protecting Human Subjects—A Series of Instructional Videotapes—Evolving Concern; Protection for Human Subjects (3 videotapes)
OPRR/OHRP

Protecting Study Volunteers in Research—A Manual for Investigative Sites
Cynthia Dunn, M.D.; Gary Chadwick, Pharm.D., MPH, CIP, 2004

Tuskegee's Truths; Rethinking the Tuskegee Syphilis Study
Susan M. Reverby (Editor), 2000

Agencies

Center for Drug Evaluation and Research (CDER)
Clinical Investigator Information
www.fda.gov/cder/about/smallbiz/clinical_investigator.htm

FDA Home Page
www.fda.gov

International Conference on Harmonisation Home Page
www.ich.org

OHRP Site
http://ohrp.osophs.dhhs.gov

World Medical Association
www.wma.net
The World Medical Association (WMA) is the organization that issued the Declaration of Helsinki and is responsible for its updates.

Bioethics Resources on the Web
www.nih.gov/sigs/bioethics
This site is maintained by the National Institutes of Health and provides links to a wide variety of bioethics resources on the web.

Human Subjects Research and IRBs
www.nih.gov/sigs/bioethics/IRB.html

ClinicalTrials.gov
www.clinicaltrials.gov/ct/gui/c/b
The U.S. National Institutes of Health, through its National Library of Medicine, has developed ClinicalTrials.gov to provide subjects, family members and members of the public current information about clinical research studies.

Other Information

Department of Health and Human Services (HHS) Protection of Human Subjects Regulations. 45 CFR 46
http://ohrp.osophs.dhhs.gov/humansubjects/guidance/45cfr46.htm

Belmont Report
http://ohrp.osophs.dhhs.gov/humansubjects/guidance/belmont.htm

Electronic Records 21 CFR 11
www.access.gpo.gov/nara/cfr/cfrhtml_00/Title_21/21cfr11_00.html
These are the FDA regulations on the use of electronic records and electronic signatures in the FDA approval process.

Applications for FDA Approval to Market a New Drug. 21 CFR 314
www.access.gpo.gov/nara/cfr/cfrhtml_00/Title_21/21cfr314_00.html
These are the FDA regulations on the application for FDA approval to market a new drug.

Biological Products. 21 CFR 600
www.access.gpo.gov/nara/cfr/cfrhtml_00/Title_21/21cfr600_00.html
These are the FDA regulations concerning biological products.

Investigational Device Exemptions. 21 CFR 812
www.access.gpo.gov/nara/cfr/cfrhtml_00/Title_21/21cfr812_00.html
These are the FDA regulations concerning the conduct of research and application for an Investigational Device Exemption (IDE) from the FDA, establishing many duties and responsibilities for investigators, sponsors and IRBs.

FDA Forms
www.fda.gov/opacom/morechoices/fdaforms/cder.html

FDA Information Sheets
www.fda.gov/oc/ohrt/irbs/default.htm

Guide to Informed Consent (FDA Information Sheets)
www.fda.gov/oc/ohrt/irbs/informedconsent.html

Continuing Review (FDA Information Sheets)
www.fda.gov/oc/ohrt/irbs/review.html

Declaration of Helsinki
www.wma.net/e/policy/17-c_e.html

Nuremberg Code
http://ohsr.od.nih.gov/nuremberg.php3

Canadian Tri-Council Policy Statement:
Ethical Conduct for Research Involving Humans
www.nserc.ca/programs/ethics/english/index.htm

Step-by-Step Instructions for Filing a Federalwide
Assurance for Domestic (U.S.) Institutions
http://ohrp.osophs.dhhs.gov/humansubjects/assurance/filasuri.htm

NIH Required Education in the Protection of
Human Research Participants
http://grants.nih.gov/grants/guide/notice-files/NOT-OD-00-039.html

Sources of Potential Investigators
www.centerwatch.com
www.clinicalinvestigators.com

APPENDIX d

Sample Forms, Logs and Checklists

Audit Preparation Checklist

1. Ensure that arrangements have been made for the audit
   - ☐ Conference room is arranged/reserved
   - ☐ Appropriate personnel have been notified and are available
   - ☐ All requested materials are available
   - ☐ The investigator will be available to meet with the auditors

2. Ensure that the following materials have been checked and are ready for the audit:
   - ☐ Copies of signed informed consent forms for all subjects entered in the study
   - ☐ Copies of all case report forms for all subjects
     - ☐ Copies of any corrections made, queries, etc.
   - ☐ Source documents for all subjects (office charts, test results, etc.)
   - ☐ Study document file
     - ☐ All study initiation records
     - ☐ List of involved study personnel and dates of involvement
     - ☐ All IRB communications
     - ☐ Sponsor communications
     - ☐ Study notes, etc.
     - ☐ Grant information should **not** be present
   - ☐ Drug dispensing records for all subjects
   - ☐ Overall drug accountability forms
   - ☐ Other materials, as requested or as appropriate

Budget Worksheet

Date:

Number of subjects to be enrolled: **Number of visits:**

Activity	Cost per procedure	Number of times procedure is done	Total cost per subject
Labor costs:			
Recruitment **			
Screening **			
Administering informed consent			
Per visit activities			
Vital signs			
Laboratory			
Interview, instructions, scheduling			
Study medication/material dispensing and accounting			
CRF completion			
Serious Adverse Event forms			
Total labor costs per subject			
Direct costs:			
Safety laboratory panel			
Urinalysis			
Diagnostic procedures			
Other laboratory tests (list):			
Total direct costs per subject			
Salary/fees:			
Investigator **			
Subinvestigator			
Study coordinator/nurse **			
Secretarial support			
Phlebotomist/lab technician			
Other			
Pharmacy fee			
Subject compensation			
Total salary/fee cost per subject			

** These figures plus labor cost for one visit of investigator and coordinator comprise screening costs.

Budget Worksheet (continued)

Administrative costs	**Total cost**
Advertising and recruitment	
Data archiving	
IRB fees	
Miscellaneous study activities and overhead	
Total administrative costs	

Total Study Budget Calculations

1. Cost per enrolled subject:
   Labor: ______________________________
   Direct: ______________________________
   Salary/fees: ______________________________
   Total: ______________________________

2. Cost per screened, not enrolled, subject (screen failure):
   Labor: ______________________________
   Salary/fees: ______________________________
   Total:______________________________

3. Subjects to be enrolled
   Cost per subject ______ **x** No. of subjects ______ = Total (A)________

   Screen failures (estimate)
   Cost per subject ______ **x** No. of subjects ______ = Total (B)________

4. Total administrative costs (Total C) = ______________________

5. Total study cost (A + B + C) = ______________________

6. Grant per subject
   Cost per subject ______ **x** No. of subjects to be enrolled ______ = Grant per subject ______

Note: If the sponsor wants a per patient grant figure, divide the total cost per study (A+B+C) by the number of subjects to be enrolled. This will give a per subject grant figure that will cover the total study expenses.

Note: The number of screen failures will need to be estimated based on previous experience, the diagnosis and the number allowed by the sponsor.

Note: Overhead may need to be listed as a percentage of the overall grant per subject.

Documents Submitted to the IRB

Protocol ____

Sponsor ____

Investigator ____

The following documents were submitted to the IRB on ____/ ____/ ____

- ☐ Protocol and amendments (if any)
- ☐ Draft informed consent form
- ☐ Investigator brochure (or package insert, if marketed drug)
- ☐ Proposed advertising or recruitment materials, if applicable
- ☐ Proposed payments to study subjects, if applicable
- ☐ Completed, signed 1572 form
- ☐ CV for the investigator and copy of current license
- ☐ IRB submission form, if applicable
- ☐ Other (list)

If any items are not applicable for this study, write "NA" next to the item.

When all relevant items have been sent, sign below.

Name ______________________________ Date ____/ ____/ ____

Elements of Consent

Required elements

- ☐ Statement that the study involves research.
    - ☐ Explanation of the purpose of the research.
    - ☐ Expected duration of subject's participation.
    - ☐ Description of procedures to be followed.
    - ☐ Identification of any procedures that are experimental.

- ☐ Description of reasonably foreseeable risks and discomforts to subject.
- ☐ Description of benefits which may be reasonably expected.
- ☐ Disclosure of alternate procedures or treatment.
- ☐ Statement re confidentiality of records.
    - ☐ Statement that FDA may inspect the records.

- ☐ Statement re compensation for any research-related injury.
- ☐ Contact person for questions about the research and subject rights.
- ☐ Contact person in the event of research-related injury.
- ☐ Statement that participation is voluntary.
- ☐ Statement that refusal to participate will not result in the penalty or loss of any benefits to which the subject is otherwise entitled.
- ☐ Statement that the subject may discontinue at any time without penalty or loss of any benefits to which the subject is otherwise entitled.

Additional elements (include as appropriate)

- ☐ Statement that the treatment may involve risks to the subject (or embryo or fetus) that are currently unforeseeable.
- ☐ Circumstances under the subject's participation may be terminated by the investigator without regard to the subject's consent.
- ☐ Any additional costs to the subject.
- ☐ Consequences for withdrawal and procedures for orderly termination.
- ☐ Statement that significant new findings will be provided to the subject.
- ☐ Approximate number of subjects involved in the study.

Enrollment Tracking Form

Protocol:__________________________ **Sponsor:**__________________________

Investigator: ____

Date	Screened	Enrolled	Completed the study	Dropouts (due to AEs)	Currently in the study
MM/DD/YY (example)	30	19	4	4 (1)	11

Error Query/Correction

Protocol____________ Protocol date ________ Sponsor ____________

Patient	Visit	Page	Field	Problem	Correction	Initials

Inventory of Returned Investigational Material

Sponsor/Address ____

____

Protocol Number ____

Protocol Title ____

Investigator/Address ____

____

Contact Person/Telephone Number ____________________________

The following investigational material is being returned.

Drug	Lot Number	Code Number	Full Containers	Partial Containers	Empty Containers	Total Containers

Comments ____

____

Inventory of Returned Investigational Material (Example)

Sponsor/Address Acme Pharma

Returned Goods Department, 1234 Main Street, Pharma City, CC 23456

Protocol Number XYZ-1234-001

Protocol Title Study of Drug A vs. Placebo in Moderate Hypertension

Investigator/Address John Smith, M.D.

BCCCR, Kalamazoo, MI 49001

Contact Person/Telephone Number Robert Doe, R.Ph. (616) 555-5555

The following investigational material is being returned.

Drug	Lot Number	Code Number	Full Containers	Partial Containers	Empty Containers	Total Containers
Blinded	12345	101	0	4	4	8
Blinded	12345	102	0	0	8	8
Blinded	12345	103	2	3	2	7-see note

Comments Patient #103 – missing one bottle – patient did not return – threw out.

Investigational Drug Dispensing Record

Protocol Number ____

Protocol Title ____

Investigator____

Subject Number/Initials ______________________________________

Treatment Code (if applicable) _________________________________

Complete the following information using a new line each time medication is dispensed or returned. Use a separate sheet for each subject.

Date Medication Dispensed or Returned	Lot Number and Identification Code	Quantity Dispensed (Number of Tablets)	Quantity Returned (Number of Tablets)	Initials	Comments

Investigational Drug Dispensing Record (Example)

Protocol Number XYZ-1234-001

Protocol Title Study of Drug A vs. Placebo in Moderate Hypertension

Sponsor Acme Pharma

Investigator John Smith, M.D.

Subject Number/Initials BBC – #101

Treatment Code (if applicable) Blinded – #101

Complete the following information using a new line each time medication is dispensed or returned. Use a separate sheet for each subject.

Date Medication Dispensed or Returned	Lot Number and Identification Code	Quantity Dispensed (Number of Tablets)	Quantity Returned (Number of Tablets)	Initials	Comments
2/20/00	Lot 12345 #101	60		KW	
3/06/00	Lot 12345 #101		4	KW	
3/06/00	Lot 12345 #101	60		KW	
2/20/00	Lot 12345 #101		0	KW	Patient forgot extra pills. Will bring next visit.

Meeting Communication Record

Protocol number____

Investigator ____

Date:

People present, including organization:

Purpose of meeting:

Synopsis of meeting discussion:

Actions taken and/or required:

Completed reports are to be filed in the study file.

Post-Study Critique Worksheet

Protocol title ______________________________

Study articles ______________________________

Phase or study type ______________________________

1. General

How many subjects were enrolled? ______________

Was the goal met? ☐ Yes ☐ No

How long did it take to enroll? ______________

Was the enrollment time goal met? ☐ Yes ☐ No

If enrollment goals were not met, please comment: ______________

____

____

____

2. Procedures/clinical assessments

Were procedures/clinical assessments difficult? ☐ Yes ☐ No

If so, describe why below.

Was sufficient staff available? ☐ Yes ☐ No

Were there other factors that make this protocol difficult to perform? If so, describe below.

Comments: ______________________________

____

____

____

3. Workload

Was the workload reasonable? ☐ Yes ☐ No

Were adequate staff available? ☐ Yes ☐ No

Were the facilities adequate? ☐ Yes ☐ No

Were problems encountered in dispensing study material? ☐ Yes ☐ No

Was the study article dispensing/accountability complicated? ☐ Yes ☐ No

Comments: ______________________________

____

____

____

4. Case report forms (CRFs)

Were the CRFs appropriate for the study? ☐ Yes ☐ No
Was enough time allowed for completing CRFs? ☐ Yes ☐ No
Were the forms "user-friendly"? ☐ Yes ☐ No
Comments: ____________________

____

____

____

5. Sponsor interactions

Were communications with the sponsor acceptable? ☐ Yes ☐ No
Was the CRA capable and easy to work with? ☐ Yes ☐ No
Comments: ____________________

____

____

____

6. Other considerations

Did our patient population benefit from the study? ☐ Yes ☐ No
Was this study desirable to do from a scientific standpoint? ☐ Yes ☐ No
What can we do to improve things the next time we do a similar study?

____

____

____

____

____

Was the overall study experience favorable? ☐ Yes ☐ No
Would you recommend working with this sponsor again? ☐ Yes ☐ No
Comments: ____________________

____

____

____

____

____

____

____

____

____

Signature Date

____

Protocol Feasibility Assessment Checklist

Please assess each item as realistically as possible in terms of our ability and capacity to do this study. All assessment forms are to be completed by:

____

Protocol title ______________________________________

Sponsor ______________________________________

Study material (drug/device/other) ______________________________

Phase or study type ______________________________________

Investigator/Coordinator ______________________________________

1. General Considerations

Have we worked with this sponsor before?	☐ Yes	☐ No
If so, was the partnership successful?	☐ Yes	☐ No
Is the number of subjects to be enrolled realistic? (N = ______)	☐ Yes	☐ No
Is the enrollment rate realistic? (Rate = ____________)	☐ Yes	☐ No
Is the enrollment period realistic? (Time = ____________)	☐ Yes	☐ No
Will our patients benefit from this study?	☐ Yes	☐ No
Is the IRB apt to have problems with any aspects of this protocol?	☐ Yes	☐ No
Is this study scientifically sound?	☐ Yes	☐ No
Do we have any competing studies?	☐ Yes	☐ No
Are there any competing studies in the community?	☐ Yes	☐ No
Can we make the necessary time commitment?	☐ Yes	☐ No
Is sufficient staff available?	☐ Yes	☐ No
Is this study interesting?	☐ Yes	☐ No

Comments: ______________________________________

____

____

____

2. Study Population

Diagnosis ____________________

Acute	☐ Yes	☐ No
Chronic	☐ Yes	☐ No
Life-threatening	☐ Yes	☐ No
Healthy volunteers	☐ Yes	☐ No
Adults capable of giving consent	☐ Yes	☐ No
Impaired adults	☐ Yes	☐ No
Minors	☐ Yes	☐ No

Comments: ____________________

____

____

____

3. Study Procedures

How many visits per subject are required?____________________

What is the visit window (e.g., visit ± 3 days)?____________________

Are procedures complicated or difficult? If so, describe below.	☐ Yes	☐ No
Are there invasive procedures (other than blood draws)? If so, describe below.	☐ Yes	☐ No
Are any outside specialists needed? If so, list:	☐ Yes	☐ No

Are there other factors that make this protocol difficult to perform? If so, describe below.

Comments: ____________________

____

____

____

4. Case Report Forms (if available)

Number of pages per subject?____________________

Time period for completing forms after each visit?____________________

Are the forms "user-friendly"?	☐ Yes	☐ No
Do laboratory values need to be transcribed?	☐ Yes	☐ No
Are patient diaries to be used?	☐ Yes	☐ No
Do the diaries need to be transcribed?	☐ Yes	☐ No
Is the study drug/other material dispensing/ accountability complicated?	☐ Yes	☐ No

Comments: ____________________

____

____

____

5. Overall Assessment

Do you recommend that the study be conducted at this site? ☐ Yes ☐ No

Comments: ____

____

____

____

____

Signature Date

____

Protocol Deviation Report

Protocol ____

Investigator ______________________________________

Subject number/identifier______________________________

Sponsor____

Date of report_____________________________________

The protocol deviation was:

Reason for the deviation:

The protocol variation was approved in advance by the sponsor: ☐ Yes ☐ No

Comments:

Signature Date

This report should be placed in the subject's study file records.

Report: Medication Blind Broken for a Study Subject

Protocol ______________________________

Sponsor______________________________

Investigator ______________________________

Subject number/identifier______________________________

Medication______________________________

Reason the medication blind was broken:

Did sponsor agree to the unblinding before it was done? If yes, give name, title and contact information for sponsor representative: ☐ Yes ☐ No

---

Comments:

File completed report in study file and in subject's chart.

Request for Study Supplies

Protocol ____

Sponsor____

Investigator____

City and State ____

Supplies needed, and number requested:

Example: Case report form books – 6
Randomized study drug – 6
Lab kits – 6

Date needed:

By April 23, 2004

Comments:

Two new subjects scheduled to start the study on April 26, 2004.
All other study drug has been allocated to current subjects.
No more case report forms available.

For more information, please contact:

CRC
Telephone number

Sample SOP Format

Name of Organization

SOP #000	Revision #	Dept. or Proces owner:	Effective date:	Page x of y

Purpose
The purpose of this SOP is to…

Scope
This SOP applies to…

The (appropriate person /title) has responsibility for…

Procedure
1. Steps listed in order
2.
3.
Etc.

Regulations
21 CFR and ICH Guideline for Good Clinical Practice details, etc.

References
To other SOPs and guidelines that are related

Attachments
If applicable

Keywords
Significant words and phrases from the SOP

Approved by	Date

Site Evaluation

The sponsor's site assessment personnel will evaluate each item below, making notes.

Investigator

- ☐ Qualifications
- ☐ Licensure
- ☐ Specialty
- ☐ Clinical trial experience
  - ☐ Number of previous trials
  - ☐ Number of similar trials
  - ☐ Enrollment in previous trials (numbers, time to enroll)
- ☐ FDA audits

Staff

- ☐ Study coordinator
- ☐ Other specialized personnel
- ☐ Training and licensure
- ☐ Experience
- ☐ Turnover
- ☐ General interest and attitude

Facility

- ☐ Appropriate for trials
- ☐ Ample storage for study supplies
- ☐ Appropriate drug storage
- ☐ Special storage equipment available (freezer, etc.)
- ☐ Special equipment available
- ☐ Active practice
- ☐ Tour offered, taken

IRB

- ☐ Local IRB available
  - ☐ Frequency and timing of meetings
  - ☐ Average time to approval
  - ☐ Responsiveness
- ☐ Use central IRB

Laboratory/Tests

- ☐ Local lab available
- ☐ Necessary tests can be done
- ☐ Timeliness
- ☐ Certification
- ☐ Have experience with central lab

Protocol feasibility

- ☐ Experience with similar studies
- ☐ Interest level
- ☐ Availability of potential subjects
- ☐ Competing studies (in practice and in community)
- ☐ Timing appropriate
- ☐ Study coordinator availability
- ☐ Can attend investigator meeting

Study Closeout

Protocol ______________________________

Sponsor ______________________________

Investigator ______________________________

Date ______________________________

- ☐ Study documents file is complete (refer to Checklist: Study Documents).
- ☐ Final report has been made to the IRB and the sponsor.
- ☐ All case report forms (CRFs) are complete and have been submitted to the sponsor.
  - ☐ All CRF corrections/queries have been addressed.
  - ☐ Any patient diaries, etc., have been submitted, as required.
- ☐ All source documentation is in order.
  - ☐ If not with study files, location of materials is noted in the document file.
- ☐ Study personnel form is complete.
- ☐ Subjects' signed informed consent forms are filed.
- ☐ Drug dispensing and disposition forms are complete.
- ☐ Study drug has been returned as per sponsor instructions.
- ☐ All other study materials (extra CRFs, etc.) have been returned to the sponsor.
- ☐ Investigator Brochure is filed with other study materials.
- ☐ All study materials are filed together as per archival procedures.
  - ☐ Location of materials is noted in site records.
- ☐ Post-study critique has been held.

Study Documents
(based on ICH GCPs)

Protocol ______________________________

Investigator ______________________________

Pre-Study

- ☐ Investigator Brochure
- ☐ Signed protocol and amendments (if any)
- ☐ Informed consent form
  - ☐ Any other information to be given to subjects
  - ☐ Any advertising materials for recruitment
- ☐ Dated, written IRB approvals for:
  - ☐ Protocol [Date:]
  - ☐ Amendments, if any [Date:]
  - ☐ Consent and any other material to be given to subjects [Date:]
  - ☐ Advertising, if any [Date:]
  - ☐ Subject compensation, if any [Date:]
- ☐ CVs for investigator, subinvestigators
- ☐ Laboratory certification and normal ranges
- ☐ Study manual, if available
- ☐ Shipping records
- ☐ Decoding procedures for blinded trials
- ☐ Financial disclosure sheets
- ☐ Contract
- ☐ Sponsor-specific documents

During the conduct of the trial

- ☐ Investigator Brochure updates
- ☐ Protocol amendments and/or revisions
- ☐ Consent revisions
- ☐ Dated, written IRB approvals of:
  - ☐ Protocol amendments [Dates:]
  - ☐ Revised consents [Dates:]
  - ☐ New or revised subject materials [Dates:]
  - ☐ New or revised advertising [Dates:]
- ☐ CVs for new investigators and/or subinvestigators
- ☐ Laboratory updates of certification and/or normal ranges
- ☐ Shipping documentation (receipt of trial materials)
- ☐ Monitoring visit log
- ☐ Communications with sponsor (letters, telephone reports, etc.)
- ☐ Signed consent forms
- ☐ Source documents

- ☐ Signed, dated, completed case report forms (CRFs)
- ☐ Documentation of CRF corrections
- ☐ Notification to sponsors and IRB of serious adverse events and related reports
- ☐ IND safety reports received from the sponsor
- ☐ Interim and/or annual reports to the IRB
- ☐ Subject screening log
- ☐ Subject identification code list
- ☐ Subject enrollment log
- ☐ Investigational product accountability
- ☐ Signature sheet (all persons making CRF entries or corrections)
- ☐ Record of retained body fluids and/or tissue samples, if any

After study completion or termination

- ☐ Drug (device) accountability
- ☐ Documentation of drug/device return or disposal
- ☐ Completed subject identification code list
- ☐ Final report to the IRB [Date:]

Comments ____

____

____

Checklist should be kept in front of study file and updated as appropriate.

Study Document File Verification Log

Study Document File Review	**Initial** / /	**Review** / /	**Review** / /	**Final** / /
Signed, IRB-approved protocol or cover sheet				
Signed, IRB-approved amendments ■ Amendment #, date ■ Amendment #, date ■ Amendment #, date				
IRB-approved informed consent document				
Signed, completed FDA 1572 form (Statement of Investigator)				
IRB approval letter, verifying approval of both the protocol and consent document				
IRB approval of advertising and subject recruitment materials, including any subject compensation				
Investigator Brochure (or package insert, for marketed products)				
Verification of laboratory certification and laboratory normal ranges				
Study Manual, if available				
Shipping records for investigation product				
Decoding procedures for blinded trials				
Financial disclosure forms				
Sponsor-specific documents and communications				
Reviewer initials				

Attach a separate sheet with comments if any problems found.

Study Monitor Visit Log

Protocol ________________ **Protocol date** ________ **Sponsor** ________________

Name	Job Title	Date(s) of Visit	Signature	Study Coordinator Initials

Use additional sheets as needed. Keep with study documents file.

Study Personnel Log

Protocol____________________ Protocol date __________ Sponsor ________________________

Name	Job Title	Initials	Start Date of Study Responsibility	End Date of Study Responsibility	Signature

Use additional sheets as needed. Update when personnel changes occur.
Keep with study documents file.

Study Subject/Chart Master List

Patient name	Chart #	Protocol Number	Subject Number/Initials

Study Subject Visit Tracking Log

Protocol ____________________ **Sponsor** ____________________

Subject	Consent Date	Baseline	Week 1	Week 2	Week 4	Final Status	Comments

Subject Identification Code List

Protocol title ______________________ **Investigator** ______________________
Protocol date ______________________ **Coordinator** ______________________

Subject Name	Address	Telephone	Soc. Security Number	Chart Number	Subject Identification

Use additional sheets as needed. Update when information (address, telephone number) for a subject changes.
Keep with study documents file.

Telephone Communication Record

Protocol ____________________ **Investigator** ____________________

Person initiating the call: ______________ Date: ____________________

Organization: ______________ Time: ____________________

Call to: ____________________

Organization: ______________ Phone number: ______________

Purpose of call:

Response/Comments:

Completed telephone reports are to be filed in the study file.

Training Verification Form

Training Program: ______________________________ **Date:** ________________

I verify that I was trained on this material, that I understood the material, and that I will follow all SOPs and guidelines included in the training.

Name (printed): ____

Signature: ______________________________________ **Date:** ________________

Training Verification Master List

Training Program: ______________________________ **Date:** ________________

The following people were trained on the attached material.

Name (printed)	Signature	Date

Attach additional sheets as necessary.
Attach a copy of the training materials to the form before filing.

Study Subject Visit Tracking Log

	Acceptable Visit Date			
Baseline Visit Date	Week 1 Visit (± 1 day)	Week 2 Visit (± 1 day)	Week 4 Visit (± 1 day)	Week 8 Visit (± 1 day)
02/01/04	02/07/04–02/9/04	02/14/04–2/16/04	02/27/04–02/29/04	3/26/04–3/28/04
02/02/04	02/08/04–02/10/04	02/15/04–2/17/04	02/28/04–03/01/04	3/27/04–3/29/04
02/03/04	02/09/04–02/11/04	02/16/04–2/18/04	02/29/04–03/02/04	3/28/04–3/30/04
02/04/04	02/10/04–02/12/04	02/17/04–2/19/04	03/01/04–03/03/04	3/29/04–3/31/04
02/05/04	02/11/04–02/13/04	02/18/04–2/20/04	03/02/04–03/04/04	3/30/04–04/01/04
02/06/04	02/12/04–02/14/04	02/19/04–2/21/04	03/03/04–03/05/04	3/31/04–04/02/04
02/07/04	02/13/04–02/15/04	02/20/04–2/22/04	03/04/04–03/06/04	04/01/04–04/03/04
02/08/04	02/14/04–02/16/04	02/21/04–2/23/04	03/05/04–03/07/04	04/02/04–04/04/04
02/09/04	02/15/04–02/17/04	02/22/04–2/24/04	03/06/04–03/08/04	04/03/04–04/05/04

APPENDIX e

Code of Federal Regulations

21 CFR 50—Protection of Human Subjects
21 CFR 54—Financial Disclosure byClinical Investigators
21 CRF 56—Institutional Review Boards
21 CFR 312—Investigational New Drug Application
21 CFR 46—Public Welfare
FDA Form 1572

TITLE 21—FOOD AND DRUGS

Chapter I: Food and Drug Administration, Department of Health and Human Services
Subchapter A: General

PART 50

Protection of Human Subjects

Authority: 21 U.S.C 321, 343, 346, 346a, 348, 350a, 350b, 352, 353, 355, 360, 360c-360f, 360h-360j, 371, 379e, 381; 42 U.S.C. 216, 241, 262, 263b-263n.

Source: 45 FR 36390, May 30, 1980, unless otherwise noted.

Subpart A—General Provisions

§50.1 Scope.

(a) This part applies to all clinical investigations regulated by the Food and Drug Administration under sections 505(i) and 520(g) of the Federal Food, Drug, and Cosmetic Act, as well as clinical investigations that support applications for research or marketing permits for products regulated by the Food and Drug Administration, including foods, including dietary supplements, that bear a nutrient content claim or a health claim, infant formulas, food and color additives, drugs for human use, medical devices for human use, biological products for human use, and electronic products. Additional specific obligations and commitments of, and standards of conduct for, persons who sponsor or monitor clinical investigations involving particular test articles may also be found in other parts (e.g., parts 312 and 812). Compliance with these parts is intended to protect the rights and safety of subjects involved in investigations filed with the Food and Drug Administration pursuant to sections 403, 406, 409, 412, 413, 502, 503, 505, 510, 513-516, 518-520, 721, and 801 of the Federal Food, Drug, and Cosmetic Act and sections 351 and 354-360F of the Public Health Service Act.

(b) References in this part to regulatory sections of the Code of Federal Regulations are to chapter I of title 21, unless otherwise noted.

[45 FR 36390, May 30, 1980; 46 FR 8979, Jan. 27, 1981, as amended at 63 FR 26697, May 13, 1998; 64 FR 399, Jan. 5, 1999; 66 FR 20597, Apr. 24, 2001]

§50.3 Definitions.

As used in this part:

(a) Act means the Federal Food, Drug, and Cosmetic Act, as amended (secs. 201—902, 52 Stat. 1040 et seq. as amended (21 U.S.C. 321—392)).

(b) Application for research or marketing permit includes:

(1) A color additive petition, described in part 71.

(2) A food additive petition, described in parts 171 and 571.

(3) Data and information about a substance submitted as part of the procedures for establishing that the substance is generally recognized as safe for use that results or may reasonably be expected to result, directly or indirectly, in its becoming a component or otherwise affecting the characteristics of any food, described in §§170.30 and 570.30.

(4) Data and information about a food additive submitted as part of the procedures for food additives permitted to be used on an interim basis pending additional study, described in §180.1.

(5) Data and information about a substance submitted as part of the procedures for establishing a tolerance for unavoidable contaminants in food and food-packaging materials, described in section 406 of the act.

(6) An investigational new drug application, described in part 312 of this chapter.

(7) A new drug application, described in

part 314.

(8) Data and information about the bioavailability or bioequivalence of drugs for human use submitted as part of the procedures for issuing, amending, or repealing a bioequivalence requirement, described in part 320.

(9) Data and information about an over-the-counter drug for human use submitted as part of the procedures for classifying these drugs as generally recognized as safe and effective and not misbranded, described in part 330.

(10) Data and information about a prescription drug for human use submitted as part of the procedures for classifying these drugs as generally recognized as safe and effective and not misbranded, described in this chapter.

(11) [Reserved]

(12) An application for a biologics license, described in part 601 of this chapter.

(13) Data and information about a biological product submitted as part of the procedures for determining that licensed biological products are safe and effective and not misbranded, described in part 601.

(14) Data and information about an in vitro diagnostic product submitted as part of the procedures for establishing, amending, or repealing a standard for these products, described in part 809.

(15) An Application for an Investigational Device Exemption, described in part 812.

(16) Data and information about a medical device submitted as part of the procedures for classifying these devices, described in section 513.

(17) Data and information about a medical device submitted as part of the procedures for establishing, amending, or repealing a standard for these devices, described in section 514.

(18) An application for premarket approval of a medical device, described in section 515.

(19) A product development protocol for a medical device, described in section 515.

(20) Data and information about an electronic product submitted as part of the procedures for establishing, amending, or repealing a standard for these products, described in section 358 of the Public Health Service Act.

(21) Data and information about an electronic product submitted as part of the procedures for obtaining a variance from any electronic product performance standard, as described in §1010.4.

(22) Data and information about an electronic product submitted as part of the procedures for granting, amending, or extending an exemption from a radiation safety performance standard, as described in §1010.5.

(23) Data and information about a clinical study of an infant formula when submitted as part of an infant formula notification under section 412(c) of the Federal Food, Drug, and Cosmetic Act.

(24) Data and information submitted in a petition for a nutrient content claim, described in §101.69 of this chapter, or for a health claim, described in §101.70 of

this chapter.

(25) Data and information from investigations involving children submitted in a new dietary ingredient notification, described in §190.6 of this chapter.

(c) Clinical investigation means any experiment that involves a test article and one or more human subjects and that either is subject to requirements for prior submission to the Food and Drug Administration under section 505(i) or 520(g) of the act, or is not subject to requirements for prior submission to the Food and Drug Administration under these sections of the act, but the results of which are intended to be submitted later to, or held for inspection by, the Food and Drug Administration as part of an application for a research or marketing permit. The term does not include experiments that are subject to the provisions of part 58 of this chapter, regarding nonclinical laboratory studies.

(d) Investigator means an individual who actually conducts a clinical investigation, i.e., under whose immediate direction the test article is administered or dispensed to, or used involving, a subject, or, in the event of an investigation conducted by a team of individuals, is the responsible leader of that team.

(e) Sponsor means a person who initiates a clinical investigation, but who does not actually conduct the investigation, i.e., the test article is administered or dispensed to or used involving, a subject under the immediate direction of another individual. A person other than an individual (e.g., corporation or agency) that uses one or more of its own employees to conduct a clinical investigation it has initiated is considered to be a sponsor (not a sponsor-investigator), and the employees are considered to be investigators.

(f) Sponsor-investigator means an individual who both initiates and actually conducts, alone or with others, a clinical investigation, i.e., under whose immediate direction the test article is administered or dispensed to, or used involving, a subject. The term does not include any person other than an individual, e.g., corporation or agency.

(g) Human subject means an individual who is or becomes a participant in research, either as a recipient of the test article or as a control. A subject may be either a healthy human or a patient.

(h) Institution means any public or private entity or agency (including Federal, State, and other agencies). The word facility as used in section 520(g) of the act is deemed to be synonymous with the term institution for purposes of this part.

(i) Institutional review board (IRB) means any board, committee, or other group formally designated by an institution to review biomedical research involving humans as subjects, to approve the initiation of and conduct periodic review of such research. The term has the same meaning as the phrase institutional review committee as used in section 520(g) of the act.

(j) Test article means any drug (including a biological product for human use), medical device for human use, human food additive, color additive, electronic product, or any other article subject to regulation under the act or under sections 351 and 354-360F of the Public Health Service Act (42 U.S.C. 262 and 263b-263n).

(k) Minimal risk means that the probability and magnitude of harm or discomfort anticipated in the research are not greater in and of themselves than those ordinarily encountered in daily life or during the performance of routine physical or psychological examinations or tests.

(l) Legally authorized representative means an individual or judicial or other body authorized under applicable law to consent on behalf of a prospective subject to the subject's particpation in the procedure(s) involved in the research.

(m) Family member means any one of the following legally competent persons: Spouse; parents; children (including adopted children); brothers, sisters, and spouses of brothers and sisters; and any individual related by blood or affinity whose close association with the subject is the equivalent of a family relationship.

(n) Assent means a child's affirmative agreement to participate in a clinical investigation. Mere failure to object may not, absent affirmative agreement, be construed as assent.

(o) Children means persons who have not attained the legal age for consent to treatments or procedures involved in clinical investigations, under the applicable law of the jurisdiction in which the clinical investigation will be conducted.

(p) Parent means a child's biological or adoptive parent.

(q) Ward means a child who is placed in the legal custody of the State or other agency, institution, or entity, consistent with applicable Federal, State, or local law.

(r) Permission means the agreement of parent(s) or guardian to the participation of their child or ward in a clinical investigation. Permission must be obtained in compliance with subpart B of this part and must include the elements of informed consent described in §50.25.

(s) Guardian means an individual who is authorized under applicable State or local law to consent on behalf of a child to general medical care when general medical care includes participation in research. For purposes of subpart D of this part, a guardian also means an individual who is authorized to consent on behalf of a child to participate in research.

[45 FR 36390, May 30, 1980, as amended at 46 FR 8950, Jan. 27, 1981; 54 FR 9038, Mar. 3, 1989; 56 FR 28028, June 18, 1991; 61 FR 51528, Oct. 2, 1996; 62 FR 39440, July 23, 1997; 64 FR 399, Jan. 5, 1999; 64 FR 56448, Oct. 20, 1999; 66 FR 20597, Apr. 24, 2001]

Subpart B—Informed Consent of Human Subjects

Source: 46 FR 8951, Jan. 27, 1981, unless otherwise noted.

§50.20 General requirements for informed consent.

Except as provided in §§50.23 and 50.24, no investigator may involve a human being as a subject in research covered by these regulations unless the investigator has obtained the legally effective informed consent of the subject or the subject's legally authorized representative. An investigator shall seek such consent only under circumstances that provide the prospective subject or the representative sufficient opportunity to consider whether or not to participate and that minimize the possibility of coercion or undue influence. The information that is given to the subject or the representative shall be in language understandable to the subject or the representative. No informed consent, whether oral or written, may include any exculpatory language through which the subject or the representative is made to waive or appear to waive any of the subject's legal rights, or releases or appears to release the investigator, the sponsor, the institution, or its agents from liability for negligence.

[46 FR 8951, Jan. 27, 1981, as amended at 64 FR 10942, Mar. 8, 1999]

§50.23 Exception from general requirements.

(a) The obtaining of informed consent shall be deemed feasible unless, before use of the test article (except as provided in paragraph (b) of this section), both the investigator and a physician who is not otherwise participating in the clinical investigation certify in writing all of the following:

(1) The human subject is confronted by a life-threatening situation necessitating the use of the test article.

(2) Informed consent cannot be obtained from the subject because of an inability to communicate with, or obtain legally effective consent from, the subject.

(3) Time is not sufficient to obtain consent from the subject's legal representative.

(4) There is available no alternative method of approved or generally recognized therapy that provides an equal or greater likelihood of saving the life of the subject.

(b) If immediate use of the test article is, in the investigator's opinion, required to preserve the life of the subject, and time is not sufficient to obtain the independent determination required in paragraph (a) of this section in advance of using the test article, the determinations of the clinical investigator shall be made and, within 5 working days after the use of the article, be reviewed and evaluated in writing by a physician who is not participating in the clinical investigation.

(c) The documentation required in paragraph (a) or (b) of this section shall be submitted to the IRB within 5 working days after the use of the test article.

(d)(1) Under 10 U.S.C. 1107(f) the President may waive the prior consent requirement for the administration of an investigational new drug to a member of the armed forces in connection with the member's participation in a particular military operation. The statute specifies that only the President may waive informed consent in this connection and the President may grant such a waiver only if the President determines in writing that obtaining consent: Is not feasible; is contrary to the best interests of the military member; or is not in the interests of national security. The statute further provides that in making a determination to waive prior informed consent on the ground that it is not feasible or the ground that it is contrary to the best interests of the military members involved, the President shall apply the standards and criteria that are set forth in the relevant

FDA regulations for a waiver of the prior informed consent requirements of section 505(i)(4) of the Federal Food, Drug, and Cosmetic Act (21 U.S.C. 355(i)(4)). Before such a determination may be made that obtaining informed consent from military personnel prior to the use of an investigational drug (including an antibiotic or biological product) in a specific protocol under an investigational new drug application (IND) sponsored by the Department of Defense (DOD) and limited to specific military personnel involved in a particular military operation is not feasible or is contrary to the best interests of the military members involved the Secretary of Defense must first request such a determination from the President, and certify and document to the President that the following standards and criteria contained in paragraphs (d)(1) through (d)(4) of this section have been met.

(i) The extent and strength of evidence of the safety and effectiveness of the investigational new drug in relation to the medical risk that could be encountered during the military operation supports the drug's administration under an IND.

(ii) The military operation presents a substantial risk that military personnel may be subject to a chemical, biological, nuclear, or other exposure likely to produce death or serious or life-threatening injury or illness.

(iii) There is no available satisfactory alternative therapeutic or preventive treatment in relation to the intended use of the investigational new drug.

(iv) Conditioning use of the investigational new drug on the voluntary participation of each member could significantly risk the safety and health of any individual member who would decline its use, the safety of other military personnel, and the accomplishment of the military mission.

(v) A duly constituted institutional review board (IRB) established and operated in accordance with the requirements of paragraphs (d)(2) and (d)(3) of this section, responsible for review of the study, has reviewed and approved the investigational new drug protocol and the administration of the investigational new drug without informed consent. DOD's request is to include the documentation required by §56.115(a)(2) of this chapter.

(vi) DOD has explained:

(A) The context in which the investigational drug will be administered, e.g., the setting or whether it will be self-administered or it will be administered by a health professional;

(B) The nature of the disease or condition for which the preventive or therapeutic treatment is intended; and

(C) To the extent there are existing data or information available, information on conditions that could alter the effects of the investigational drug.

(vii) DOD's recordkeeping system is capable of tracking and will be used to track the proposed treatment from supplier to the individual recipient.

(viii) Each member involved in the military operation will be given, prior to the administration of the investigational new drug, a specific written information sheet (including information required by 10 U.S.C. 1107(d)) concerning the investigational new drug, the risks and benefits of its use, potential side effects, and other pertinent information about the appropriate use of the product.

(ix) Medical records of members involved in the military operation will accurately document the receipt by members of the notification required by paragraph (d)(1)(viii) of this section.

(x) Medical records of members involved in the military operation will accurately document the receipt by members of any investigational new drugs in accordance with FDA regulations including part 312 of this chapter.

(xi) DOD will provide adequate followup to assess whether there are beneficial or adverse health consequences that result from the use of the investigational product.

(xii) DOD is pursuing drug development, including a time line, and marketing approval with due diligence.

(xiii) FDA has concluded that the investigational new drug protocol may proceed subject to a decision by the President on the informed consent waiver request.

(xiv) DOD will provide training to the appropriate medical personnel and potential recipients on the specific investigational new drug to be administered prior to its use.

(xv) DOD has stated and justified the time period for which the waiver is needed, not to exceed one year, unless separately renewed under these standards and criteria.

(xvi) DOD shall have a continuing obligation to report to the FDA and to the President any changed circumstances relating to these standards and criteria (including the time period referred to in paragraph (d)(1)(xv) of this section) or that otherwise might affect the determination to use an investigational new drug without informed consent.

(xvii) DOD is to provide public notice as soon as practicable and consistent with classification requirements through notice in the FEDERAL REGISTER describing each waiver of informed consent determination, a summary of the most updated scientific information on the products used, and other pertinent information.

(xviii) Use of the investigational drug without informed consent otherwise conforms with applicable law.

(2) The duly constituted institutional review board, described in paragraph (d)(1)(v) of this section, must include at least 3 nonaffiliated members who shall not be employees or officers of the Federal Government (other than for purposes of membership on the IRB) and shall be required to obtain any necessary security clearances. This IRB shall review the proposed IND protocol at a convened meeting at which a majority of the members are present including at least one member whose primary concerns are in nonscientific areas and, if feasible, including a majority of the nonaffiliated members. The information required by §56.115(a)(2) of this chapter is to be provided to the Secretary of Defense for further review.

(3) The duly constituted institutional review board, described in paragraph (d)(1)(v) of this section, must review and

approve:

(i) The required information sheet;

(ii) The adequacy of the plan to disseminate information, including distribution of the information sheet to potential recipients, on the investigational product (e.g., in forms other than written);

(iii) The adequacy of the information and plans for its dissemination to health care providers, including potential side effects, contraindications, potential interactions, and other pertinent considerations; and

(iv) An informed consent form as required by part 50 of this chapter, in those circumstances in which DOD determines that informed consent may be obtained from some or all personnel involved.

(4) DOD is to submit to FDA summaries of institutional review board meetings at which the proposed protocol has been reviewed.

(5) Nothing in these criteria or standards is intended to preempt or limit FDA's and DOD's authority or obligations under applicable statutes and regulations.

[46 FR 8951, Jan. 27, 1981, as amended at 55 FR 52817, Dec. 21, 1990; 64 FR 399, Jan. 5, 1999; 64 FR 54188, Oct. 5, 1999]

§50.24 Exception from informed consent requirements for emergency research.

(a) The IRB responsible for the review, approval, and continuing review of the clinical investigation described in this section may approve that investigation without requiring that informed consent of all research subjects be obtained if the IRB (with the concurrence of a licensed physician who is a member of or consultant to the IRB and who is not otherwise participating in the clinical investigation) finds and documents each of the following:

(1) The human subjects are in a life-threatening situation, available treatments are unproven or unsatisfactory, and the collection of valid scientific evidence, which may include evidence obtained through randomized placebo-controlled investigations, is necessary to determine the safety and effectiveness of particular interventions.

(2) Obtaining informed consent is not feasible because:

(i) The subjects will not be able to give their informed consent as a result of their medical condition;

(ii) The intervention under investigation must be administered before consent from the subjects' legally authorized representatives is feasible; and

(iii) There is no reasonable way to identify prospectively the individuals likely to become eligible for participation in the clinical investigation.

(3) Participation in the research holds out the prospect of direct benefit to the subjects because:

(i) Subjects are facing a life-threatening situation that necessitates intervention;

(ii) Appropriate animal and other preclinical studies have been conducted, and the information derived from those studies and related evidence support the potential for the intervention to provide a direct benefit to the individual subjects; and

(iii) Risks associated with the investigation are reasonable in relation to what is known about the medical condition of the potential class of subjects, the risks and benefits of standard therapy, if any, and what is known about the risks and benefits of the proposed intervention or activity.

(4) The clinical investigation could not practicably be carried out without the waiver.

(5) The proposed investigational plan defines the length of the potential therapeutic window based on scientific evidence, and the investigator has committed to attempting to contact a legally authorized representative for each subject within that window of time and, if feasible, to asking the legally authorized representative contacted for consent within that window rather than proceeding without consent. The investigator will summarize efforts made to contact legally authorized representatives and make this information available to the IRB at the time of continuing review.

(6) The IRB has reviewed and approved informed consent procedures and an informed consent document consistent with §50.25. These procedures and the informed consent document are to be used with subjects or their legally authorized representatives in situations where use of such procedures and documents is feasible. The IRB has reviewed and approved procedures and information to be used when providing an opportunity for a family member to object to a subject's participation in the clinical investigation consistent with paragraph (a)(7)(v) of this section.

(7) Additional protections of the rights and welfare of the subjects will be provided, including, at least:

(i) Consultation (including, where appropriate, consultation carried out by the IRB) with representatives of the communities in which the clinical investigation will be conducted and from which the subjects will be drawn;

(ii) Public disclosure to the communities in which the clinical investigation will be conducted and from which the subjects will be drawn, prior to initiation of the clinical investigation, of plans for the investigation and its risks and expected benefits;

(iii) Public disclosure of sufficient information following completion of the clinical investigation to apprise the community and researchers of the study, including the demographic characteristics of the research population, and its results;

(iv) Establishment of an independent data monitoring committee to exercise oversight of the clinical investigation; and

(v) If obtaining informed consent is not feasible and a legally authorized representative is not reasonably available, the investigator has committed, if feasible, to attempting to contact within the therapeutic window the subject's family member who is not a legally authorized representative, and asking whether he or she objects to the subject's participation in the clinical investigation. The investigator will summarize efforts made to contact family members and make this information available to the IRB at the time of continuing review.

(b) The IRB is responsible for ensuring that procedures are in place to inform, at the earliest feasible opportunity, each subject, or if the subject remains incapacitated, a legally authorized representative of the subject, or if such a representative is not reasonably available, a family member, of the subject's inclusion in the clinical investigation, the details of the investigation and other information contained in the informed consent document. The IRB shall also ensure that there is a procedure to inform the subject, or if the subject remains incapacitated, a legally authorized representative of the subject, or if such a representative is not reasonably available, a family member, that he or she may discontinue the subject's participation at any time without penalty or loss of benefits to which the subject is otherwise entitled. If a legally authorized representative or family member is told about the clinical investigation and the subject's condition improves, the subject is also to be informed as soon as feasible. If a subject is entered into a clinical investigation with waived consent and the subject dies before a legally authorized representative or family member can be contacted, information about the clinical investigation is to be provided to the subject's legally authorized representative or family member, if feasible.

(c) The IRB determinations required by paragraph (a) of this section and the documentation required by paragraph (e) of this section are to be retained by the IRB for at least 3 years after completion of the clinical investigation, and the records shall be accessible for inspection and copying by FDA in accordance with §56.115(b) of this chapter.

(d) Protocols involving an exception to the informed consent requirement under this section must be performed under a separate investigational new drug application (IND) or investigational device exemption (IDE) that clearly identifies such protocols as protocols that may include subjects who are unable to consent. The submission of those protocols in a separate IND/IDE is required even if an IND for the same drug product or an IDE for the same device already exists. Applications for investigations under this section may not be submitted as amendments under §§312.30 or 812.35 of this chapter.

(e) If an IRB determines that it cannot approve a clinical investigation because the investigation does not meet the criteria in the exception provided under paragraph (a) of this section or because of other relevant ethical concerns, the IRB must document its findings and provide these findings promptly in writing to the clinical investigator and to the sponsor of the clinical investigation. The sponsor of the clinical investigation must promptly disclose this information to FDA and to the sponsor's clinical investigators who are participating or are asked to participate in this or a substantially equivalent clinical investigation of the sponsor, and to other IRB's that have been, or are, asked to review this or a substantially equivalent investigation by that sponsor.

[61 FR 51528, Oct. 2, 1996]

§50.25 Elements of informed consent.

(a) Basic elements of informed consent. In seeking informed consent, the following information shall be provided to each subject:

(1) A statement that the study involves research, an explanation of the purposes of the research and the expected duration of the subject's participation, a description of the procedures to be followed, and identification of any procedures which are experimental.

(2) A description of any reasonably foreseeable risks or discomforts to the subject.

(3) A description of any benefits to the subject or to others which may reasonably be expected from the research.

(4) A disclosure of appropriate alternative procedures or courses of treatment, if any, that might be advantageous to the subject.

(5) A statement describing the extent, if any, to which confidentiality of records identifying the subject will be maintained and that notes the possibility that the Food and Drug Administration may inspect the records.

(6) For research involving more than minimal risk, an explanation as to whether any compensation and an explanation as to whether any medical treatments are available if injury occurs and, if so, what they consist of, or where further information may be obtained.

(7) An explanation of whom to contact for answers to pertinent questions about the research and research subjects' rights, and whom to contact in the event of a research-related injury to the subject.

(8) A statement that participation is voluntary, that refusal to participate will involve no penalty or loss of benefits to which the subject is otherwise entitled, and that the subject may discontinue participation at any time without penalty or loss of benefits to which the subject is otherwise entitled.

(b) Additional elements of informed consent. When appropriate, one or more of the following elements of information shall also be provided to each subject:

(1) A statement that the particular treatment or procedure may involve risks to the subject (or to the embryo or fetus, if the subject is or may become pregnant) which are currently unforeseeable.

(2) Anticipated circumstances under which the subject's participation may be terminated by the investigator without regard to the subject's consent.

(3) Any additional costs to the subject that may result from participation in the research.

(4) The consequences of a subject's decision to withdraw from the research and procedures for orderly termination of participation by the subject.

(5) A statement that significant new findings developed during the course of the research which may relate to the subject's willingness to continue participation will be provided to the subject.

(6) The approximate number of subjects involved in the study.

(c) The informed consent requirements in these regulations are not intended to preempt any applicable Federal, State, or local laws which require additional information to be disclosed for informed consent to be legally effective.

(d) Nothing in these regulations is intended to limit the authority of a physician to provide emergency medical care to the extent the physician is permitted to do so under applicable Federal, State, or local law.

§50.27 Documentation of informed consent.

(a) Except as provided in §56.109(c), informed consent shall be documented by the use of a written consent form approved by the IRB and signed and dated by the subject or the subject's legally authorized representative at the time of consent. A copy shall be given to the person signing the form.

(b) Except as provided in §56.109(c), the consent form may be either of the following:

(1) A written consent document that embodies the elements of informed consent required by §50.25. This form may be read to the subject or the subject's legally authorized representative, but, in any event, the investigator shall give either the subject or the representative adequate opportunity to read it before it is signed.

(2) A short form written consent document stating that the elements of informed consent required by §50.25 have been presented orally to the subject or the subject's legally authorized representative. When this method is used, there shall be a witness to the oral presentation. Also, the IRB shall approve a written summary of what is to be said to the subject or the representative. Only the short form itself is to be signed by the subject or the representative. However, the witness shall sign both the short form and a copy of the summary, and the person actually obtaining the consent shall sign a copy of the summary. A copy of the summary shall be given to the subject or the representative in addition to a copy of the short form.

[46 FR 8951, Jan. 27, 1981, as amended at 61 FR 57280, Nov. 5, 1996]

Subpart C [Reserved]

Subpart D—Additional Safeguards for Children in Clinical Investigations

Source: 66 FR 20598, Apr. 24, 2001, unless otherwise noted.

§50.50 IRB duties.

In addition to other responsibilities assigned to IRBs under this part and part 56 of this chapter, each IRB must review clinical investigations involving children as subjects covered by this subpart D and approve only those clinical investigations that satisfy the criteria described in §50.51, §50.52, or §50.53 and the conditions of all other applicable sections of this subpart D.

§50.51 Clinical investigations not involving greater than minimal risk.

Any clinical investigation within the scope described in §§50.1 and 56.101 of this chapter in which no greater than minimal risk to children is presented may involve children as subjects only if the IRB finds and documents that adequate provisions are made for soliciting the assent of the children and the permission of their parents or guardians as set forth in §50.55.

§50.52 Clinical investigations involving greater than minimal risk but presenting the prospect of direct benefit to individual subjects.

Any clinical investigation within the scope described in §§50.1 and 56.101 of this chapter in which more than minimal risk to children is presented by an intervention or procedure that holds out the prospect of direct benefit for the individual subject, or by a monitoring procedure that is likely to contribute to the subject's well-being, may involve children as subjects only if the IRB finds and documents that:

(a) The risk is justified by the anticipated benefit to the subjects;

(b) The relation of the anticipated benefit to the risk is at least as favorable to the subjects as that presented by available alternative approaches; and

(c) Adequate provisions are made for soliciting the assent of the children and permission of their parents or guardians as set forth in §50.55.

§50.53 Clinical investigations involving greater than minimal risk and no prospect of direct benefit to individual subjects, but likely to yield generalizable knowledge about the subjects' disorder or condition.

Any clinical investigation within the scope described in §§50.1 and56.101 of this chapter in which more than minimal risk to children is presented by an intervention or procedure that does not hold out the prospect of direct benefit for the individual subject, or by a monitoring procedure that is not likely to contribute to the well-being of the subject, may involve children as subjects only if the IRB finds and documents that:

(a) The risk represents a minor increase over minimal risk;

(b) The intervention or procedure presents experiences to subjects that are reasonably commensurate with those inherent in their actual or expected medical, dental, psychological, social, or educational situations;

(c) The intervention or procedure is likely to yield generalizable knowledge about the subjects' disorder or condition that is of vital importance for the understanding or amelioration of the subjects' disorder or condition; and

(d) Adequate provisions are made for soliciting the assent of the children and permission of their parents or guardians as set forth in §50.55.

§50.54 Clinical investigations not otherwise approvable that present an opportunity to understand, prevent, or alleviate a serious problem affecting the health or welfare of children.

If an IRB does not believe that a clinical investigation within the scope described in §§50.1 and 56.101 of this chapter and involving children as subjects meets the requirements of §50.51, §50.52, or §50.53, the clinical investigation may proceed only if:

(a) The IRB finds and documents that the clinical investigation presents a reasonable opportunity to further the understanding, prevention, or alleviation of a serious problem affecting the health or welfare of children; and

(b) The Commissioner of Food and Drugs, after consultation with a panel of experts in pertinent disciplines (for example: science, medicine, education, ethics, law) and following opportunity for public review and comment, determines either:

(1) That the clinical investigation in fact satisfies the conditions of §50.51, §50.52, or §50.53, as applicable, or

(2) That the following conditions are met:

(i) The clinical investigation presents a reasonable opportunity to further the understanding, prevention, or alleviation of a serious problem affecting the health or welfare of children;

(ii) The clinical investigation will be conducted in accordance with sound ethical principles; and

(iii) Adequate provisions are made for soliciting the assent of children and the permission of their parents or guardians as set forth in §50.55.

§50.55 Requirements for permission by parents or guardians and for assent by children.

(a) In addition to the determinations required under other applicable sections of this subpart D, the IRB must determine that adequate provisions are made for soliciting the assent of the children when in the judgment of the IRB the children are capable of providing assent.

(b) In determining whether children are capable of providing assent, the IRB must take into account the ages, maturity, and psychological state of the children involved. This judgment may be made for all children to be involved in clinical investigations under a particular protocol, or for each child, as the IRB deems appropriate.

(c) The assent of the children is not a necessary condition for proceeding with the clinical investigation if the IRB determines:

(1) That the capability of some or all of the children is so limited that they cannot reasonably be consulted, or

(2) That the intervention or procedure involved in the clinical investigation holds out a prospect of direct benefit that is important to the health or well-being of the children and is available only in the context of the clinical investigation.

(d) Even where the IRB determines that the subjects are capable of assenting, the IRB may still waive the assent requirement if it finds and documents that:

(1) The clinical investigation involves no more than minimal risk to the subjects;

(2) The waiver will not adversely affect the rights and welfare of the subjects;

(3) The clinical investigation could not practicably be carried out without the waiver; and

(4) Whenever appropriate, the subjects will be provided with additional pertinent information after participation.

(e) In addition to the determinations required under other applicable sections of this subpart D, the IRB must determine that the permission of each child's parents or guardian is granted.

(1) Where parental permission is to be obtained, the IRB may find that the permission of one parent is sufficient, if consistent with State law, for clinical investigations to be conducted under §50.51 or §50.52.

(2) Where clinical investigations are covered by §50.53 or §50.54 and permission is to be obtained from parents, both parents must give their permission unless one parent is deceased, unknown, incompetent, or not reasonably available, or when only one parent has legal responsibility for the care and custody of the child if consistent with State law.

(f) Permission by parents or guardians must be documented in accordance with and to the extent required by §50.27.

(g) When the IRB determines that assent is required, it must also determine whether and how assent must be documented.

§50.56 Wards.

(a) Children who are wards of the State or any other agency, institution, or entity can be included in clinical investigations approved under §50.53 or §50.54 only if such clinical investigations are:

(1) Related to their status as wards; or

(2) Conducted in schools, camps, hospitals, institutions, or similar settings in which the majority of children involved as subjects are not wards.

(b) If the clinical investigation is approved under paragraph (a) of this section, the IRB must require appointment of an advocate for each child who is a ward.

(1) The advocate will serve in addition to any other individual acting on behalf of the child as guardian or in loco parentis.

(2) One individual may serve as advocate for more than one child.

(3) The advocate must be an individual who has the background and experience to act in, and agrees to act in, the best interest of the child for the duration of the child's participation in the clinical investigation.

(4) The advocate must not be associated in any way (except in the role as advocate or member of the IRB) with the clinical investigation, the investigator(s), or the guardian organization.

TITLE 21—FOOD AND DRUGS

Chapter I: Food and Drug Administration, Department of Health and Human Services

Subchapter A: General

PART 54

Financial Disclosure by Clinical Investigators

Authority: 21 U.S.C. 321, 331, 351, 352, 353, 355, 360, 360c-360j, 371, 372, 373, 374, 375, 376, 379; 42 U.S.C. 262.

Source: 63 FR 5250, Feb. 2, 1998, unless otherwise noted.

§54.1 Purpose.

(a) The Food and Drug Administration (FDA) evaluates clinical studies submitted in marketing applications, required by law, for new human drugs and biological products and marketing applications and reclassification petitions for medical devices.

(b) The agency reviews data generated in these clinical studies to determine whether the applications are approvable under the statutory requirements. FDA may consider clinical studies inadequate and the data inadequate if, among other things, appropriate steps have not been taken in the design, conduct, reporting, and analysis of the studies to minimize bias. One potential source of bias in clinical studies is a financial interest of the clinical investigator in the outcome of the study because of the way payment is arranged (e.g., a royalty) or because the investigator has a proprietary interest in the product (e.g., a patent) or because the investigator has an equity interest in the sponsor of the covered study. This section and conforming regulations require an applicant whose submission relies in part on clinical data to disclose certain financial arrangements between sponsor(s) of the covered studies and the clinical investigators and certain interests of the clinical investigators in the product under study or in the sponsor of the covered studies. FDA will use this information, in conjunction with information about the design and purpose of the study, as well as information obtained through on-site inspections, in the agency's assessment of the reliability of the data.

§54.2 Definitions.

For the purposes of this part:

(a) Compensation affected by the outcome of clinical studies means compensation that could be higher for a favorable outcome than for an unfavorable outcome, such as compensation that is explicitly greater for a favorable result or compensation to the investigator in the form of an equity interest in the sponsor of a covered study or in the form of compensation tied to sales of the product, such as a royalty interest.

(b) Significant equity interest in the sponsor of a covered study means any ownership interest, stock options, or other financial interest whose value cannot be readily determined through reference to public prices (generally, interests in a nonpublicly traded corporation), or any equity interest in a publicly traded corporation that exceeds $50,000 during the time the clinical investigator is carrying out the study and for 1 year following completion of the study.

(c) Proprietary interest in the tested product means property or other financial interest in the product including, but not limited to, a patent, trademark, copyright or licensing agreement.

(d) Clinical investigator means only a listed or identified investigator or subinvestigator who is directly involved in the treatment or evaluation of research subjects. The term also includes the spouse and each dependent child of the investigator.

(e) Covered clinical study means any study of a drug or device in humans submitted in a marketing application or reclassification petition subject to this part that the applicant or FDA relies on to establish that the product is effective (including studies that show equivalence to an effective product) or any study in which a single investigator makes a significant contribution to the demonstration of safety. This would, in general, not include phase l tolerance studies or pharmacokinetic studies, most clinical pharmacology studies (unless they are critical to an efficacy determination), large open safety studies conducted at multiple sites, treatment protocols, and parallel track protocols. An applicant may consult with FDA as to which clinical studies constitute "covered clinical studies" for purposes of complying with financial disclosure requirements.

(f) Significant payments of other sorts means payments made by the sponsor of a covered study to the investigator or the institution to support activities of the investigator that have a monetary value of more than $25,000, exclusive of the costs of conducting the clinical study or other clinical studies, (e.g., a grant to fund ongoing research, compensation in the form of equipment or retainers for ongoing consultation or honoraria) during the time the clinical investigator is carrying out the study and for 1 year following the completion of the study.

(g) Applicant means the party who submits a marketing application to FDA for approval of a drug, device, or biologic product. The applicant is responsible for submitting the appropriate certification and disclosure statements required in this part.

(h) Sponsor of the covered clinical study means the party supporting a particular study at the time it was carried out.

[63 FR 5250, Feb. 2, 1998, as amended at 63 FR 72181, Dec. 31, 1998]

§54.3 Scope.

The requirements in this part apply to any applicant who submits a marketing application for a human drug, biological product, or device and who submits covered clinical studies. The applicant is responsible for making the appropriate certification or disclosure statement where the applicant either contracted with one or more clinical investigators to conduct the studies or submitted studies conducted by others not under contract to the applicant.

§54.4 Certification and disclosure requirements.

For purposes of this part, an applicant must submit a list of all clinical investigators who conducted covered clinical studies to determine whether the applicant's product meets FDA's marketing requirements, identifying those clinical investigators who are full-time or part-time employees of the sponsor of each covered study. The applicant must also completely and accurately disclose or certify information concerning the financial interests of a clinical investigator who is not a full-time or part-time employee of the sponsor for each covered clinical study. Clinical investigators subject to investigational new drug or investigational device exemption regulations must provide the sponsor of the study with sufficient accurate information needed to allow subsequent disclosure or certification. The applicant is required to submit for each clinical investigator who participates in a covered study, either a certification that none of the financial arrangements described in §54.2 exist, or disclose the nature of those arrangements to the agency. Where the applicant acts with due diligence to obtain the information required in this section but is unable to do so, the applicant shall certify that despite the applicant's due diligence in attempting to obtain the information, the applicant was unable to obtain the information and shall include the reason.

(a) The applicant (of an application submitted under sections 505, 506, 510(k), 513, or 515 of the Federal Food, Drug, and Cosmetic Act, or section 351 of the Public Health Service Act) that relies in whole or in part on clinical studies shall submit, for each clinical investigator who participated in a covered clinical study, either a certification described in paragraph (a)(1) of this section or a disclosure statement described in paragraph (a)(3) of this section.

(1) Certification: The applicant covered by this section shall submit for all clinical investigators (as defined in §54.2(d)), to whom the certification applies, a completed Form FDA 3454 attesting to the absence of financial interests and arrangements described in paragraph (a)(3) of this section. The form shall be dated and signed by the chief financial officer or other responsible corporate official or representative.

(2) If the certification covers less than all covered clinical data in the application, the applicant shall include in the certification a list of the studies covered by this certification.

(3) Disclosure Statement: For any clinical investigator defined in §54.2(d) for whom the applicant does not submit the certification described in paragraph (a)(1) of this section, the applicant shall submit a completed Form FDA 3455 disclosing completely and accurately the following:

(i) Any financial arrangement entered into between the sponsor of the covered study and the clinical investigator involved in the conduct of a covered clinical trial, whereby the value of the compensation to the clinical investigator for conducting the study could be influenced by the outcome of the study;

(ii) Any significant payments of other sorts from the sponsor of the covered study, such as a grant to fund ongoing research, compensation in the form of equipment, retainer for ongoing consultation, or honoraria;

(iii) Any proprietary interest in the tested product held by any clinical investigator involved in a study;

(iv) Any significant equity interest in the sponsor of the covered study held by any clinical investigator involved in any clinical study; and

(v) Any steps taken to minimize the potential for bias resulting from any of the disclosed arrangements, interests, or payments.

(b) The clinical investigator shall provide to the sponsor of the covered study sufficient accurate financial information to allow the sponsor to submit complete and accurate certification or disclosure statements as required in paragraph (a) of this section. The investigator shall promptly update this information if any relevant changes occur in the course of the investigation or for 1 year following completion of the study.

(c) Refusal to file application. FDA may refuse to file any marketing application described in paragraph (a) of this section that does not contain the information required by this section or a certification by the applicant that the applicant has acted with due diligence to obtain the information but was unable to do so and stating the reason.

[63 FR 5250, Feb. 2, 1998; 63 FR 35134, June 29, 1998, as amended at 64 FR 399, Jan. 5, 1999]

§54.5 Agency evaluation of financial interests.

(a) Evaluation of disclosure statement. FDA will evaluate the information disclosed under §54.4(a)(2) about each covered clinical study in an application to determine the impact of any disclosed financial interests on the reliability of the study. FDA may consider both the size and nature of a disclosed financial interest (including the potential increase in the value of the interest if the product is approved) and steps that have been taken to minimize the potential for bias.

(b) Effect of study design. In assessing the potential of an investigator's financial interests to bias a study, FDA will take into account the design and purpose of the study. Study designs that utilize such approaches as multiple investigators (most of whom do not have a disclosable interest), blinding, objective endpoints, or measurement of endpoints by someone other than the investigator may adequately protect against any bias created by a disclosable financial interest.

(c) Agency actions to ensure reliability of data. If FDA determines that the financial interests of any clinical investigator raise a serious question about the integrity of the data, FDA will take any action it deems necessary to ensure the reliability of the data including:

(1) Initiating agency audits of the data derived from the clinical investigator in question;

(2) Requesting that the applicant submit further analyses of data, e.g., to evaluate the effect of the clinical investigator's data on overall study outcome;

(3) Requesting that the applicant conduct additional independent studies to confirm the results of the questioned study; and

(4) Refusing to treat the covered clinical study as providing data that can be the basis for an agency action.

§54.6 Recordkeeping and record retention.

(a) Financial records of clinical investigators to be retained. An applicant who has submitted a marketing application containing covered clinical studies shall keep on file certain information pertaining to the financial interests of clinical investigators who conducted studies on which the application relies and who are not full or part-time employees of the applicant, as follows:

(1) Complete records showing any financial interest or arrangement as described in §54.4(a)(3)(i) paid to such clinical investigators by the sponsor of the covered study.

(2) Complete records showing significant payments of other sorts, as described in §54.4(a)(3)(ii), made by the sponsor of the covered clinical study to the clinical investigator.

(3) Complete records showing any financial interests held by clinical investigators as set forth in §54.4(a)(3)(iii) and (a)(3)(iv).

(b) Requirements for maintenance of clinical investigators' financial records.

(1) For any application submitted for a covered product, an applicant shall retain records as described in paragraph (a) of this section for 2 years after the date of approval of the application.

(2) The person maintaining these records shall, upon request from any properly authorized officer or employee of FDA, at reasonable times, permit such officer or

employee to have access to and copy and verify these records.

Chapter I: Food and Drug Administration, Department of Health and Human Services
Subchapter A: General

PART 56

Institutional Review Boards

Authority: 21 U.S.C. 321, 343, 346, 346a, 348, 350a, 350b, 351, 352, 353, 355, 360, 360c-360f, 360h-360j, 371, 379e, 381; 42 U.S.C. 216, 241, 262, 263b-263n.

Source: 46 FR 8975, Jan. 27, 1981, unless otherwise noted.

Subpart A—General Provisions

§56.101 Scope.

(a) This part contains the general standards for the composition, operation, and responsibility of an Institutional Review Board (IRB) that reviews clinical investigations regulated by the Food and Drug Administration under sections 505(i) and 520(g) of the act, as well as clinical investigations that support applications for research or marketing permits for products regulated by the Food and Drug Administration, including foods, including dietary supplements, that bear a nutrient content claim or a health claim, infant formulas, food and color additives, drugs for human use, medical devices for human use, biological products for human use, and electronic products. Compliance with this part is intended to protect the rights and welfare of human subjects involved in such investigations.

(b) References in this part to regulatory sections of the Code of Federal Regulations are to chapter I of title 21, unless otherwise noted.

[46 FR 8975, Jan. 27, 1981, as amended at 64 FR 399, Jan. 5, 1999; 66 FR 20599, Apr. 24, 2001]

§56.102 Definitions.

As used in this part:

(a) Act means the Federal Food, Drug, and Cosmetic Act, as amended (secs. 201-902, 52 Stat. 1040 et seq., as amended (21 U.S.C. 321-392)).

(b) Application for research or marketing permit includes:

(1) A color additive petition, described in part 71.

(2) Data and information regarding a substance submitted as part of the procedures for establishing that a substance is generally recognized as safe for a use which results or may reasonably be expected to result, directly or indirectly, in its becoming a component or otherwise affecting the characteristics of any food, described in §170.35.

(3) A food additive petition, described in part 171.

(4) Data and information regarding a food additive submitted as part of the procedures regarding food additives permitted to be used on an interim basis pending additional study, described in §180.1.

(5) Data and information regarding a substance submitted as part of the procedures for establishing a tolerance for unavoidable contaminants in food and food-packaging materials, described in section 406 of the act.

(6) An investigational new drug application, described in part 312 of this chapter.

(7) A new drug application, described in part 314.

(8) Data and information regarding the bioavailability or bioequivalence of drugs for human use submitted as part of the procedures for issuing, amending, or repealing a bioequivalence requirement, described in part 320.

(9) Data and information regarding an over-the-counter drug for human use submitted as part of the procedures for classify-

ing such drugs as generally recognized as safe and effective and not misbranded, described in part 330.

(10) An application for a biologics license, described in part 601 of this chapter.

(11) Data and information regarding a biological product submitted as part of the procedures for determining that licensed biological products are safe and effective and not misbranded, as described in part 601 of this chapter.

(12) An Application for an Investigational Device Exemption, described in parts 812 and 813.

(13) Data and information regarding a medical device for human use submitted as part of the procedures for classifying such devices, described in part 860.

(14) Data and information regarding a medical device for human use submitted as part of the procedures for establishing, amending, or repealing a standard for such device, described in part 861.

(15) An application for premarket approval of a medical device for human use, described in section 515 of the act.

(16) A product development protocol for a medical device for human use, described in section 515 of the act.

(17) Data and information regarding an electronic product submitted as part of the procedures for establishing, amending, or repealing a standard for such products, described in section 358 of the Public Health Service Act.

(18) Data and information regarding an electronic product submitted as part of the procedures for obtaining a variance from any electronic product performance standard, as described in §1010.4.

(19) Data and information regarding an electronic product submitted as part of the procedures for granting, amending, or extending an exemption from a radiation safety performance standard, as described in §1010.5.

(20) Data and information regarding an electronic product submitted as part of the procedures for obtaining an exemption from notification of a radiation safety defect or failure of compliance with a radiation safety performance standard, described in subpart D of part 1003.

(21) Data and information about a clinical study of an infant formula when submitted as part of an infant formula notification under section 412(c) of the Federal Food, Drug, and Cosmetic Act.

(22) Data and information submitted in a petition for a nutrient content claim, described in §101.69 of this chapter, and for a health claim, described in §101.70 of this chapter.

(23) Data and information from investigations involving children submitted in a new dietary ingredient notification, described in §190.6 of this chapter.

(c) Clinical investigation means any experiment that involves a test article and one or more human subjects, and that either must meet the requirements for prior submission to the Food and Drug Administration under section 505(i) or 520(g) of the act, or need not meet the requirements for prior submission to the Food and Drug Administration under these sections of the act, but the results of which are intended to be later submitted to, or held for inspection by, the Food and Drug Administration as part of an application for a research or marketing permit. The term does not include experiments that must meet the provisions of part 58, regarding nonclinical laboratory studies. The terms research, clinical research, clinical study, study, and clinical investigation are deemed to be synonymous for purposes of this part.

(d) Emergency use means the use of a test article on a human subject in a life-threatening situation in which no standard acceptable treatment is available, and in which there is not sufficient time to obtain IRB approval.

(e) Human subject means an individual who is or becomes a participant in research, either as a recipient of the test article or as a control. A subject may be either a healthy individual or a patient.

(f) Institution means any public or private entity or agency (including Federal, State, and other agencies). The term facility as used in section 520(g) of the act is deemed to be synonymous with the term institution for purposes of this part.

(g) Institutional Review Board (IRB) means any board, committee, or other group formally designated by an institution to review, to approve the initiation of, and to conduct periodic review of, biomedical research involving human subjects. The primary purpose of such review is to assure the protection of the rights and welfare of the human subjects. The term has the same meaning as the phrase institutional review committee as used in section 520(g) of the act.

(h) Investigator means an individual who actually conducts a clinical investigation (i.e., under whose immediate direction the test article is administered or dispensed to, or used involving, a subject) or, in the event of an investigation conducted by a team of individuals, is the responsible leader of that team.

(i) Minimal risk means that the probability and magnitude of harm or discomfort anticipated in the research are not greater in and of themselves than those ordinarily encountered in daily life or during the performance of routine physical or psychological examinations or tests.

(j) Sponsor means a person or other entity that initiates a clinical investigation, but that does not actually conduct the investigation, i.e., the test article is administered or dispensed to, or used involving, a subject under the immediate direction of another individual. A person other than an individual (e.g., a corporation or agency) that uses one or more of its own employees to conduct an investigation that it has initiated is considered to be a sponsor (not a sponsor-investigator), and the employees are considered to be investigators.

(k) Sponsor-investigator means an individual who both initiates and actually conducts, alone or with others, a clinical investigation, i.e., under whose immediate direction the test article is administered or dispensed to, or used involving, a subject. The term does not include any person other than an individual, e.g., it does not include a corporation or agency. The obligations of a sponsor-investigator under this part include both those of a sponsor and those of an investigator.

(l) Test article means any drug for human use, biological product for human use, medical device for human use, human food additive, color additive, electronic product, or any other article subject to regulation under the act or under sections 351 or 354-360F of the Public Health Service Act.

(m) IRB approval means the determination of the IRB that the clinical investigation has been reviewed and may be conducted at an institution within the constraints set forth by the IRB and by other institutional and Federal requirements.

[46 FR 8975, Jan. 27, 1981, as amended at 54 FR 9038, Mar. 3, 1989; 56 FR 28028, June 18, 1991; 64 FR 399, Jan. 5, 1999; 64 FR 56448, Oct. 20, 1999; 65 FR 52302, Aug. 29, 2000; 66 FR 20599, Apr. 24, 2001]

§56.103 Circumstances in which IRB review is required.

(a) Except as provided in §§56.104 and 56.105, any clinical investigation which must meet the requirements for prior submission (as required in parts 312, 812, and 813) to the Food and Drug Administration shall not be initiated unless that investigation has been reviewed and approved by, and remains subject to continuing review by, an IRB meeting the requirements of this part.

(b) Except as provided in §§56.104 and 56.105, the Food and Drug Administration may decide not to consider in support of an application for a research or marketing permit any data or information that has been derived from a clinical investigation that has not been approved by, and that was not subject to initial and continuing review by, an IRB meeting the requirements of this part. The determination that a clinical investigation may not be considered in support of an application for a research or marketing permit does not, however, relieve the applicant for such a permit of any obligation under any other applicable regulations to submit the results of the investigation to the Food and Drug Administration.

(c) Compliance with these regulations will in no way render inapplicable pertinent Federal, State, or local laws or regulations.

[46 FR 8975, Jan. 27, 1981; 46 FR 14340, Feb. 27, 1981]

§56.104 Exemptions from IRB requirement.

The following categories of clinical investigations are exempt from the requirements of this part for IRB review:

(a) Any investigation which commenced before July 27, 1981 and was subject to requirements for IRB review under FDA regulations before that date, provided that the investigation remains subject to review of an IRB which meets the FDA requirements in effect before July 27, 1981.

(b) Any investigation commenced before July 27, 1981 and was not otherwise subject to requirements for IRB review under Food and Drug Administration regulations before that date.

(c) Emergency use of a test article, provided that such emergency use is reported to the IRB within 5 working days. Any subsequent use of the test article at the institution is subject to IRB review.

(d) Taste and food quality evaluations and consumer acceptance studies, if wholesome foods without additives are consumed or if a food is consumed that contains a food ingredient at or below the level and for a use found to be safe, or agricultural, chemical, or environmental contaminant at or below the level found to be safe, by the Food and Drug Administration or approved by the Environmental Protection Agency or the Food Safety and Inspection Service of the U.S. Department of Agriculture.

[46 FR 8975, Jan. 27, 1981, as amended at 56 FR 28028, June 18, 1991]

§56.105 Waiver of IRB requirement.

On the application of a sponsor or sponsor-investigator, the Food and Drug Administration may waive any of the requirements contained in these regulations, including the requirements for IRB review, for specific research activities or for classes of research activities, otherwise covered by these regulations.

Subpart B—Organization and Personnel

§56.107 IRB membership.

(a) Each IRB shall have at least five members, with varying backgrounds to promote complete and adequate review of research activities commonly conducted by the institution. The IRB shall be sufficiently qualified through the experience and expertise of its members, and the diversity of the members, including consideration of race, gender, cultural backgrounds, and sensitivity to such issues as community attitudes, to promote respect for its advice and counsel in safeguarding the rights and welfare of human subjects. In addition to possessing the professional competence necessary to review the specific research activities, the IRB shall be able to ascertain the acceptability of proposed research in terms of institutional commitments and regulations, applicable law, and standards or professional conduct and practice. The IRB shall therefore include persons knowledgeable in these areas. If an IRB regularly reviews research that involves a vulnerable catgory of subjects, such as children, prisoners, pregnant women, or handicapped or mentally disabled persons, consideration shall be given to the inclusion of one or more individuals who are knowledgeable about and experienced in working with those subjects.

(b) Every nondiscriminatory effort will be made to ensure that no IRB consists entirely of men or entirely of women, including the instituton's consideration of qualified persons of both sexes, so long as no selection is made to the IRB on the basis of gender. No IRB may consist entirely of members of one profession.

(c) Each IRB shall include at least one member whose primary concerns are in the scientific area and at least one member whose primary concerns are in nonscientific areas.

(d) Each IRB shall include at least one member who is not otherwise affiliated with the institution and who is not part of the immediate family of a person who is affiliated with the institution.

(e) No IRB may have a member participate in the IRB's initial or continuing review of any project in which the member has a conflicting interest, except to provide information requested by the IRB.

(f) An IRB may, in its discretion, invite individuals with competence in special areas to assist in the review of complex issues which require expertise beyond or in addition to that available on the IRB. These individuals may not vote with the IRB.

[46 FR 8975, Jan 27, 1981, as amended at 56 FR 28028, June 18, 1991; 56 FR 29756, June 28, 1991]

Subpart C—IRB Functions and Operations

§56.108 IRB functions and operations.

In order to fulfill the requirements of these regulations, each IRB shall:

(a) Follow written procedures: (1) For conducting its initial and continuing review of research and for reporting its findings and actions to the investigator and the institution; (2) for determining which projects require review more often than annually and which projects need verification from sources other than the investigator that no material changes have occurred since previous IRB review; (3) for ensuring prompt reporting to the IRB of changes in research activity; and (4) for ensuring that changes in approved research, during the period for which IRB approval has already been given, may not be initiated without IRB review and approval except where necessary to eliminate apparent immediate hazards to the human subjects.

(b) Follow written procedures for ensuring prompt reporting to the IRB, appropriate institutional officials, and the Food and Drug Administration of: (1) Any unanticipated problems involving risks to human subjects or others; (2) any instance of serious or continuing noncompliance with these regulations or the requirements or determinations of the IRB; or (3) any suspension or termination of IRB approval.

(c) Except when an expedited review procedure is used (see §56.110), review proposed research at convened meetings at which a majority of the members of the IRB are present, including at least one member whose primary concerns are in nonscientific areas. In order for the research to be approved, it shall receive the approval of a majority of those members present at the meeting.

[46 FR 8975, Jan. 27, 1981, as amended at 56 FR 28028, June 18, 1991; 67 FR 9585, Mar. 4, 2002]

§56.109 IRB review of research.

(a) An IRB shall review and have authority to approve, require modifications in (to secure approval), or disapprove all research activities covered by these regulations.

(b) An IRB shall require that information given to subjects as part of informed consent is in accordance with §50.25. The IRB may require that information, in addition to that specifically mentioned in §50.25, be given to the subjects when in the IRB's judgment the information would meaningfully add to the protection of the rights and welfare of subjects.

(c) An IRB shall require documentation of informed consent in accordance with §50.27 of this chapter, except as follows:

(1) The IRB may, for some or all subjects, waive the requirement that the subject, or the subject's legally authorized representative, sign a written consent form if it finds that the research presents no more than minimal risk of harm to subjects and involves no procedures for which written consent is normally required outside the research context; or

(2) The IRB may, for some or all subjects, find that the requirements in §50.24 of this chapter for an exception from informed consent for emergency research are met.

(d) In cases where the documentation requirement is waived under paragraph (c)(1) of this section, the IRB may require the investigator to provide subjects with a written statement regarding the research.

(e) An IRB shall notify investigators and the institution in writing of its decision to approve or disapprove the proposed research activity, or of modifications required to secure IRB approval of the research activity. If the IRB decides to disapprove a research activity, it shall include in its written notification a statement of the reasons for its decision and give the investigator an opportunity to respond in person or in writing. For investigations involving an exception to informed consent under §50.24 of this chapter, an IRB shall promptly notify in writing the investigator and the sponsor of the research when an IRB determines that it cannot approve the research because it does not meet the criteria in the exception provided under §50.24(a) of this chapter or because of other relevant ethical concerns. The written notification shall include a statement of the reasons for the IRB's determination.

(f) An IRB shall conduct continuing review of research covered by these regulations at intervals appropriate to the degree of risk, but not less than once per year, and shall have authority to observe or have a third party observe the consent process and the research.

(g) An IRB shall provide in writing to the sponsor of research involving an exception to informed consent under §50.24 of this chapter a copy of information that has been publicly disclosed under §50.24(a)(7)(ii) and (a)(7)(iii) of this chapter. The IRB shall provide this information to the sponsor promptly so that the sponsor is aware that such disclosure has occurred. Upon receipt, the sponsor shall provide copies of the information disclosed to FDA.

(h) When some or all of the subjects in a study are children, an IRB must determine that the research study is in compliance with part 50, subpart D of this chapter, at the time of its initial review of the research. When some or all of the subjects in a study that is ongoing on April 30, 2001 are children, an IRB must conduct a review of the research to determine compliance with part 50, subpart D of this chapter, either at the time of continuing review or, at the discretion of the IRB, at an earlier date.

[46 FR 8975, Jan. 27, 1981, as amended at 61 FR 51529, Oct. 2, 1996; 66 FR 20599, Apr. 24, 2001]

§56.110 Expedited review procedures for certain kinds of research involving no more than minimal risk, and for minor changes in approved research.

(a) The Food and Drug Administration has established, and published in the FEDERAL REGISTER, a list of categories of research that may be reviewed by the IRB through an expedited review procedure. The list will be amended, as appropriate, through periodic republication in the FEDERAL REGISTER.

(b) An IRB may use the expedited review procedure to review either or both of the following: (1) Some or all of the research appearing on the list and found by the reviewer(s) to involve no more than minimal risk, (2) minor changes in previously approved research during the period (of 1 year or less) for which approval is authorized. Under an expedited review procedure, the review may be carried out by the IRB chairperson or by one or more experienced reviewers designated by the IRB chairperson from among the members of the IRB. In reviewing the research, the reviewers may exercise all of the authorities of the IRB except that the reviewers may not disapprove the research. A research activity may be disapproved only after review in accordance with the nonexpedited review procedure set forth in §56.108(c).

(c) Each IRB which uses an expedited review procedure shall adopt a method for keeping all members advised of research proposals which have been approved under the procedure.

(d) The Food and Drug Administration may restrict, suspend, or terminate an institution's or IRB's use of the expedited review procedure when necessary to protect the rights or welfare of subjects.

[46 FR 8975, Jan. 27, 1981, as amended at 56 FR 28029, June 18, 1991]

§56.111 Criteria for IRB approval of research.

(a) In order to approve research covered by these regulations the IRB shall determine that all of the following requirements are satisfied:

(1) Risks to subjects are minimized: (i) By using procedures which are consistent with sound research design and which do not unnecessarily expose subjects to risk, and (ii) whenever appropriate, by using procedures already being performed on the subjects for diagnostic or treatment purposes.

(2) Risks to subjects are reasonable in relation to anticipated benefits, if any, to subjects, and the importance of the knowledge that may be expected to result. In evaluating risks and benefits, the IRB should consider only those risks and benefits that may result from the research (as distinguished from risks and benefits of therapies that subjects would receive even if not participating in the research). The IRB should not consider possible long-range effects of applying knowledge gained in the research (for example, the possible effects of the research on public policy) as among those research risks that fall within the purview of its responsibility.

(3) Selection of subjects is equitable. In making this assessment the IRB should take into account the purposes of the research and the setting in which the research will be conducted and should be particularly cognizant of the special problems of research involving vulnerable populations, such as children, prisoners, pregnant women, handicapped, or mentally disabled persons, or economically or educationally disadvantaged persons.

(4) Informed consent will be sought from each prospective subject or the subject's legally authorized representative, in accordance with and to the extent required by part 50.

(5) Informed consent will be appropriately documented, in accordance with and to the extent required by §50.27.

(6) Where appropriate, the research plan makes adequate provision for monitoring the data collected to ensure the safety of subjects.

(7) Where appropriate, there are adequate provisions to protect the privacy of subjects and to maintain the confidentiality of data.

(b) When some or all of the subjects, such as children, prisoners, pregnant women, handicapped, or mentally disabled persons, or economically or educationally disadvantaged persons, are likely to be vulnerable to coercion or undue influence additional safeguards have been included in the study to protect the rights and welfare of these subjects.

(c) In order to approve research in which some or all of the subjects are children, an IRB must determine that all research is in compliance with part 50, subpart D of this chapter.

[46 FR 8975, Jan. 27, 1981, as amended at 56 FR 28029, June 18, 1991; 66 FR 20599, Apr. 24, 2001]

§56.112 Review by institution.

Research covered by these regulations that has been approved by an IRB may be subject to further appropriate review and approval or disapproval by officials of the institution. However, those officials may not approve the research if it has not been approved by an IRB.

§56.113 Suspension or termination of IRB approval of research.

An IRB shall have authority to suspend or terminate approval of research that is not being conducted in accordance with the IRB's requirements or that has been associated with unexpected serious harm to subjects. Any suspension or termination of approval shall include a statement of the reasons for the IRB's action and shall be reported promptly to the investigator, appropriate institutional officials, and the Food and Drug Administration.

§56.114 Cooperative research.

In complying with these regulations, institutions involved in multi-institutional studies may use joint review, reliance upon the review of another qualified IRB, or similar arrangements aimed at avoidance of duplication of effort.

Subpart D—Records and Reports

§56.115 IRB records.

(a) An institution, or where appropriate an IRB, shall prepare and maintain adequate documentation of IRB activities, including the following:

(1) Copies of all research proposals reviewed, scientific evaluations, if any, that accompany the proposals, approved sample consent documents, progress reports submitted by investigators, and reports of injuries to subjects.

(2) Minutes of IRB meetings which shall be in sufficient detail to show attendance at the meetings; actions taken by the IRB; the vote on these actions including the number of members voting for, against, and abstaining; the basis for requiring changes in or disapproving research; and a written summary of the discussion of controverted issues and their resolution.

(3) Records of continuing review activities.

(4) Copies of all correspondence between the IRB and the investigators.

(5) A list of IRB members identified by name; earned degrees; representative capacity; indications of experience such as board

certifications, licenses, etc., sufficient to describe each member's chief anticipated contributions to IRB deliberations; and any employment or other relationship between each member and the institution; for example: full-time employee, part-time employee, a member of governing panel or board, stockholder, paid or unpaid consultant.

(6) Written procedures for the IRB as required by §56.108 (a) and (b).

(7) Statements of significant new findings provided to subjects, as required by §50.25.

(b) The records required by this regulation shall be retained for at least 3 years after completion of the research, and the records shall be accessible for inspection and copying by authorized representatives of the Food and Drug Administration at reasonable times and in a reasonable manner.

(c) The Food and Drug Administration may refuse to consider a clinical investigation in support of an application for a research or marketing permit if the institution or the IRB that reviewed the investigation refuses to allow an inspection under this section.

[46 FR 8975, Jan. 27, 1981, as amended at 56 FR 28029, June 18, 1991; 67 FR 9585, Mar. 4, 2002]

Subpart E—Administrative Actions for Noncompliance

§56.120 Lesser administrative actions.

(a) If apparent noncompliance with these regulations in the operation of an IRB is observed by an FDA investigator during an inspection, the inspector will present an oral or written summary of observations to an appropriate representative of the IRB. The Food and Drug Administra-tion may subsequently send a letter describing the noncompliance to the IRB and to the parent institution. The agency will require that the IRB or the parent institution respond to this letter within a time period specified by FDA and describe the corrective actions that will be taken by the IRB, the institution, or both to achieve compliance with these regulations.

(b) On the basis of the IRB's or the institution's response, FDA may schedule a reinspection to confirm the adequacy of corrective actions. In addition, until the IRB or the parent institution takes appropriate corrective action, the agency may:

(1) Withhold approval of new studies subject to the requirements of this part that are conducted at the institution or reviewed by the IRB;

(2) Direct that no new subjects be added to ongoing studies subject to this part;

(3) Terminate ongoing studies subject to this part when doing so would not endanger the subjects; or

(4) When the apparent noncompliance creates a significant threat to the rights and welfare of human subjects, notify relevant State and Federal regulatory agencies and other parties with a direct interest in the agency's action of the deficiencies in the operation of the IRB.

(c) The parent institution is presumed to be responsible for the operation of an IRB, and the Food and Drug Administration will ordinarily direct any administrative action under this subpart against the institution.

However, depending on the evidence of responsibility for deficiencies, determined during the investigation, the Food and Drug Administration may restrict its administrative actions to the IRB or to a component of the parent institution determined to be responsible for formal designation of the IRB.

§56.121 Disqualification of an IRB or an institution.

(a) Whenever the IRB or the institution has failed to take adequate steps to correct the noncompliance stated in the letter sent by the agency under §56.120(a), and the Commissioner of Food and Drugs determines that this noncompliance may justify the disqualification of the IRB or of the parent institution, the Commissioner will institute proceedings in accordance with the requirements for a regulatory hearing set forth in part 16.

(b) The Commissioner may disqualify an IRB or the parent institution if the Commissioner determines that:

(1) The IRB has refused or repeatedly failed to comply with any of the regulations set forth in this part, and

(2) The noncompliance adversely affects the rights or welfare of the human subjects in a clinical investigation.

(c) If the Commissioner determines that disqualification is appropriate, the Commissioner will issue an order that explains the basis for the determination and that prescribes any actions to be taken with regard to ongoing clinical research conducted under the review of the IRB. The Food and Drug Administration will send notice of the disqualification to the IRB and the parent institution. Other parties with a direct interest, such as sponsors and clinical investigators, may also be sent a notice of the disqualification. In addition, the agency may elect to publish a notice of its action in the FEDERAL REGISTER.

(d) The Food and Drug Administration will not approve an application for a research permit for a clinical investigation that is to be under the review of a disqualified IRB or that is to be conducted at a disqualified institution, and it may refuse to consider in support of a marketing permit the data from a clinical investigation that was reviewed by a disqualified IRB as conducted at a disqualified institution, unless the IRB or the parent institution is reinstated as provided in §56.123.

§56.122 Public disclosure of information regarding revocation.

A determination that the Food and Drug Administration has disqualified an institution and the administrative record regarding that determination are disclosable to the public under part 20.

§56.123 Reinstatement of an IRB or an institution.

An IRB or an institution may be reinstated if the Commissioner determines, upon an evaluation of a written submission from the IRB or institution that explains the corrective action that the institution or IRB plans to take, that the IRB or institution has provided adequate assurance that it will operate in compliance with the standards set forth in this part. Notification of reinstatement shall be provided to all persons notified under §56.121(c).

§56.124 Actions alternative or additional to disqualification.

Disqualification of an IRB or of an institution is independent of, and neither in lieu of nor a precondition to, other proceedings or actions authorized by the act. The Food and Drug Administration may, at any time, through the Department of Justice institute any appropriate judicial proceedings (civil or criminal) and any other appropriate regulatory action, in addition to or in lieu of, and before, at the time of, or after, disqualification. The agency may also refer pertinent matters to another Federal, State, or local government agency for any action that that agency determines to be appropriate.

TITLE 21—FOOD AND DRUGS

Chapter I: Food and Drug Administration, Department of Health and Human Services
Subchapter D: Drugs for Human Use

PART 312

Investigational New Drug Application

Subpart D—Responsibilities of Sponsors and Investigators

312.50 General responsibilities of sponsors
312.52 Transfer of obligations to a contract research organization
312.53 Selecting investigators and monitors
312.54 Emergency research under §50.24 of this chapter
312.55 Informing investigators
312.56 Review of ongoing investigations
312.57 Recordkeeping and record retention
312.58 Inspection of sponsor's records and reports
312.59 Disposition of unused supply of investigational drug
312.60 General responsibilities of investigators
312.61 Control of the investigational drug
312.62 Investigator recordkeeping and record retention
312.64 Investigator reports
312.66 Assurance of IRB review
312.68 Inspection of investigator's records and reports
312.69 Handling of controlled substances
312.70 Disqualification of a clinical investigator

Subpart E—Drugs Intended to Treat Life-threatening and Severely-debilitating Illnesses

312.80 Purpose
312.81 Scope
312.82 Early consultation
312.83 Treatment protocols
312.84 Risk-benefit analysis in review of marketing applications for drugs to treat life-threatening and severely-debilitating illnesses
312.85 Phase 4 studies
312.86 Focused FDA regulatory research
312.87 Active monitoring of conduct and evaluation of clinical trials
312.88 Safeguards for patient safety

Subpart F—Miscellaneous

312.110 Import and export requirements
312.120 Foreign clinical studies not conducted under an IND
312.130 Availability for public disclosure of data and information in an IND
312.140 Address for correspondence
312.145 Guidance documents

Subpart G—Drugs for Investigational Use in Laboratory Research Animals or in Vitro Tests

312.160 Drugs for investigational use in laboratory research animals orin vitro tests

Authority: 21 U.S.C. 321, 331, 351, 352, 353, 355, 371; 42 U.S.C. 262.
Source: 52 FR 8831, Mar. 19, 1987, unless otherwise noted.

Subpart A—General Provisions

§312.1 Scope.

(a) This part contains procedures and requirements governing the use of investigational new drugs, including procedures and requirements for the submission to, and review by, the Food and Drug Administration of investigational new drug applications (IND's). An investigational new drug for which an IND is in effect in accordance with this part is exempt from the premarketing approval requirements that are otherwise applicable and may be shipped lawfully for the purpose of conducting clinical investigations of that drug.

(b) References in this part to regulations in the Code of Federal Regulations are to chapter I of title 21, unless otherwise noted.

§312.2 Applicability.

(a) Applicability. Except as provided in this section, this part applies to all clinical investigations of products that are subject to section 505 of the Federal Food, Drug, and Cosmetic Act or to the licensing provisions of the Public Health Service Act (58 Stat. 632, as amended (42 U.S.C. 201 et seq.)).

(b) Exemptions. (1) The clinical investigation of a drug product that is lawfully marketed in the United States is exempt from the requirements of this part if all the following apply:

(i) The investigation is not intended to be reported to FDA as a well-controlled study in support of a new indication for use nor intended to be used to support any other significant change in the labeling for the drug;

(ii) If the drug that is undergoing investigation is lawfully marketed as a prescription drug product, the investigation is not intended to support a significant change in the advertising for the product;

(iii) The investigation does not involve a route of administration or dosage level or use in a patient population or other factor that significantly increases the risks (or decreases the acceptability of the risks) associated with the use of the drug product;

(iv) The investigation is conducted in compliance with the requirements for institutional review set forth in part 56 and with the requirements for informed consent set forth in part 50; and

(v) The investigation is conducted in compliance with the requirements of §312.7.

(2)(i) A clinical investigation involving an in vitro diagnostic biological product listed in paragraph (b)(2)(ii) of this section is exempt from the requirements of this part if (a) it is intended to be used in a diagnostic procedure that confirms the diagnosis made by another, medically established, diagnostic product or procedure and (b) it is shipped in compliance with §312.160.

(ii) In accordance with paragraph (b)(2)(i) of this section, the following products are exempt from the requirements of this part: (a) blood grouping serum; (b) reagent red blood cells; and (c) anti-human globulin.

(3) A drug intended solely for tests in vitro or in laboratory research animals is exempt from the requirements of this part if shipped in accordance with §312.160.

(4) FDA will not accept an application for an investigation that is exempt under the provisions of paragraph (b)(1) of this section.

(5) A clinical investigation involving use of a placebo is exempt from the requirements of this part if the investigation does not otherwise require submission of an IND.

(6) A clinical investigation involving an exception from informed consent under §50.24 of this chapter is not exempt from the requirements of this part.

(c) Bioavailability studies. The applicability of this part to in vivo bioavailability studies in humans is subject to the provisions of §320.31.

(d) Unlabeled indication. This part does not apply to the use in the practice of medicine for an unlabeled indication of a new drug product approved under part 314 or of a licensed biological product.

(e) Guidance. FDA may, on its own initiative, issue guidance on the applicability of this part to particular investigational uses of drugs. On request, FDA will advise on the applicability of this part to a planned clinical investigation.

[52 FR 8831, Mar. 19, 1987, as amended at 61 FR 51529, Oct. 2, 1996; 64 FR 401, Jan. 5, 1999]

§312.3 Definitions and interpretations.

(a) The definitions and interpretations of terms contained in section 201 of the Act apply to those terms when used in this part:

(b) The following definitions of terms also apply to this part:

Act means the Federal Food, Drug, and Cosmetic Act (secs. 201-902, 52 Stat. 1040 et seq., as amended (21 U.S.C. 301-392)).

Clinical investigation means any experiment in which a drug is administered or dispensed to, or used involving, one or more human subjects. For the purposes of this part, an experiment is any use of a drug except for the use of a marketed drug in the course of medical practice.

Contract research organization means a person that assumes, as an independent contractor with the sponsor, one or more of the obligations of a sponsor, e.g., design of a protocol, selection or monitoring of investigations, evaluation of reports, and preparation of materials to be submitted to the Food and Drug Administration.

FDA means the Food and Drug Administration.

IND means an investigational new drug application. For purposes of this part, "IND" is synonymous with "Notice of Claimed Investigational Exemption for a New Drug."

Investigational new drug means a new drug or biological drug that is used in a clinical investigation. The term also includes a biological product that is used in vitro for diagnostic purposes. The terms "investigational drug" and "investigational new drug" are deemed to be synonymous for purposes of this part.

Investigator means an individual who actually conducts a clinical investigation (i.e., under whose immediate direction the drug is administered or dispensed to a subject). In the event an investigation is conducted by a team of individuals, the investigator is the responsible leader of the team. "Subinvestigator" includes any other individual member of that team.

Marketing application means an application for a new drug submitted under section 505(b) of the act or a biologics license application for a biological product submitted under the Public Health Service Act.

Sponsor means a person who takes responsibility for and initiates a clinical investigation. The sponsor may be an individual or pharmaceutical company, governmental agency, academic institution, private organization, or other organization. The sponsor does not actually conduct the investigation unless the sponsor is a sponsor-investigator. A person other than an individual that uses one or more of its own employees to conduct an investigation that it has initiated is a sponsor, not a sponsor-investigator, and the employees are investigators.

Sponsor-Investigator means an individual who both initiates and conducts an investigation, and under whose immediate direction the investigational drug is administered or dispensed. The term does not include any person other than an individual. The requirements applicable to a sponsor-investigator under this part include both those applicable to an investigator and a sponsor.

Subject means a human who participates in an investigation, either as a recipient of the investigational new drug or as a control. A subject may be a healthy human or a patient with a disease.

[52 FR 8831, Mar. 19, 1987, as amended at 64 FR 401, Jan. 5, 1999; 64 FR 56449, Oct. 20, 1999]

§312.6 Labeling of an investigational new drug.

(a) The immediate package of an investigational new drug intended for human use shall bear a label with the statement "Caution: New Drug—Limited by Federal (or United States) law to investigational use."

(b) The label or labeling of an investigational new drug shall not bear any statement that is false or misleading in any particular and shall not represent that the investigational new drug is safe or effective for the purposes for which it is being investigated.

§312.7 Promotion and charging for investigational drugs.

(a) Promotion of an investigational new drug. A sponsor or investigator, or any person acting on behalf of a sponsor or investigator, shall not represent in a promotional context that an investigational new drug is safe or effective for the purposes for which it is under investigation or otherwise promote the drug. This provision is not intended to restrict the full exchange of scientific information concerning the drug, including dissemination of scientific findings in scientific or lay media. Rather, its intent is to restrict promotional claims of safety or effectiveness of the drug for a use for which it is under investigation and to preclude commercialization of the drug before it is approved for commercial distribution.

(b) Commercial distribution of an investigational new drug. A sponsor or investigator shall not commercially distribute or test market an investigational new drug.

(c) Prolonging an investigation. A sponsor shall not unduly prolong an investigation after finding that the results of the investigation appear to establish sufficient data to support a marketing application.

(d) Charging for and commercialization of investigational drugs—(1) Clinical trials under an IND. Charging for an investigational drug in a clinical trial under an IND is not permitted without the prior written approval of FDA. In requesting such approval, the sponsor shall provide a full written explanation of why charging is necessary in order for the sponsor to undertake or continue the clinical trial, e.g., why distribution of the drug to test subjects should not be considered part of the normal cost of doing business.

(2) Treatment protocol or treatment IND. A sponsor or investigator may charge for an investigational drug for a treatment use under a treatment protocol or treatment IND provided: (i) There is adequate enrollment in the ongoing clinical investigations under the authorized IND; (ii) charging does not constitute commercial marketing of a new drug for which a marketing application has not been approved; (iii) the drug is not being commercially promoted or advertised; and (iv) the sponsor of the drug is actively pursuing marketing approval with due diligence. FDA must be notified in writing in advance of commencing any such charges, in an information amendment submitted under §312.31. Authorization for charging goes into effect automatically 30 days after receipt by FDA of the information amendment, unless the sponsor is notified to the contrary.

(3) Noncommercialization of investigational drug. Under this section, the sponsor may not commercialize an investigational drug by charging a price larger than that necessary to recover costs of manufacture, research, development, and handling of the investigational drug.

(4) Withdrawal of authorization. Authorization to charge for an investigational drug under this section may be withdrawn by FDA if the agency finds that the conditions underlying the authorization are no longer satisfied.

[52 FR 8831, Mar. 19, 1987, as amended at 52 FR 19476, May 22, 1987; 67 FR 9585, Mar. 4, 2002]

§312.10 Waivers.

(a) A sponsor may request FDA to waive applicable requirement under this part. A waiver request may be submitted either in an IND or in an information amendment to an IND. In an emergency, a request may be made by telephone or other rapid communication means. A waiver request is required to contain at least one of the following:

(1) An explanation why the sponsor's compliance with the requirement is unnecessary or cannot be achieved;

(2) A description of an alternative submission or course of action that satisfies the purpose of the requirement; or

(3) Other information justifying a waiver.

(b) FDA may grant a waiver if it finds that the sponsor's noncompliance would not pose a significant and unreasonable risk to human subjects of the investigation and that one of the following is met:

(1) The sponsor's compliance with the requirement is unnecessary for the agency to evaluate the application, or compliance cannot be achieved;

(2) The sponsor's proposed alternative satisfies the requirement; or

(3) The applicant's submission otherwise justifies a waiver.

[52 FR 8831, Mar. 19, 1987, as amended at 52 FR 23031, June 17, 1987; 67 FR 9585, Mar. 4, 2002]

Subpart B—Investigational New Drug Application (IND)

§312.20 Requirement for an IND.

(a) A sponsor shall submit an IND to FDA if the sponsor intends to conduct a clinical investigation with an investigational new drug that is subject to §312.2(a).

(b) A sponsor shall not begin a clinical investigation subject to §312.2(a) until the investigation is subject to an IND which is in effect in accordance with §312.40.

(c) A sponsor shall submit a separate IND for any clinical investigation involving an exception from informed consent under §50.24 of this chapter. Such a clinical investigation is not permitted to proceed without the prior written authorization from FDA. FDA shall provide a written determination 30 days after FDA receives the IND or earlier.

[52 FR 8831, Mar. 19, 1987, as amended at 61 FR 51529, Oct. 2, 1996; 62 FR 32479, June 16, 1997]

§312.21 Phases of an investigation.

An IND may be submitted for one or more phases of an investigation. The clinical investigation of a previously untested drug is generally divided into three phases. Although in general the phases are conducted sequentially, they may overlap. These three phases of an investigation are a follows:

(a) Phase 1. (1) Phase 1 includes the initial introduction of an investigational new drug into humans. Phase 1 studies are typically closely monitored and may be conducted in patients or normal volunteer subjects. These studies are designed to determine the metabolism and pharmacologic actions of the drug in humans, the side effects associated with increasing doses, and, if possible, to gain early evidence on effectiveness. During Phase 1, sufficient information about the drug's pharmacokinetics and pharmacological effects should be obtained to permit the design of well-controlled, scientifically valid, Phase 2 studies. The total number of subjects and patients included in Phase 1 studies varies with the drug, but is generally in the range of 20 to 80.

(2) Phase 1 studies also include studies of drug metabolism, structure-activity relationships, and mechanism of action in humans, as well as studies in which investigational drugs are used as research tools to explore biological phenomena or disease processes.

(b) Phase 2. Phase 2 includes the controlled clinical studies conducted to evaluate the effectiveness of the drug for a particular indication or indications in patients with the disease or condition under study and to determine the common short-term side effects and risks associated with the drug. Phase 2 studies are typically well controlled, closely monitored, and conducted in a relatively small number of patients, usually involving no more than several hundred subjects.

(c) Phase 3. Phase 3 studies are expanded controlled and uncontrolled trials. They are performed after preliminary evidence suggesting effectiveness of the drug has been obtained, and are intended to gather the additional information about effectiveness and safety that is needed to evaluate the overall benefit-risk relationship of the drug and to provide an adequate basis for physician labeling. Phase 3 studies usually include from several hundred to several thousand subjects.

§312.22 General principles of the IND submission.

(a) FDA's primary objectives in reviewing an IND are, in all phases of the investigation, to assure the safety and rights of subjects, and, in Phase 2 and 3, to help assure that the quality of the scientific evaluation of drugs is adequate to permit an evaluation of the drug's effectiveness and safety. Therefore, although FDA's review of Phase 1 submissions will focus on assessing the safety of Phase 1 investigations, FDA's review of Phases 2 and 3 submissions will also include an assessment of the scientific quality of the clinical investigations and the likelihood that the investigations will yield data capable of meeting statutory standards for marketing approval.

(b) The amount of information on a particular drug that must be submitted in an IND to assure the accomplishment of the objectives described in paragraph (a) of this section depends upon such factors as the novelty of the drug, the extent to which it has been studied previously, the known or suspected risks, and the developmental phase of the drug.

(c) The central focus of the initial IND submission should be on the general investigational plan and the protocols for specific human studies. Subsequent amendments to the IND that contain new or revised protocols should build logically on previous submissions and should be supported by additional information, including the results of animal toxicology studies or other human studies as appropriate. Annual reports to the IND should serve as the focus for reporting the status of studies being conducted under the IND and should update the general investigational plan for the coming year.

(d) The IND format set forth in §312.23 should be followed routinely by sponsors in the interest of fostering an efficient review of applications. Sponsors are expected to exercise considerable discretion, however, regarding the content of information submitted in each section, depending upon the kind of drug being studied and the nature of the available information. Section 312.23 outlines the information needed for a commercially sponsored IND for a new molecular entity. A sponsor-investigator who uses, as a research tool, an investigational new drug that is already subject to a manufacturer's IND or marketing application should follow the same general format, but ordinarily may, if authorized by the manufacturer, refer to the manufacturer's IND or marketing application in providing the technical information supporting the proposed clinical investigation. A sponsor-investigator who uses an investigational drug not subject to a manufacturer's IND or marketing application is ordinarily required to submit all technical information supporting the IND, unless such information may be referenced from the scientific literature.

§312.23 IND content and format.

(a) A sponsor who intends to conduct a clinical investigation subject to this part shall submit an "Investigational New Drug Application" (IND) including, in the following order:

(1) Cover sheet (Form FDA-1571). A cover sheet for the application containing the following:

(i) The name, address, and telephone number of the sponsor, the date of the application, and the name of the investigational new drug.

(ii) Identification of the phase or phases of the clinical investigation to be conducted.

(iii) A commitment not to begin clinical investigations until an IND covering the investigations is in effect.

(iv) A commitment that an Institutional Review Board (IRB) that complies with the requirements set forth in part 56 will be responsible for the initial and continuing review and approval of each of the studies in the proposed clinical investigation and that the investigator will report to the IRB proposed changes in the research activity in accordance with the requirements of part 56.

(v) A commitment to conduct the investigation in accordance with all other applicable regulatory requirements.

(vi) The name and title of the person responsible for monitoring the conduct and progress of the clinical investigations.

(vii) The name(s) and title(s) of the person(s) responsible under §312.32 for review and evaluation of information relevant to the safety of the drug.

(viii) If a sponsor has transferred any obligations for the conduct of any clinical study to a contract research organization, a statement containing the name and address of the contract research organization, identification of the clinical study, and a listing of the obligations transferred. If all obligations governing the conduct of the study have been transferred, a general statement of this transfer—in lieu of a listing of the specific obligations transferred—may be submitted.

(ix) The signature of the sponsor or the sponsor's authorized representative. If the person signing the application does not reside or have a place of business within the United States, the IND is required to contain the name and address of, and be countersigned by, an attorney, agent, or other authorized official who resides or maintains a place of business within the United States.

(2) A table of contents.

(3) Introductory statement and general investigational plan. (i) A brief introductory statement giving the name of the drug and all active ingredients, the drug's pharmacological class, the structural formula of the drug (if known), the formulation of the dosage form(s) to be used, the route of administration, and the broad objectives and planned duration of the proposed clinical investigation(s).

(ii) A brief summary of previous human experience with the drug, with reference to other IND's if pertinent, and to investigational or marketing experience in other countries that may be relevant to the safety of the proposed clinical investigation(s).

(iii) If the drug has been withdrawn from investigation or marketing in any country for any reason related to safety or effectiveness, identification of the country(ies) where the drug was withdrawn and the reasons for the withdrawal.

(iv) A brief description of the overall plan for investigating the drug product for the following year. The plan should include the following: (a) The rationale for the drug or the research study; (b) the indication(s) to be studied; (c) the general approach to be followed in evaluating the drug; (d) the kinds of clinical trials to be conducted in the first year following the submission (if plans are not developed for the entire year, the sponsor should so indicate); (e) the estimated number of patients to be given the drug in those studies; and (f) any risks of particular severity or seriousness anticipated on the basis of the toxicological data in animals or prior studies in humans with the drug or related drugs.

(4) [Reserved]

(5) Investigator's brochure. If required under §312.55, a copy of the investigator's brochure, containing the following information:

(i) A brief description of the drug substance and the formulation, including the structural formula, if known.

(ii) A summary of the pharmacological and toxicological effects of the drug in animals and, to the extent known, in humans.

(iii) A summary of the pharmacokinetics and biological disposition of the drug in animals and, if known, in humans.

(iv) A summary of information relating to safety and effectiveness in humans obtained from prior clinical studies. (Reprints of published articles on such studies may be appended when useful.)

(v) A description of possible risks and side effects to be anticipated on the basis of prior experience with the drug under investigation or with related drugs, and of precautions or special monitoring to be done as part of the investigational use of the drug.

(6) Protocols. (i) A protocol for each planned study. (Protocols for studies not submitted initially in the IND should be submitted in accordance with §312.30(a).) In general, protocols for Phase 1 studies may be less detailed and more flexible than protocols for Phase 2 and 3 studies. Phase 1 protocols should be directed primarily at providing an outline of the investigation—an estimate of the number of patients to be involved, a description of safety exclusions, and a description of the dosing plan including duration, dose, or method to be used in determining dose—and should specify in detail only those elements of the study that are critical to safety, such as necessary monitoring of vital signs and blood chemistries. Modifications of the experimental design of Phase 1 studies that do not affect critical safety assessments are required to be reported to FDA only in the annual report.

(ii) In Phases 2 and 3, detailed protocols describing all aspects of the study should be submitted. A protocol for a Phase 2 or 3 investigation should be designed in such a way that, if the sponsor anticipates that some deviation from the study design may become necessary as the investigation progresses, alternatives or contingencies to provide for such deviation are built into the protocols at the outset. For example, a protocol for a controlled short-term study might include a plan for an early crossover of nonresponders to an alternative therapy.

(iii) A protocol is required to contain the following, with the specific elements and detail of the protocol reflecting the above distinctions depending on the phase of study:

(a) A statement of the objectives and purpose of the study.

(b) The name and address and a statement of the qualifications (curriculum vitae or other statement of qualifications) of each investigator, and the name of each subinvestigator (e.g., research fellow, resident) working under the supervision of the investigator; the name and address of the research facilities to be used; and the name and address of each reviewing Institutional Review Board.

(c) The criteria for patient selection and for exclusion of patients and an estimate of the number of patients to be studied.

(d) A description of the design of the study, including the kind of control group to be used, if any, and a description of methods to be used to minimize bias on the part of subjects, investigators, and analysts.

(e) The method for determining the dose(s) to be administered, the planned maximum dosage, and the duration of individual patient exposure to the drug.

(f) A description of the observations and measurements to be made to fulfill the objectives of the study.

(g) A description of clinical procedures, laboratory tests, or other measures to be taken to monitor the effects of the drug in human subjects and to minimize risk.

(7) Chemistry, manufacturing, and control information. (i) As appropriate for the particular investigations covered by the IND, a section describing the composition, manufacture, and control of the drug substance and the drug product. Although in each phase of the investigation sufficient information is required to be submitted to assure the proper identification, quality, purity, and strength of the investigational drug, the amount of information needed to make that assurance will vary with the phase of the investigation, the proposed duration of the investigation, the dosage form, and the amount of information otherwise available. FDA recognizes that modifications to the method of preparation of the new drug substance and dosage form and changes in the dosage form itself are likely as the investigation progresses. Therefore, the emphasis in an initial Phase 1 submission should generally be placed on the identification and control of the raw materials and the new drug substance. Final specifications for the drug substance and drug product are not expected until the end of the investigational process.

(ii) It should be emphasized that the amount of information to be submitted depends upon the scope of the proposed clinical investigation. For example, although stability data are required in all phases of the IND to demonstrate that the new drug substance and drug product are within acceptable chemical and physical limits for the planned duration of the proposed clinical investigation, if very short-term tests are proposed, the supporting stability data can be correspondingly limited.

(iii) As drug development proceeds and as the scale or production is changed from the pilot-scale production appropriate for the limited initial clinical investigations to the larger-scale production needed for expanded clinical trials, the sponsor should submit information amendments to supplement the initial information submitted on the chemistry, manufacturing, and control processes with information appropriate to the expanded scope of the investigation.

(iv) Reflecting the distinctions described in this paragraph (a)(7), and based on the phase(s) to be studied, the submission is required to contain the following:

(a) Drug substance. A description of the drug substance, including its physical, chemical, or biological characteristics; the name and address of its manufacturer; the general method of preparation of the drug substance; the acceptable limits and analytical methods used to assure the identity, strength, quality, and purity of the drug substance; and information sufficient to support stability of the drug substance during the toxicological studies and the planned clinical studies. Reference to the current edition of the United States Pharmacopeia—National Formulary may satisfy relevant requirements in this paragraph.

(b) Drug product. A list of all components, which may include reasonable alternatives for inactive compounds, used in the manufacture of the investigational drug product, including both those components intended to appear in the drug product and those which may not appear but which are used in the manufacturing process, and, where applicable, the quantitative composition of the investigational drug product, including any reasonable variations that may be expected during the investigational stage; the name and address of the drug product manufacturer; a brief general description of the manufacturing and packaging procedure as appropriate for the product; the acceptable limits and analytical methods used to assure the identity, strength, quality, and purity of the drug product; and information sufficient to assure the product's stability during the planned clinical studies. Reference to the current edition of the United States Pharmacopeia—National Formulary may satisfy certain requirements in this paragraph.

(c) A brief general description of the composition, manufacture, and control of any placebo used in a controlled clinical trial.

(d) Labeling. A copy of all labels and labeling to be provided to each investigator.

(e) Environmental analysis requirements. A claim for categorical exclusion under §25.30 or 25.31 or an environmental assessment under §25.40.

(8) Pharmacology and toxicology information. Adequate information about pharmacological and toxicological studies of the drug involving laboratory animals or in vitro, on the basis of which the sponsor has concluded that it is reasonably safe to conduct the proposed clinical investigations. The kind, duration, and scope of animal and other tests required varies with the duration and nature of the proposed clinical investigations. Guidance documents are available from FDA that describe ways in which these requirements may be met. Such information is required to include the identification and qualifications of the individuals who evaluated the results of such studies and concluded that it is reasonably safe to begin the proposed investigations and a statement of where the investigations were conducted and where the records are available for inspection. As drug development proceeds, the sponsor is required to submit informational amendments, as appropriate, with additional information pertinent to safety.

(i) Pharmacology and drug disposition. A section describing the pharmacological effects and mechanism(s) of action of the drug in animals, and information on the absorption, distribution, metabolism, and excretion of the drug, if known.

(ii) Toxicology. (a) An integrated summary of the toxicological effects of the drug in animals and in vitro. Depending on the nature of the drug and the phase of the investigation, the description is to include the results of acute, subacute, and chronic toxicity tests; tests of the drug's effects on reproduction and the developing fetus; any special toxicity test related to the drug's particular mode of administration or conditions of use (e.g., inhalation, dermal, or ocular toxicology); and any in vitro studies intended to evaluate drug toxicity.

(b) For each toxicology study that is intended primarily to support the safety of the proposed clinical investigation, a full tabulation of data suitable for detailed review.

(iii) For each nonclinical laboratory study subject to the good laboratory practice regulations under part 58, a statement that the study was conducted in compliance with the good laboratory practice regulations in part 58, or, if the study was not conducted in compliance with those regulations, a brief statement of the reason for the noncompliance.

(9) Previous human experience with the investigational drug. A summary of previous human experience known to the applicant, if any, with the investigational drug. The information is required to include the following:

(i) If the investigational drug has been investigated or marketed previously, either in the United States or other countries, detailed information about such experience that is relevant to the safety of the proposed investigation or to the investigation's rationale. If the durg has been the subject of controlled trials, detailed information on such trials that is relevant to an assessment of the drug's effectiveness for the proposed investigational use(s) should also be provided. Any published material that is relevant to the safety of the proposed investigation or to an assessment of the drug's effectiveness for its proposed investigational use should be provided in full. Published material that is less directly relevant may be supplied by a bibliography.

(ii) If the drug is a combination of drugs previously investigated or marketed, the information required under paragraph (a)(9)(i) of this section should be provided for each active drug component. However, if any component in such combination is subject to an approved marketing application or is otherwise lawfully marketed in the United States, the sponsor is not required to submit published material concerning that active drug component unless such material relates directly to the proposed investigational use (including publications relevant to component-component interaction).

(iii) If the drug has been marketed outside the United States, a list of the countries in which the drug has been marketed and a list of the countries in which the drug has been withdrawn from marketing for reasons potentially related to safety or effectiveness.

(10) Additional information. In certain applications, as described below, information on special topics may be needed. Such information shall be submitted in this section as follows:

(i) Drug dependence and abuse potential. If the drug is a psychotropic substance or otherwise has abuse potential, a section describing relevant clinical studies and experience and studies in test animals.

(ii) Radioactive drugs. If the drug is a radioactive drug, sufficient data from animal or human studies to allow a reasonable calculation of radiation-absorbed dose to the whole body and critical organs upon administration to a human subject. Phase 1 studies of radioactive drugs must include studies which will obtain sufficient data for dosimetry calculations.

(iii) Pediatric studies. Plans for assessing pediatric safety and effectiveness.

(iv) Other information. A brief statement of any other information that would aid evaluation of the proposed clinical investigations with respect to their safety or their design and potential as controlled clinical trials to support marketing of the drug.

(11) Relevant information. If requested by FDA, any other relevant information needed for review of the application.

(b) Information previously submitted. The sponsor ordinarily is not required to resubmit information previously submitted, but may incorporate the information by reference. A reference to information submitted previously must identify the file by name, reference number, volume, and page number where the information can be found. A reference to information submitted to the agency by a person other than the sponsor is required to contain a written statement that authorizes the reference and that is signed by the person who submitted the information.

(c) Material in a foreign language. The sponsor shall submit an accurate and complete English translation of each part of the IND that is not in English. The sponsor shall also submit a copy of each original literature publication for which an English translation is submitted.

(d) Number of copies. The sponsor shall submit an original and two copies of all submissions to the IND file, including the original submission and all amendments and reports.

(e) Numbering of IND submissions. Each submission relating to an IND is required to be numbered serially using a single, three-digit serial number. The initial IND is required to be numbered 000; each subsequent submission (e.g., amendment, report, or correspondence) is required to be numbered chronologically in sequence.

(f) Identification of exception from informed consent. If the investigation involves an exception from informed consent under §50.24 of this chapter, the sponsor shall prominently identify on the cover sheet that the investigation is subject to the requirements in §50.24 of this chapter.

[52 FR 8831, Mar. 19, 1987, as amended at 52 FR 23031, June 17, 1987; 53 FR 1918, Jan. 25, 1988; 61 FR 51529, Oct. 2, 1996; 62 FR 40599, July 29, 1997; 63 FR 66669, Dec. 2, 1998; 65 FR 56479, Sept. 19, 2000; 67 FR 9585, Mar. 4, 2002]

§312.30 Protocol amendments.

Once an IND is in effect, a sponsor shall amend it as needed to ensure that the clinical investigations are conducted according to protocols included in the application. This section sets forth the provisions under which new protocols may be submitted and changes in previously submitted protocols may be made. Whenever a sponsor intends to conduct a clinical investigation with an exception from informed consent for emergency research as set forth in §50.24 of this chapter, the sponsor shall submit a separate IND for such investigation.

(a) New protocol. Whenever a sponsor intends to conduct a study that is not covered by a protocol already contained in the IND, the sponsor shall submit to FDA a protocol amendment containing the protocol for the study. Such study may begin provided two conditions are met: (1) The sponsor has submitted the protocol to FDA for its review; and (2) the protocol has been approved by the Institutional Review Board (IRB) with responsibility for review and approval of the study in accordance with the requirements of part 56. The sponsor may comply with these two conditions in either order.

(b) Changes in a protocol. (1) A sponsor shall submit a protocol amendment describing any change in a Phase 1 protocol that significantly affects the safety of subjects or any change in a Phase 2 or 3 protocol that significantly affects the safety of subjects, the scope of the investigation, or the scientific quality of the study. Examples of changes requiring an amendment under this paragraph include:

(i) Any increase in drug dosage or duration of exposure of individual subjects to the drug beyond that in the current protocol, or any significant increase in the number of subjects under study.

(ii) Any significant change in the design of a protocol (such as the addition or dropping of a control group).

(iii) The addition of a new test or procedure that is intended to improve monitoring for, or reduce the risk of, a side effect or adverse event; or the dropping of a test intended to monitor safety.

(2)(i) A protocol change under paragraph (b)(1) of this section may be made provided two conditions are met:

(a) The sponsor has submitted the change to FDA for its review; and

(b) The change has been approved by the IRB with responsibility for review and approval of the study. The sponsor may comply with these two conditions in either order.

(ii) Notwithstanding paragraph (b)(2)(i) of this section, a protocol change intended to eliminate an apparent immediate hazard to subjects may be implemented immediately provided FDA is subsequently notified by protocol amendment and the reviewing IRB is notified in accordance with §56.104(c).

(c) New investigator. A sponsor shall submit a protocol amendment when a new investigator is added to carry out a previously submitted protocol, except that a protocol amendment is not required when a licensed practitioner is added in the case of a treatment protocol under §312.34. Once the investigator is added to the study, the investigational drug may be shipped to the investigator and the investigator may begin participating in the study. The sponsor shall notify FDA of the new investigator within 30 days of the investigator being added.

(d) Content and format. A protocol amendment is required to be prominently identified as such (i.e., "Protocol Amendment: New Protocol", "Protocol Amendment: Change in Protocol", or "Protocol Amendment: New Investigator"), and to contain the following:

(1)(i) In the case of a new protocol, a copy of the new protocol and a brief description of the most clinically significant differences between it and previous protocols.

(ii) In the case of a change in protocol, a brief description of the change and reference (date and number) to the submission that contained the protocol.

(iii) In the case of a new investigator, the investigator's name, the qualifications to conduct the investigation, reference to the previously submitted protocol, and all additional information about the investigator's study as is required under §312.23(a)(6)(iii)(b).

(2) Reference, if necessary, to specific technical information in the IND or in a concurrently submitted information amendment to the IND that the sponsor relies on to support any clinically significant change in the new or amended protocol. If the reference is made to supporting information already in the IND, the sponsor shall identify by name, reference number, volume, and page number the location of the information.

(3) If the sponsor desires FDA to comment on the submission, a request for such comment and the specific questions FDA's response should address.

(e) When submitted. A sponsor shall submit a protocol amendment for a new protocol or a change in protocol before its implementation. Protocol amendments to add a new investigator or to provide additional information about investigators may be grouped and submitted at 30-day intervals. When several submissions of new protocols or protocol changes are anticipated during a short period, the sponsor is encouraged, to the extent feasible, to include these all in a single submission.

[52 FR 8831, Mar. 19, 1987, as amended at 52 FR 23031, June 17, 1987; 53 FR 1918, Jan. 25, 1988; 61 FR 51530, Oct. 2, 1996; 67 FR 9585, Mar. 4, 2002]

§312.31 Information amendments.

(a) Requirement for information amendment. A sponsor shall report in an information amendment essential information on the IND that is not within the scope of a protocol amendment, IND safety reports, or annual report. Examples of information requiring an information amendment include:

(1) New toxicology, chemistry, or other technical information; or

(2) A report regarding the discontinuance of a clinical investigation.

(b) Content and format of an information amendment. An information amendment is required to bear prominent identification of its contents (e.g., "Information Amendment: Chemistry, Manufacturing, and Control", "Infor-mation Amendment: Pharmacology-Toxicol-ogy", "Information Amendment: Clinical"), and to contain the following:

(1) A statement of the nature and purpose of the amendment.

(2) An organized submission of the data in a format appropriate for scientific review.

(3) If the sponsor desires FDA to comment on an information amendment, a request for such comment.

(c) When submitted. Information amendments to the IND should be submitted as necessary but, to the extent feasible, not more than every 30 days.

[52 FR 8831, Mar. 19, 1987, as amended at 52 FR 23031, June 17, 1987; 53 FR 1918, Jan. 25, 1988; 67 FR 9585, Mar. 4, 2002]

§312.32 IND safety reports.

(a) Definitions. The following definitions of terms apply to this section:-

Associated with the use of the drug. There is a reasonable possibility that the experience may have been caused by the drug.

Disability. A substantial disruption of a person's ability to conduct normal life functions.

Life-threatening adverse drug experience. Any adverse drug experience that places the patient or subject, in the view of the investigator, at immediate risk of death from the reaction as it occurred, i.e., it does not include a reaction that, had it occurred in a more severe form, might have caused death.

Serious adverse drug experience: Any adverse drug experience occurring at any dose that results in any of the following outcomes: Death, a life-threatening adverse drug experience, inpatient hospitalization or prolongation of existing hospitalization, a persistent or significant disability/incapacity, or a congenital anomaly/birth defect. Important medical events that may not result in death, be life-threatening, or require hospitalization may be considered a serious adverse drug experience when, based upon appropriate medical judgment, they may jeopardize the patient or subject and may require medical or surgical intervention to prevent one of the outcomes listed in this definition. Examples of such medical events include allergic bronchospasm requiring intensive treatment in an emergency room or at home, blood dyscrasias or convulsions that do not result in inpatient hospitalization, or the development of drug dependency or drug abuse.

Unexpected adverse drug experience: Any adverse drug experience, the specificity or severity of which is not consistent with the current investigator brochure; or, if an investigator brochure is not required or available, the specificity or severity of which is not consistent with the risk information described in the general investigational plan or elsewhere in the current application, as amended. For example, under this definition, hepatic necrosis would be unexpected (by virtue of greater severity) if the investigator brochure only referred to elevated hepatic enzymes or hepatitis. Similarly, cerebral thromboembolism and cerebral vasculitis would be unexpected (by virtue of greater specificity) if the investigator brochure only listed cerebral vascular accidents. "Unexpected," as used in this definition, refers to an adverse drug experience that has not been previously observed (e.g., included in the investigator brochure) rather than from the perspective of such experience not being anticipated from the pharmacological properties of the pharmaceutical product.

(b) Review of safety information. The sponsor shall promptly review all information relevant to the safety of the drug obtained or otherwise received by the sponsor from any source, foreign or domestic, including information derived from any clinical or epidemiological investigations, animal investigations, commercial marketing experience, reports in the scientific literature, and unpublished scientific papers, as well as reports from foreign regulatory authorities that have not already been previously reported to the agency by the sponsor.

(c) IND safety reports. (1) Written reports—(i) The sponsor shall notify FDA and all participating investigators in a written IND safety report of:

(A) Any adverse experience associated with the use of the drug that is both serious and unexpected; or

(B) Any finding from tests in laboratory animals that suggests a significant risk for human subjects including reports of mutagenicity, teratogenicity, or carcinogenicity. Each notification shall be made as soon as possible and in no event later than 15 calendar days after the sponsor's initial receipt of the information. Each written notification may be submitted on FDA Form 3500A or in a narrative format (foreign events may be submitted either on an FDA Form 3500A or, if preferred, on a CIOMS I form; reports from animal or epidemiological studies shall be submitted in a narrative format) and shall bear prominent identification of its contents, i.e., "IND Safety Report." Each written notification to FDA shall be transmitted to the FDA new drug review division in the Center for Drug Evaluation and Research or the product review division in the Center for Biologics Evaluation and Research that has responsibility for review of the IND. If FDA determines that additional data are needed, the agency may require further data to be submitted.

(ii) In each written IND safety report, the sponsor shall identify all safety reports previously filed with the IND concerning a similar adverse experience, and shall analyze the significance of the adverse experience in light of the previouos, similar reports.

(2) Telephone and facsimile transmission safety reports. The sponsor shall also notify FDA by telephone or by facsimile transmission of any unexpected fatal or life-threatening experience associated with the use of the drug as soon as possible but in no event later than 7 calendar days after the sponsor's initial receipt of the information. Each telephone call or facsimile transmission to FDA shall be transmitted to the FDA new drug review division in the Center for Drug Evaluation and Research or the product review division in the Center for Biologics Evaluation and Research that has responsibility for review of the IND.

(3) Reporting format or frequency. FDA may request a sponsor to submit IND safety reports in a format or at a frequency different than that required under this paragraph. The sponsor may also propose and adopt a different reporting format or frequency if the change is agreed to in advance by the director of the new drug review division in the Center for Drug Evaluation and Research or the director of the products review division in the Center for Biologics Evaluation and Research which is responsible for review of the IND.

(4) A sponsor of a clinical study of a marketed drug is not required to make a safety report for any adverse experience associated with use of the drug that is not from the clinical study itself.

(d) Followup. (1) The sponsor shall promptly investigate all safety information received by it.

(2) Followup information to a safety report shall be submitted as soon as the relevant information is available.

(3) If the results of a sponsor's investigation show that an adverse drug experience not initially determined to be reportable under paragraph (c) of this section is so reportable, the sponsor shall report such experience in a written safety report as soon as possible, but in no event later than 15 calendar days after the determination is made.

(4) Results of a sponsor's investigation of other safety information shall be submitted,

as appropriate, in an information amendment or annual report.

(e) Disclaimer. A safety report or other information submitted by a sponsor under this part (and any release by FDA of that report or information) does not necessarily reflect a conclusion by the sponsor or FDA that the report or information constitutes an admission that the drug caused or contributed to an adverse experience. A sponsor need not admit, and may deny, that the report or information submitted by the sponsor constitutes an admission that the drug caused or contributed to an adverse experience.

[52 FR 8831, Mar. 19, 1987, as amended at 52 FR 23031, June 17, 1987; 55 FR 11579, Mar. 29, 1990; 62 FR 52250, Oct. 7, 1997; 67 FR 9585, Mar. 4, 2002]

§312.33 Annual reports.

A sponsor shall within 60 days of the anniversary date that the IND went into effect, submit a brief report of the progress of the investigation that includes:

(a) Individual study information. A brief summary of the status of each study in progress and each study completed during the previous year. The summary is required to include the following information for each study:

(1) The title of the study (with any appropriate study identifiers such as protocol number), its purpose, a brief statement identifying the patient population, and a statement as to whether the study is completed.

(2) The total number of subjects initially planned for inclusion in the study; the number entered into the study to date, tabulated by age group, gender, and race; the number whose participation in the study was completed as planned; and the number who dropped out of the study for any reason.

(3) If the study has been completed, or if interim results are known, a brief description of any available study results.

(b) Summary information. Information obtained during the previous year's clinical and nonclinical investigations, including:

(1) A narrative or tabular summary showing the most frequent and most serious adverse experiences by body system.

(2) A summary of all IND safety reports submitted during the past year.

(3) A list of subjects who died during participation in the investigation, with the cause of death for each subject.

(4) A list of subjects who dropped out during the course of the investigation in association with any adverse experience, whether or not thought to be drug related.

(5) A brief description of what, if anything, was obtained that is pertinent to an understanding of the drug's actions, including, for example, information about dose response, information from controlled trails, and information about bioavailability.

(6) A list of the preclinical studies (including animal studies) completed or in progress during the past year and a summary of the major preclinical findings.

(7) A summary of any significant manufacturing or microbiological changes made during the past year.

(c) A description of the general investigational plan for the coming year to replace that submitted 1 year earlier. The general investigational plan shall contain the information required under §312.23(a)(3)(iv).

(d) If the investigator brochure has been revised, a description of the revision and a copy of the new brochure.

(e) A description of any significant Phase 1 protocol modifications made during the previous year and not previously reported to the IND in a protocol amendment.

(f) A brief summary of significant foreign marketing developments with the drug during the past year, such as approval of marketing in any country or withdrawal or suspension from marketing in any country.

(g) If desired by the sponsor, a log of any outstanding business with respect to the IND for which the sponsor requests or expects a reply, comment, or meeting.

[52 FR 8831, Mar. 19, 1987, as amended at 52 FR 23031, June 17, 1987; 63 FR 6862, Feb. 11, 1998; 67 FR 9585, Mar. 4, 2002]

§312.34 Treatment use of an investigational new drug.

(a) General. A drug that is not approved for marketing may be under clinical investigation for a serious or immediately life-threatening disease condition in patients for whom no comparable or satisfactory alternative drug or other therapy is available. During the clinical investigation of the drug, it may be appropriate to use the drug in the treatment of patients not in the clinical trials, in accordance with a treatment protocol or treatment IND. The purpose of this section is to facilitate the availability of promising new drugs to desperately ill patients as early in the drug development process as possible, before general marketing begins, and to obtain additional data on the drug's safety and effectiveness. In the case of a serious disease, a drug ordinarily may be made available for treatment use under this section during Phase 3 investigations or after all clinical trials have been completed; however, in appropriate circumstances, a drug may be made available for treatment use during Phase 2. In the case of an immediately life-threatening disease, a drug may be made available for treatment use under this section earlier than Phase 3, but ordinarily not earlier than Phase 2. For purposes of this section, the "treatment use" of a drug includes the use of a drug for diagnostic purposes. If a protocol for an investigational drug meets the criteria of this section, the protocol is to be submitted as a treatment protocol under the provisions of this section.

(b) Criteria. (1) FDA shall permit an investigational drug to be used for a treatment use under a treatment protocol or treatment IND if:

(i) The drug is intended to treat a serious or immediately life-threatening disease;

(ii) There is no comparable or satisfactory alternative drug or other therapy available to treat that stage of the disease in the intended patient population;

(iii) The drug is under investigation in a controlled clinical trial under an IND in effect for the trial, or all clinical trials have been completed; and

(iv) The sponsor of the controlled clinical trial is actively pursuing marketing approval of the investigational drug with due diligence.

(2) Serious disease. For a drug intended to treat a serious disease, the Commissioner may deny a request for treatment use under a treatment protocol or treatment IND if there is insufficient evidence of safety and effectiveness to support such use.

(3) Immediately life-threatening disease. (i) For a drug intended to treat an immediately life-threatening disease, the Commissioner may deny a request for treatment use of an investigational drug under a treatment protocol or treatment IND if the available scientific evidence, taken as a whole, fails to provide a reasonable basis for concluding that the drug:

(A) May be effective for its intended use in its intended patient population; or

(B) Would not expose the patients to whom the drug is to be administered to an unreasonable and significant additional risk of illness or injury.

(ii) For the purpose of this section, an "immediately life-threatening" disease means a stage of a disease in which there is a reasonable likelihood that death will occur within a matter of months or in which premature death is likely without early treatment.

(c) Safeguards. Treatment use of an investigational drug is conditioned on the sponsor and investigators complying with the safeguards of the IND process, including the regulations governing informed consent (21 CFR part 50) and institutional review boards (21 CFR part 56) and the applicable provisions of part 312, including distribution of the drug through qualified experts, maintenance of adequate manufacturing facilities, and submission of IND safety reports.

(d) Clinical hold. FDA may place on clinical hold a proposed or ongoing treatment protocol or treatment IND in accordance with §312.42.

[52 FR 19476, May 22, 1987, as amended at 57 FR 13248, Apr. 15, 1992]

§312.35 Submissions for treatment use.

(a) Treatment protocol submitted by IND sponsor. Any sponsor of a clinical investigation of a drug who intends to sponsor a treatment use for the drug shall submit to FDA a treatment protocol under §312.34 if the sponsor believes the criteria of §312.34 are satisfied. If a protocol is not submitted under §312.34, but FDA believes that the protocol should have been submitted under this section, FDA may deem the protocol to be submitted under §312.34. A treatment use under a treatment protocol may begin 30 days after FDA receives the protocol or on earlier notification by FDA that the treatment use described in the protocol may begin.

(1) A treatment protocol is required to contain the following:

(i) The intended use of the drug.

(ii) An explanation of the rationale for use of the drug, including, as appropriate, either a list of what available regimens ordinarily should be tried before using the investigational drug or an explanation of why the use of the investigational drug is preferable to the use of available marketed treatments.

(iii) A brief description of the criteria for patient selection.

(iv) The method of administration of the drug and the dosages.

(v) A description of clinical procedures, laboratory tests, or other measures to monitor the effects of the drug and to minimize risk.

(2) A treatment protocol is to be supported by the following:

(i) Informational brochure for supplying to each treating physician.

(ii) The technical information that is relevant to safety and effectiveness of the drug for the intended treatment purpose. Information contained in the sponsor's IND may be incorporated by reference.

(iii) A commitment by the sponsor to assure compliance of all participating investigators with the informed consent requirements of 21 CFR part 50.

(3) A licensed practioner who receives an investigational drug for treatment use under a treatment protocol is an "investigator" under the protocol and is responsible for meeting all applicable investigator responsibilities under this part and 21 CFR parts 50 and 56.

(b) Treatment IND submitted by licensed practitioner. (1) If a licensed medical practitioner wants to obtain an investigational drug subject to a controlled clinical trial for a treatment use, the practitioner should first attempt to obtain the drug from the sponsor of the controlled trial under a treatment protocol. If the sponsor of the controlled clinical investigation of the drug will not establish a treatment protocol for the drug under paragraph (a) of this section, the licensed medical practitioner may seek to obtain the drug from the sponsor and submit a treatment IND to FDA requesting authorization to use the investigational drug for treatment use. A treatment use under a treatment IND may begin 30 days after FDA receives the IND or on earlier notification by FDA that the treatment use under the IND may begin. A treatment IND is required to contain the following:

(i) A cover sheet (Form FDA 1571) meeting §312.23(g)(1).

(ii) Information (when not provided by the sponsor) on the drug's chemistry, manufacturing, and controls, and prior clinical and nonclinical experience with the drug submitted in accordance with §312.23. A sponsor of a clinical investigation subject to an IND who supplies an investigational drug to a licensed medical practitioner for purposes of a separate treatment clinical investigation shall be deemed to authorize the incorporation-by-reference of the technical information contained in the sponsor's IND into the medical practitioner's treatment IND.

(iii) A statement of the steps taken by the practitioner to obtain the drug under a treatment protocol from the drug sponsor.

(iv) A treatment protocol containing the same information listed in paragraph (a)(1) of this section.

(v) A statement of the practitioner's qualifications to use the investigational drug for the intended treatment use.

(vi) The practitioner's statement of familiarity with information on the drug's safety and effectiveness derived from previous clinical and nonclinical experience with the drug.

(vii) Agreement to report to FDA safety information in accordance with §312.32.

(2) A licensed practitioner who submits a treatment IND under this section is the sponsor-investigator for such IND and is

responsible for meeting all applicable sponsor and investigator responsibilities under this part and 21 CFR parts 50 and 56.

[52 FR 19477, May 22, 1987, as amended at 57 FR 13249, Apr. 15, 1992; 67 FR 9585, Mar. 4, 2002]

§312.36 Emergency use of an investigational new drug (IND).

Need for an investigational drug may arise in an emergency situation that does not allow time for submission of an IND in accordance with §312.23 or §312.34. In such a case, FDA may authorize shipment of the drug for a specified use in advance of submission of an IND. A request for such authorization may be transmitted to FDA by telephone or other rapid communication means. For investigational biological drugs regulated by the Center for Biologics Evaluation and Research, the request should be directed to the Office of Communication, Training and Manufacturers Assistance (HFM–40), Center for Biologics Evaluation and Research, 301–827–2000. For all other investigational drugs, the request for authorization should be directed to the Division of Drug Information (HFD–240), Center for Drug Evaluation and Research, 301–827–4570. After normal working hours, eastern standard time, the request should be directed to the FDA Office of Emergency Operations (HFA–615), 301–443–1240. Except in extraordinary circumstances, such authorization will be conditioned on the sponsor making an appropriate IND submission as soon as practicable after receiving the authorization.

[69 FR 17927, Apr. 6, 2004]

§312.38 Withdrawal of an IND.

(a) At any time a sponsor may withdraw an effective IND without prejudice.

(b) If an IND is withdrawn, FDA shall be so notified, all clinical investigations conducted under the IND shall be ended, all current investigators notified, and all stocks of the drug returned to the sponsor or otherwise disposed of at the request of the sponsor in accordance with §312.59.

(c) If an IND is withdrawn because of a safety reason, the sponsor shall promptly so inform FDA, all participating investigators, and all reviewing Institutional Review Boards, together with the reasons for such withdrawal.

[52 FR 8831, Mar. 19, 1987, as amended at 52 FR 23031, June 17, 1987; 67 FR 9586, Mar. 4, 2002]

Subpart C—Administrative Actions

§312.40 General requirements for use of an investigational new drug in a clinical investigation.

(a) An investigational new drug may be used in a clinical investigation if the following conditions are met:

(1) The sponsor of the investigation submits an IND for the drug to FDA; the IND is in effect under paragraph (b) of this section; and the sponsor complies with all applicable requirements in this part and parts 50 and 56 with respect to the conduct of the clinical investigations; and

(2) Each participating investigator conducts his or her investigation in compliance with the requirements of this part and parts 50 and 56.

(b) An IND goes into effect:

(1) Thirty days after FDA receives the IND, unless FDA notifies the sponsor that the investigations described in the IND are subject to a clinical hold under §312.42; or

(2) On earlier notification by FDA that the clinical investigations in the IND may begin. FDA will notify the sponsor in writing of the date it receives the IND.

(c) A sponsor may ship an investigational new drug to investigators named in the IND:

(1) Thirty days after FDA receives the IND; or

(2) On earlier FDA authorization to ship the drug.

(d) An investigator may not administer an investigational new drug to human subjects until the IND goes into effect under paragraph (b) of this section.

§312.41 Comment and advice on an IND.

(a) FDA may at any time during the course of the investigation communicate with the sponsor orally or in writing about deficiencies in the IND or about FDA's need for more data or information.

(b) On the sponsor's request, FDA will provide advice on specific matters relating to an IND. Examples of such advice may include advice on the adequacy of technical data to support an investigational plan, on the design of a clinical trial, and on whether proposed investigations are likely to produce the data and information that is needed to meet requirements for a marketing application.

(c) Unless the communication is accompanied by a clinical hold order under §312.42, FDA communications with a sponsor under this section are solely advisory and do not require any modification in the planned or ongoing clinical investigations or response to the agency.

[52 FR 8831, Mar. 19, 1987, as amended at 52 FR 23031, June 17, 1987; 67 FR 9586, Mar. 4, 2002]

§312.42 Clinical holds and requests for modification.

(a) General. A clinical hold is an order issued by FDA to the sponsor to delay a proposed clinical investigation or to suspend an ongoing investigation. The clinical hold order may apply to one or more of the investigations covered by an IND. When a proposed study is placed on clinical hold, subjects may not be given the investigational drug. When an ongoing study is placed on clinical hold, no new subjects may be recruited to the study and placed on the investigational drug; patients already in the study should be taken off therapy involving the investigational drug unless specifically permitted by FDA in the interest of patient safety.

(b) Grounds for imposition of clinical hold—(1) Clinical hold of a Phase 1 study under an IND. FDA may place a proposed or ongoing Phase 1 investigation on clinical hold if it finds that:

(i) Human subjects are or would be exposed to an unreasonable and significant risk of illness or injury;

(ii) The clinical investigators named in the IND are not qualified by reason of their scientific training and experience to conduct the investigation described in the IND;

(iii) The investigator brochure is misleading, erroneous, or materially incomplete; or

(iv) The IND does not contain sufficient information required under §312.23 to assess the risks to subjects of the proposed studies.

(v) The IND is for the study of an investigational drug intended to treat a life-threatening disease or condition that affects both genders, and men or women with reproductive potential who have the disease or condition being studied are excluded from eligibility because of a risk or potential risk from use of the investigational drug of reproductive toxicity (i.e., affecting reproductive organs) or developmental toxicity (i.e., affecting potential offspring). The phrase "women with reproductive potential" does not include pregnant women. For purposes of this paragraph, "life-threatening illnesses or diseases" are defined as "diseases or conditions where the likelihood of death is high unless the course of the disease is interrupted." The clinical hold would not apply under this paragraph to clinical studies conducted:

(A) Under special circumstances, such as studies pertinent only to one gender (e.g., studies evaluating the excretion of a drug in semen or the effects on menstrual function);

(B) Only in men or women, as long as a study that does not exclude members of the other gender with reproductive potential is being conducted concurrently, has been conducted, or will take place within a reasonable time agreed upon by the agency; or

(C) Only in subjects who do not suffer from the disease or condition for which the drug is being studied.

(2) Clinical hold of a Phase 2 or 3 study under an IND. FDA may place a proposed or ongoing Phase 2 or 3 investigation on clinical hold if it finds that:

(i) Any of the conditions in paragraphs (b)(1)(i) through (b)(1)(v) of this section apply; or

(ii) The plan or protocol for the investigation is clearly deficient in design to meet its stated objectives.

(3) Clinical hold of a treatment IND or treatment protocol.

(i) Proposed use. FDA may place a proposed treatment IND or treatment protocol on clinical hold if it is determined that:

(A) The pertinent criteria in §312.34(b) for permitting the treatment use to begin are not satisfied; or

(B) The treatment protocol or treatment IND does not contain the information required under §312.35 (a) or (b) to make the specified determination under §312.34(b).

(ii) Ongoing use. FDA may place an ongoing treatment protocol or treatment IND on clinical hold if it is determined that:

(A) There becomes available a comparable or satisfactory alternative drug or other therapy to treat that stage of the disease in the intended patient population for which the investigational drug is being used;

(B) The investigational drug is not under investigation in a controlled clinical trial under an IND in effect for the trial and not all controlled clinical trials necessary to support a marketing application have been completed, or a clinical study under the IND has been placed on clinical hold:

(C) The sponsor of the controlled clinical trial is not pursuing marketing approval with due diligence;

(D) If the treatment IND or treatment protocol is intended for a serious disease, there is insufficient evidence of safety and effectiveness to support such use; or

(E) If the treatment protocol or treatment IND was based on an immediately life-threatening disease, the available scientific evidence, taken as a whole, fails to provide a reasonable basis for concluding that the drug:

(1) May be effective for its intended use in its intended population; or

(2) Would not expose the patients to whom the drug is to be administered to an unreasonable and significant additional risk of illness or injury.

(iii) FDA may place a proposed or ongoing treatment IND or treatment protocol on clinical hold if it finds that any of the conditions in paragraph (b)(4)(i) through (b)(4)(viii) of this section apply.

(4) Clinical hold of any study that is not designed to be adequate and well-controlled. FDA may place a proposed or ongoing investigation that is not designed to be adequate and well-controlled on clinical hold if it finds that:

(i) Any of the conditions in paragraph (b)(1) or (b)(2) of this section apply; or

(ii) There is reasonable evidence the investigation that is not designed to be adequate and well-controlled is impeding enrollment in, or otherwise interfering with the conduct or completion of, a study that is designed to be an adequate and well-controlled investigation of the same or another investigational drug; or

(iii) Insufficient quantities of the investigational drug exist to adequately conduct both the investigation that is not designed to be adequate and well-controlled and the investigations that are designed to be adequate and well-controlled; or

(iv) The drug has been studied in one or more adequate and well-controlled investigations that strongly suggest lack of effectiveness; or

(v) Another drug under investigation or approved for the same indication and available to the same patient population has demonstrated a better potential benefit/risk balance; or

(vi) The drug has received marketing approval for the same indication in the same patient population; or

(vii) The sponsor of the study that is designed to be an adequate and well-controlled investigation is not actively pursuing marketing approval of the investigational drug with due diligence; or

(viii) The Commissioner determines that it would not be in the public interest for the study to be conducted or continued. FDA ordinarily intends that clinical holds under paragraphs (b)(4)(ii), (b)(4)(iii) and (b)(4)(v) of this section would only apply to additional enrollment in nonconcurrently controlled trials rather than eliminating continued access to individuals already receiving the investigational drug.

(5) Clinical hold of any investigation involving an exception from informed consent under §50.24 of this chapter. FDA may place a proposed or ongoing investigation involving an exception from informed consent under §50.24 of this chapter on clinical hold if it is determined that:

(i) Any of the conditions in paragraphs (b)(1) or (b)(2) of this section apply; or

(ii) The pertinent criteria in §50.24 of this chapter for such an investigation to begin or continue are not submitted or not satisfied.

(6) Clinical hold of any investigation involving an exception from informed consent under §50.23(d) of this chapter. FDA may place a proposed or ongoing investigation involving an exception from informed consent under §50.23(d) of this chapter on clinical hold if it is determined that:

(i) Any of the conditions in paragraphs (b)(1) or (b)(2) of this section apply; or

(ii) A determination by the President to waive the prior consent requirement for the administration of an investigational new drug has not been made.

(c) Discussion of deficiency. Whenever FDA concludes that a deficiency exists in a clinical investigation that may be grounds for the imposition of clinical hold FDA will, unless patients are exposed to immediate and serious risk, attempt to discuss and satisfactorily resolve the matter with the sponsor before issuing the clinical hold order.

(d) Imposition of clinical hold. The clinical hold order may be made by telephone or other means of rapid communication or in writing. The clinical hold order will identify the studies under the IND to which the hold applies, and will briefly explain the basis for the action. The clinical hold order will be made by or on behalf of the Division Director with responsibility for review of the IND. As soon as possible, and no more than 30 days after imposition of the clinical hold, the Division Director will provide the sponsor a written explanation of the basis for the hold.

(e) Resumption of clinical investigations. An investigation may only resume after FDA (usually the Division Director, or the Director's designee, with responsibility for review of the IND) has notified the sponsor that the investigation may proceed. Resumption of the affected investigation(s) will be authorized when the sponsor corrects the deficiency(ies) previously cited or otherwise satisfies the agency that the investigation(s) can proceed. FDA may notify a sponsor of its determination regarding the clinical hold by telephone or other means of rapid communication. If a sponsor of an IND that has been placed on clinical hold requests in writing that the clinical hold be removed and submits a complete response to the issue(s) identified in the clinical hold order, FDA shall respond in writing to the sponsor within 30-calendar days of receipt of the request and the complete response. FDA's response will either remove or maintain the clinical hold, and will state the reasons for such determination. Notwithstanding the 30-calendar day response time, a sponsor may not proceed with a clinical trial on which a clinical hold has been imposed until the sponsor has been notified by FDA that the hold has been lifted.

(f) Appeal. If the sponsor disagrees with the reasons cited for the clinical hold, the sponsor may request reconsideration of the decision in accordance with §312.48.

(g) Conversion of IND on clinical hold to inactive status. If all investigations covered by an IND remain on clinical hold for 1 year or more, the IND may be placed on inactive status by FDA under §312.45.

[52 FR 8831, Mar. 19, 1987, as amended at 52 FR 19477, May 22, 1987; 57 FR 13249, Apr. 15, 1992; 61 FR 51530, Oct. 2, 1996; 63 FR 68678, Dec. 14, 1998; 64 FR 54189, Oct. 5, 1999; 65 FR 34971, June 1, 2000]

§312.44 Termination.

(a) General. This section describes the procedures under which FDA may terminate an IND. If an IND is terminated, the sponsor shall end all clinical investigations conducted under the IND and recall or otherwise provide for the disposition of all unused supplies of the drug. A termination action may be based on deficiencies in the IND or in the conduct of an investigation under an IND. Except as provided in paragraph (d) of this section, a termination shall be preceded by a proposal to terminate by FDA and an opportunity for the sponsor to respond. FDA will, in general, only initiate an action under this section after first attempting to resolve differences informally or, when appropriate, through the clinical hold procedures described in §312.42.

(b) Grounds for termination—(1) Phase 1. FDA may propose to terminate an IND during Phase 1 if it finds that:

(i) Human subjects would be exposed to an unreasonable and significant risk of illness or unjury.

(ii) The IND does not contain sufficient information required under §312.23 to assess the safety to subjects of the clinical investigations.

(iii) The methods, facilities, and controls used for the manufacturing, processing, and packing of the investigational drug are inadequate to establish and maintain appropriate standards of identity, strength, quality, and purity as needed for subject safety.

(iv) The clinical investigations are being conducted in a manner substantially different than that described in the protocols submitted in the IND.

(v) The drug is being promoted or distributed for commercial purposes not justified by the requirements of the investigation or permitted by §312.7.

(vi) The IND, or any amendment or report to the IND, contains an untrue statement of a material fact or omits material information required by this part.

(vii) The sponsor fails promptly to investigate and inform the Food and Drug Administration and all investigators of serious and unexpected adverse experiences in accordance with §312.32 or fails to make any other report required under this part.

(viii) The sponsor fails to submit an accurate annual report of the investigations in accordance with §312.33.

(ix) The sponsor fails to comply with any other applicable requirement of this part, part 50, or part 56.

(x) The IND has remained on inactive status for 5 years or more.

(xi) The sponsor fails to delay a proposed investigation under the IND or to suspend an ongoing investigation that has been placed on clinical hold under §312.42(b)(4).

(2) Phase 2 or 3. FDA may propose to terminate an IND during Phase 2 or Phase 3 if FDA finds that:

(i) Any of the conditions in paragraphs (b)(1)(i) through (b)(1)(xi) of this section apply; or

(ii) The investigational plan or protocol(s) is not reasonable as a bona fide scientific plan to determine whether or not the drug is safe and effective for use; or

(iii) There is convincing evidence that the drug is not effective for the purpose for which it is being investigated.

(3) FDA may propose to terminate a treatment IND if it finds that:

(i) Any of the conditions in paragraphs (b)(1)(i) through (x) of this section apply; or

(ii) Any of the conditions in §312.42(b)(3) apply.

(c) Opportunity for sponsor response. (1) If FDA proposes to terminate an IND, FDA will notify the sponsor in writing, and invite correction or explanation within a period of 30 days.

(2) On such notification, the sponsor may provide a written explanation or correction or may request a conference with FDA to provide the requested explanation or correction. If the sponsor does not respond to the notification within the allocated time, the IND shall be terminated.

(3) If the sponsor responds but FDA does not accept the explanation or correction submitted, FDA shall inform the sponsor in writing of the reason for the nonacceptance and provide the sponsor with an opportunity for a regulatory hearing before FDA under part 16 on the question of whether the IND should be terminated. The sponsor's request for a regulatory hearing must be made within 10 days of the sponsor's receipt of FDA's notification of nonacceptance.

(d) Immediate termination of IND. Notwith-standing paragraphs (a) through (c) of this section, if at any time FDA concludes that continuation of the investigation presents an immediate and substantial danger to the health of individuals, the agency shall immediately, by written notice to the sponsor from the Director of the Center for Drug Evaluation and Research or the Director of the Center for Biologics Evaluation and Research, terminate the IND. An IND so terminated is subject to reinstatement by the Director on the basis of additional submissions that eliminate such danger. If an IND is terminated under this paragraph, the agency will afford the sponsor an opportunity for a regulatory hearing under part 16 on the question of whether the IND should be reinstated.

[52 FR 8831, Mar. 19, 1987, as amended at 52 FR 23031, June 17, 1987; 55 FR 11579, Mar. 29, 1990; 57 FR 13249, Apr. 15, 1992; 67 FR 9586, Mar. 4, 2002]

§312.45 Inactive status.

(a) If no subjects are entered into clinical studies for a period of 2 years or more under an IND, or if all investigations under an IND remain on clinical hold for 1 year or more, the IND may be placed by FDA on inactive status. This action may be taken by FDA either on request of the sponsor or on FDA's own initiative. If FDA seeks to act on its own initiative under this section, it shall first notify the sponsor in writing of the proposed inactive status. Upon receipt of such notification, the sponsor shall have 30 days to respond as to why the IND should continue to remain active.

(b) If an IND is placed on inactive status, all investigators shall be so notified and all stocks of the drug shall be returned or otherwise disposed of in accordance with §312.59.

(c) A sponsor is not required to submit annual reports to an IND on inactive status. An inactive IND is, however, still in effect for purposes of the public disclosure of data and information under §312.130.

(d) A sponsor who intends to resume clinical investigation under an IND placed on inactive status shall submit a protocol amendment under §312.30 containing the proposed general investigational plan for the coming year and appropriate protocols. If the protocol amendment relies on information previously submitted, the plan shall reference such information. Additional information supporting the proposed investigation, if any, shall be submitted in an information amendment. Notwithstanding the provisions of §312.30, clinical investigations under an IND on inactive status may only resume (1) 30 days after FDA receives the protocol amendment, unless FDA notifies the sponsor that the investigations described in the amendment are subject to a clinical hold under §312.42, or (2) on earlier notification by FDA that the clinical investigations described in the protocol amendment may begin.

(e) An IND that remains on inactive status for 5 years or more may be terminated under §312.44.

[52 FR 8831, Mar. 19, 1987, as amended at 52 FR 23031, June 17, 1987; 67 FR 9586, Mar. 4, 2002]

§312.47 Meetings.

(a) General. Meetings between a sponsor and the agency are frequently useful in resolving questions and issues raised during the course of a clinical investigation. FDA encourages such meetings to the extent that they aid in the evaluation of the drug and in the solution of scientific problems concerning the drug, to the extent that FDA's resources permit. The general principle underlying the conduct of such meetings is that there should be free, full, and open communication about any scientific or medical question that may arise during the clinical investigation. These meetings shall be conducted and documented in accordance with part 10.

(b) "End-of-Phase 2" meetings and meetings held before submission of a marketing application. At specific times during the drug investigation process, meetings between FDA and a sponsor can be especially helpful in minimizing wasteful expenditures of time and money and thus in speeding the drug development and evaluation process. In particular, FDA has found that meetings at the end of Phase 2 of an investigation (end-of-Phase 2 meetings) are of considerable assistance in planning later studies and that meetings held near completion of Phase 3 and before submission of a marketing application ("pre-NDA" meetings) are helpful in developing methods of presentation and submission of data in the marketing application that facilitate review and allow timely FDA response.

(1) End-of-Phase 2 meetings—(i) Purpose. The purpose of an end-of-phase 2 meeting is to determine the safety of proceeding to Phase 3, to evaluate the Phase 3 plan and protocols and the adequacy of current studies and plans to assess pediatric safety and effectiveness, and to identify any additional information necessary to support a marketing application for the uses under investigation.

(ii) Eligibility for meeting. While the end-of-Phase 2 meeting is designed primarily for IND's involving new molecular entities or major new uses of marketed drugs, a sponsor of any IND may request and obtain an end-of-Phase 2 meeting.

(iii) Timing. To be most useful to the sponsor, end-of-Phase 2 meetings should be held before major commitments of effort and resources to specific Phase 3 tests are made. The scheduling of an end-of-Phase 2 meeting is not, however, intended to delay the transition of an investigation from Phase 2 to Phase 3.

(iv) Advance information. At least 1 month in advance of an end-of-Phase 2 meeting, the sponsor should submit background information on the sponsor's plan for Phase 3, including summaries of the Phase 1 and 2 investigations, the specific protocols for Phase 3 clinical studies, plans for any additional nonclinical studies, plans for pediatric studies, including a time line for protocol finalization, enrollment, completion, and data analysis, or information to support any planned request for waiver or deferral of pediatric studies, and, if available, tentative labeling for the drug. The recommended contents of such a submission are described more fully in FDA Staff Manual Guide 4850.7 that is publicly available under FDA's public information regulations in part 20.

(v) Conduct of meeting. Arrangements for an end-of-Phase 2 meeting are to be made with the division in FDA's Center for Drug Evaluation and Research or the Center for Biologics Evaluation and Research which is responsible for review of the IND. The meeting will be scheduled by FDA at a time convenient to both FDA and the sponsor. Both the sponsor and FDA may bring consultants to the meeting. The meeting should be directed primarily at establishing agreement between FDA and the sponsor of the overall plan for Phase 3 and the objectives and design of particular studies. The adequacy of the technical information to support Phase 3 studies and/or a marketing application may also be discussed. FDA will also provide its best judgment, at that time, of the pediatric studies that will be required for the drug product and whether their submission will be deferred until after approval. Agreements reached at the meeting on these matters will be recorded in minutes of the conference that will be taken by FDA in accordance with §10.65 and provided to the sponsor. The minutes along with any other written material provided to the sponsor will serve as a permanent record of any agreements reached. Barring a significant scientific development that requires otherwise, studies conducted in accordance with the agreement shall be presumed to be sufficient in objective and design for the purpose of obtaining marketing approval for the drug.

(2) "Pre-NDA" and "pre-BLA" meetings. FDA has found that delays associated with the initial review of a marketing application may be reduced by exchanges of informa-

tion about a proposed marketing application. The primary purpose of this kind of exchange is to uncover any major unresolved problems, to identify those studies that the sponsor is relying on as adequate and well-controlled to establish the drug's effectiveness, to identify the status of ongoing or needed studies adequate to assess pediatric safety and effectiveness, to acquaint FDA reviewers with the general information to be submitted in the marketing application (including technical information), to discuss appropriate methods for statistical analysis of the data, and to discuss the best approach to the presentation and formatting of data in the marketing application. Arrangements for such a meeting are to be initiated by the sponsor with the division responsible for review of the IND. To permit FDA to provide the sponsor with the most useful advice on preparing a marketing application, the sponsor should submit to FDA's reviewing division at least 1 month in advance of the meeting the following information:

(i) A brief summary of the clinical studies to be submitted in the application.

(ii) A proposed format for organizing the submission, including methods for presenting the data.

(iii) Information on the status of needed or ongoing pediatric studies.

(iv) Any other information for discussion at the meeting.

[52 FR 8831, Mar. 19, 1987, as amended at 52 FR 23031, June 17, 1987; 55 FR 11580, Mar. 29, 1990; 63 FR 66669, Dec. 2, 1998; 67 FR 9586, Mar. 4, 2002]

§312.48 Dispute resolution.

(a) General. The Food and Drug Administration is committed to resolving differences between sponsors and FDA reviewing divisions with respect to requirements for IND's as quickly and amicably as possible through the cooperative exchange of information and views.

(b) Administrative and procedural issues. When administrative or procedural disputes arise, the sponsor should first attempt to resolve the matter with the division in FDA's Center for Drug Evaluation and Research or Center for Biologics Evaluation and Research which is responsible for review of the IND, beginning with the consumer safety officer assigned to the application. If the dispute is not resolved, the sponsor may raise the matter with the person designated as ombudsman, whose function shall be to investigate what has happened and to facilitate a timely and equitable resolution. Appropriate issues to raise with the ombudsman include resolving difficulties in scheduling meetings and obtaining timely replies to inquiries. Further details on this procedure are contained in FDA Staff Manual Guide 4820.7 that is publicly available under FDA's public information regulations in part 20.

(c) Scientific and medical disputes. (1) When scientific or medical disputes arise during the drug investigation process, sponsors should discuss the matter directly with the responsible reviewing officials. If necessary, sponsors may request a meeting with the appropriate reviewing officials and management representatives in order to seek a resolution. Requests for such meetings shall be directed to the director of the division in FDA's Center for Drug Evaluation and Research or Center for Biologics Evaluation and Research which is responsible for review of the IND. FDA will make every attempt to grant requests for meetings that involve important issues and that can be scheduled at mutually convenient times.

(2) The "end-of-Phase 2" and "pre-NDA" meetings described in §312.47(b) will also provide a timely forum for discussing and resolving scientific and medical issues on which the sponsor disagrees with the agency.

(3) In requesting a meeting designed to resolve a scientific or medical dispute, applicants may suggest that FDA seek the advice of outside experts, in which case FDA may, in its discretion, invite to the meeting one or more of its advisory committee members or other consultants, as designated by the agency. Applicants may rely on, and may bring to any meeting, their own consultants. For major scientific and medical policy issues not resolved by informal meetings, FDA may refer the matter to one of its standing advisory committees for its consideration and recommendations.

[52 FR 8831, Mar. 19, 1987, as amended at 55 FR 11580, Mar. 29, 1990]

Subpart D—Responsibilities of Sponsors and Investigators

§312.50 General responsibilities of sponsors.

Sponsors are responsibile for selecting qualified investigators, providing them with the information they need to conduct an investigation properly, ensuring proper monitoring of the investigation(s), ensuring that the investigation(s) is conducted in accordance with the general investigational plan and protocols contained in the IND, maintaining an effective IND with respect to the investigations, and ensuring that FDA and all participating investigators are promptly informed of significant new adverse effects or risks with respect to the drug. Additional specific responsibilities of sponsors are described elsewhere in this part.

§312.52 Transfer of obligations to a contract research organization.

(a) A sponsor may transfer responsibility for any or all of the obligations set forth in this part to a contract research organization. Any such transfer shall be described in writing. If not all obligations are transferred, the writing is required to describe each of the obligations being assumed by the contract research organization. If all obligations are transferred, a general statement that all obligations have been transferred is acceptable. Any obligation not covered by the written description shall be deemed not to have been transferred.

(b) A contract research organization that assumes any obligation of a sponsor shall comply with the specific regulations in this chapter applicable to this obligation and shall be subject to the same regulatory action as a sponsor for failure to comply with any obligation assumed under these regulations. Thus, all references to "sponsor" in this part apply to a contract research organization to the extent that it assumes one or more obligations of the sponsor.

§312.53 Selecting investigators and monitors.

(a) Selecting investigators. A sponsor shall select only investigators qualified by training and experience as appropriate experts to investigate the drug.

(b) Control of drug. A sponsor shall ship investigational new drugs only to investigators participating in the investigation.

(c) Obtaining information from the investigator. Before permitting an investigator to begin participation in an investigation, the sponsor shall obtain the following:

(1) A signed investigator statement (Form FDA-1572) containing:

(i) The name and address of the investigator;

(ii) The name and code number, if any, of the protocol(s) in the IND identifying the study(ies) to be conducted by the investigator;

(iii) The name and address of any medical school, hospital, or other research facility where the clinical investigation(s) will be conducted;

(iv) The name and address of any clinical laboratory facilities to be used in the study;

(v) The name and address of the IRB that is responsible for review and approval of the study(ies);

(vi) A commitment by the investigator that he or she:

(a) Will conduct the study(ies) in accordance with the relevant, current protocol(s) and will only make changes in a protocol after notifying the sponsor, except when necessary to protect the safety, the rights, or welfare of subjects;

(b) Will comply with all requirements regarding the obligations of clinical investigators and all other pertinent requirements in this part;

(c) Will personally conduct or supervise the described investigation(s);

(d) Will inform any potential subjects that the drugs are being used for investigational purposes and will ensure that the requirements relating to obtaining informed consent (21 CFR part 50) and institutional review board review and approval (21 CFR part 56) are met;

(e) Will report to the sponsor adverse experiences that occur in the course of the investigation(s) in accordance with §312.64;

(f) Has read and understands the information in the investigator's brochure, including the potential risks and side effects of the drug; and

(g) Will ensure that all associates, colleagues, and employees assisting in the conduct of the study(ies) are informed about their obligations in meeting the above commitments.

(vii) A commitment by the investigator that, for an investigation subject to an institutional review requirement under part 56, an IRB that complies with the requirements of that part will be responsible for the initial and continuing review and approval of the clinical investigation and that the investigator will promptly report to the IRB all changes in the research activity and all unanticipated problems involving risks to human subjects or others, and will not make any changes in the research without IRB approval, except where necessary to eliminate apparent immediate hazards to the human subjects.

(viii) A list of the names of the subinvestigators (e.g., research fellows, residents) who will be assisting the investigator in the conduct of the investigation(s).

(2) Curriculum vitae. A curriculum vitae or other statement of qualifications of the investigator showing the education, training, and experience that qualifies the investigator as an expert in the clinical investigation of the drug for the use under investigation.

(3) Clinical protocol. (i) For Phase 1 investigations, a general outline of the planned investigation including the estimated duration of the study and the maximum number of subjects that will be involved.

(ii) For Phase 2 or 3 investigations, an outline of the study protocol including an approximation of the number of subjects to be treated with the drug and the number to be employed as controls, if any; the clinical uses to be investigated; characteristics of subjects by age, sex, and condition; the kind of clinical observations and laboratory tests to be conducted; the estimated duration of the study; and copies or a description of case report forms to be used.

(4) Financial disclosure information. Sufficient accurate financial information to allow the sponsor to submit complete and accurate certification or disclosure statements required under part 54 of this chapter. The sponsor shall obtain a commitment from the clinical investigator to promptly update this information if any relevant changes occur during the course of the investigation and for 1 year following the completion of the study.

(d) Selecting monitors. A sponsor shall select a monitor qualified by training and experience to monitor the progress of the investigation.

[52 FR 8831, Mar. 19, 1987, as amended at 52 FR 23031, June 17, 1987; 61 FR 57280, Nov. 5, 1996; 63 FR 5252, Feb. 2, 1998; 67 FR 9586, Mar. 4, 2002]

§312.54 Emergency research under §50.24 of this chapter.

(a) The sponsor shall monitor the progress of all investigations involving an exception from informed consent under §50.24 of this chapter. When the sponsor receives from the IRB information concerning the public disclosures required by §50.24(a)(7)(ii) and (a)(7)(iii) of this chapter, the sponsor promptly shall submit to the IND file and to Docket Number 95S-0158 in the Dockets Management Branch (HFA-305), Food and Drug Administration, 5630 Fishers Lane, rm. 1061, Rockville, MD 20852, copies of the information that was disclosed, identified by the IND number.

(b) The sponsor also shall monitor such investigations to identify when an IRB determines that it cannot approve the research because it does not meet the criteria in the exception in §50.24(a) of this chapter or because of other relevant ethical concerns. The sponsor promptly shall provide this information in writing to FDA, investigators who are asked to participate in this or a substantially equivalent clinical investigation, and other IRB's that are asked to review this or a substantially equivalent investigation.

[61 FR 51530, Oct. 2, 1996, as amended at 68 FR 24879, May 9, 2003]

§312.55 Informing investigators.

(a) Before the investigation begins, a sponsor (other than a sponsor-investigator) shall give each participating clinical investigator an investigator brochure containing the information described in §312.23(a)(5).

(b) The sponsor shall, as the overall investigation proceeds, keep each participating investigator informed of new observations discovered by or reported to the sponsor on the drug, particularly with respect to adverse effects and safe use. Such information may be distributed to investigators by means of periodically revised investigator brochures, reprints or published studies, reports or letters to clinical investigators, or other appropriate means. Important safety information is required to be relayed to investigators in accordance with §312.32.

[52 FR 8831, Mar. 19, 1987, as amended at 52 FR 23031, June 17, 1987; 67 FR 9586, Mar. 4, 2002]

§312.56 Review of ongoing investigations.

(a) The sponsor shall monitor the progress of all clinical investigations being conducted under its IND.

(b) A sponsor who discovers that an investigator is not complying with the signed agreement (Form FDA-1572), the general investigational plan, or the requirements of this part or other applicable parts shall promptly either secure compliance or discontinue shipments of the investigational new drug to the investigator and end the investigator's participation in the investigation. If the investigator's participation in the investigation is ended, the sponsor shall require that the investigator dispose of or return the investigational drug in accordance with the requirements of §312.59 and shall notify FDA.

(c) The sponsor shall review and evaluate the evidence relating to the safety and effectiveness of the drug as it is obtained from the investigator. The sponsors shall make such reports to FDA regarding information relevant to the safety of the drug as are required under §312.32. The sponsor shall make annual reports on the progress of the investigation in accordance with §312.33.

(d) A sponsor who determines that its investigational drug presents an unreasonable and significant risk to subjects shall discontinue those investigations that present the risk, notify FDA, all institutional review boards, and all investigators who have at any time participated in the investigation of the discontinuance, assure the disposition of all stocks of the drug outstanding as required by §312.59, and furnish FDA with a full report of the sponsor's actions. The sponsor shall discontinue the investigation as soon as possible, and in no event later than 5 working days after making the determination that the investigation should be discontinued. Upon request, FDA will confer with a sponsor on the need to discontinue an investigation.

[52 FR 8831, Mar. 19, 1987, as amended at 52 FR 23031, June 17, 1987; 67 FR 9586, Mar. 4, 2002]

§312.57 Recordkeeping and record retention.

(a) A sponsor shall maintain adequate records showing the receipt, shipment, or other disposition of the investigational drug. These records are required to include, as appropriate, the name of the investigator to whom the drug is shipped, and the date, quantity, and batch or code mark of each such shipment.

(b) A sponsor shall maintain complete and accurate records showing any financial interest in §54.4(a)(3)(i), (a)(3)(ii), (a)(3)(iii), and (a)(3)(iv) of this chapter paid to clinical investigators by the sponsor of the covered study. A sponsor shall also maintain complete and accurate records concerning all other financial interests of investigators subject to part 54 of this chapter.

(c) A sponsor shall retain the records and reports required by this part for 2 years after a marketing application is approved for the drug; or, if an application is not approved for the drug, until 2 years after shipment and delivery of the drug for investigational use is discontinued and FDA has been so notified.

(d) A sponsor shall retain reserve samples of any test article and reference standard identified in, and used in any of the bioequivalence or bioavailability studies described in, §320.38 or §320.63 of this chapter, and release the reserve samples to FDA upon request, in accordance with, and for the period specified in §320.38.

[52 FR 8831, Mar. 19, 1987, as amended at 52 FR 23031, June 17, 1987; 58 FR 25926, Apr. 28, 1993; 63 FR 5252, Feb. 2, 1998; 67 FR 9586, Mar. 4, 2002]

§312.58 Inspection of sponsor's records and reports.

(a) FDA inspection. A sponsor shall upon request from any properly authorized officer or employee of the Food and Drug Administration, at reasonable times, permit such officer or employee to have access to and copy and verify any records and reports relating to a clinical investigation conducted under this part. Upon written request by FDA, the sponsor shall submit the records or reports (or copies of them) to FDA. The sponsor shall discontinue shipments of the drug to any investigator who has failed to maintain or make available records or reports of the investigation as required by this part.

(b) Controlled substances. If an investigational new drug is a substance listed in any schedule of the Controlled Substances Act (21 U.S.C. 801; 21 CFR part 1308), records concerning shipment, delivery, receipt, and disposition of the drug, which are required to be kept under this part or other applicable parts of this chapter shall, upon the request of a properly authorized employee of the Drug Enforcement Administration of the U.S. Department of Justice, be made available by the investigator or sponsor to whom the request is made, for inspection and copying. In addition, the sponsor shall assure that adequate precautions are taken, including storage of the investigational drug in a securely locked, substantially constructed cabinet, or other securely locked, substantially constructed enclosure, access to which is limited, to prevent theft or diversion of the substance into illegal channels of distribution.

§312.59 Disposition of unused supply of investigational drug.

The sponsor shall assure the return of all unused supplies of the investigational drug from each individual investigator whose participation in the investigation is discontinued or terminated. The sponsor may authorize alternative disposition of unused supplies of the investigational drug provided this alternative disposition does not expose humans to risks from the drug. The sponsor shall maintain written records of any disposition of the drug in accordance with §312.57.

[52 FR 8831, Mar. 19, 1987, as amended at 52 FR 23031, June 17, 1987; 67 FR 9586, Mar. 4, 2002]

§312.60 General responsibilities of investigators.

An investigator is responsible for ensuring that an investigation is conducted according to the signed investigator statement, the investigational plan, and applicable regulations; for protecting the rights, safety, and welfare of subjects under the investigator's care; and for the control of drugs under investigation. An investigator shall, in accordance with the provisions of part 50 of this chapter, obtain the informed consent of each human subject to whom the drug is administered, except as provided in §§50.23 or 50.24 of this chapter. Additional specific responsibilities of clinical investigators are set forth in this part and in parts 50 and 56 of this chapter.

[52 FR 8831, Mar. 19, 1987, as amended at 61 FR 51530, Oct. 2, 1996]

§312.61 Control of the investigational drug.

An investigator shall administer the drug only to subjects under the investigator's personal supervision or under the supervision of a subinvestigator responsible to the investigator. The investigator shall not supply the investigational drug to any person not authorized under this part to receive it.

§312.62 Investigator recordkeeping and record retention.

(a) Disposition of drug. An investigator is required to maintain adequate records of the disposition of the drug, including dates, quantity, and use by subjects. If the investigation is terminated, suspended, discontinued, or completed, the investigator shall return the unused supplies of the drug to the sponsor, or otherwise provide for disposition of the unused supplies of the drug under §312.59.

(b) Case histories. An investigator is required to prepare and maintain adequate and accurate case histories that record all observations and other data pertinent to the investigation on each individual administered the investigational drug or employed as a control in the investigation. Case histories include the case report forms and supporting data including, for example, signed and dated consent forms and medical records including, for example, progress notes of the physician, the individual's hospital chart(s), and the nurses' notes. The case history for each individual shall document that informed consent was obtained prior to participation in the study.

(c) Record retention. An investigator shall retain records required to be maintained under this part for a period of 2 years following the date a marketing application is approved for the drug for the indication for which it is being investigated; or, if no application is to be filed or if the application is not approved for such indication, until 2 years after the investigation is discontinued and FDA is notified.

[52 FR 8831, Mar. 19, 1987, as amended at 52 FR 23031, June 17, 1987; 61 FR 57280, Nov. 5, 1996; 67 FR 9586, Mar. 4, 2002]

§312.64 Investigator reports.

(a) Progress reports. The investigator shall furnish all reports to the sponsor of the drug who is responsible for collecting and evaluating the results obtained. The sponsor is required under §312.33 to submit annual reports to FDA on the progress of the clinical investigations.

(b) Safety reports. An investigator shall promptly report to the sponsor any adverse effect that may reasonably be regarded as caused by, or probably caused by, the drug. If the adverse effect is alarming, the investigator shall report the adverse effect immediately.

(c) Final report. An investigator shall provide the sponsor with an adequate report shortly after completion of the investigator's participation in the investigation.

(d) Financial disclosure reports. The clinical investigator shall provide the sponsor with sufficient accurate financial information to allow an applicant to submit complete and accurate certification or disclosure statements as required under part 54 of this chapter. The clinical investigator shall promptly update this information if any relevant changes occur during the course of the investigation and for 1 year following the completion of the study.

[52 FR 8831, Mar. 19, 1987, as amended at 52 FR 23031, June 17, 1987; 63 FR 5252, Feb. 2, 1998; 67 FR 9586, Mar. 4, 2002]

§312.66 Assurance of IRB review.

An investigator shall assure that an IRB that complies with the requirements set forth in part 56 will be responsible for the initial and continuing review and approval of the proposed clinical study. The investigator shall also assure that he or she will promptly report to the IRB all changes in the research activity and all unanticipated problems involving risk to human subjects or others, and that he or she will not make any changes in the research without IRB approval, except where necessary to eliminate apparent immediate hazards to human subjects.

[52 FR 8831, Mar. 19, 1987, as amended at 52 FR 23031, June 17, 1987; 67 FR 9586, Mar. 4, 2002]

§312.68 Inspection of investigator's records and reports.

An investigator shall upon request from any properly authorized officer or employee of FDA, at reasonable times, permit such officer or employee to have access to, and copy and verify any records or reports made by the investigator pursuant to §312.62. The investigator is not required to divulge subject names unless the records of particular individuals require a more detailed study of the cases, or unless there is reason to believe that the records do not represent actual case studies, or do not represent actual results obtained.

§312.69 Handling of controlled substances.

If the investigational drug is subject to the Controlled Substances Act, the investigator shall take adequate precautions, including storage of the investigational drug in a securely locked, substantially constructed cabinet, or other securely locked, substantially constructed enclosure, access to which is limited, to prevent theft or diversion of the substance into illegal channels of distribution.

§312.70 Disqualification of a clinical investigator.

(a) If FDA has information indicating that an investigator (including a sponsor-investigator) has repeatedly or deliberately failed to comply with the requirements of this part, part 50, or part 56 of this chapter, or has submitted to FDA or to the sponsor false information in any required report, the Center for Drug Evaluation and Research or the Center for Biologics Evaluation and Research will furnish the investigator written notice of the matter complained of and offer the investigator an opportunity to explain the matter in writing, or, at the option of the investigator, in an informal conference. If an explanation is offered but not accepted by the Center for Drug Evaluation and Research or the Center for Biologics Evaluation and Research, the investigator will be given an opportunity for a regulatory hearing under part 16 on the question of whether the investigator is entitled to receive investigational new drugs.

(b) After evaluating all available information, including any explanation presented by the investigator, if the Commissioner determines that the investigator has repeatedly or deliberately failed to comply with the requirements of this part, part 50, or part 56 of this chapter, or has deliberately or repeatedly submitted false information to FDA or to the sponsor in any required report, the Commissioner will notify the investigator and the sponsor of any investigation in which the investigator has been named as a participant that the investigator is not entitled to receive investigational drugs. The notification will provide a statement of basis for such determination.

(c) Each IND and each approved application submitted under part 314 containing data reported by an investigator who has been determined to be ineligible to receive investigational drugs will be examined to determine whether the investigator has submitted unreliable data that are essential to the continuation of the investigation or essential to the approval of any marketing application.

(d) If the Commissioner determines, after the unreliable data submitted by the investigator are eliminated from consideration, that the data remaining are inadequate to support a conclusion that it is reasonably safe to continue the investigation, the Commissioner will notify the sponsor who shall have an opportunity for a regulatory hearing under part 16. If a danger to the public health exists, however, the Commissioner shall terminate the IND immediately and notify the sponsor of the determination. In such case, the sponsor shall have an opportunity for a regulatory hearing before FDA under part 16 on the question of whether the IND should be reinstated.

(e) If the Commissioner determines, after the unreliable data submitted by the investigator are eliminated from consideration, that the continued approval of the drug product for which the data were submitted cannot be justified, the Commissioner will proceed to withdraw approval of the drug product in accordance with the applicable provisions of the act.

(f) An investigator who has been determined to be ineligible to receive investigational drugs may be reinstated as eligible when the Commissioner determines that the investigator has presented adequate assurances that the investigator will employ investigatioal drugs solely in compliance with the provisions of this part and of parts 50 and 56.

[52 FR 8831, Mar. 19, 1987, as amended at 52 FR 23031, June 17, 1987; 55 FR 11580, Mar. 29, 1990; 62 FR 46876, Sept. 5, 1997; 67 FR 9586, Mar. 4, 2002]

Subpart E—Drugs Intended to Treat Life-threatening and Severely-debilitating Illnesses

Authority: 21 U.S.C. 351, 352, 353, 355, 371; 42 U.S.C. 262.

Source: 53 FR 41523, Oct. 21, 1988, unless otherwise noted.

§312.80 Purpose.

The purpose of this section is to establish procedures designed to expedite the development, evaluation, and marketing of new therapies intended to treat persons with life-threatening and severely-debilitating illnesses, especially where no satisfactory alternative therapy exists. As stated §314.105(c) of this chapter, while the statutory standards of safety and effectiveness apply to all drugs, the many kinds of drugs that are subject to them, and the wide range of uses for those drugs, demand flexibility in applying the standards. The Food and Drug Administration (FDA) has determined that it is appropriate to exercise the broadest flexibility in applying the statutory standards, while preserving appropriate guarantees for safety and effectiveness. These procedures reflect the recognition that physicians and patients are generally willing to accept greater risks or side effects from products that treat life-threatening and severely-debilitating illnesses, than they would accept from products that treat less serious illnesses. These procedures also reflect the recognition that the benefits of the drug need to be evaluated in light of the severity of the disease being treated. The procedure outlined in this section should be interpreted consistent with that purpose.

§312.81 Scope.

This section applies to new drug and biological products that are being studied for their safety and effectiveness in treating life-threatening or severely-debilitating diseases.

(a) For purposes of this section, the term "life-threatening" means:

(1) Diseases or conditions where the likelihood of death is high unless the course of the disease is interrupted; and

(2) Diseases or conditions with potentially fatal outcomes, where the end point of clinical trial analysis is survival.

(b) For purposes of this section, the term "severely debilitating" means diseases or conditions that cause major irreversible morbidity.

(c) Sponsors are encouraged to consult with FDA on the applicability of these procedures to specific products.

[53 FR 41523, Oct. 21, 1988, as amended at 64 FR 401, Jan. 5, 1999]

§312.82 Early consultation.

For products intended to treat life-threatening or severely-debilitating illnesses, sponsors may request to meet with FDA-reviewing officials early in the drug development process to review and reach agreement on the design of necessary preclinical and clinical studies. Where appropriate, FDA will invite to such meetings one or more outside expert scientific consultants or advisory committee members. To the extent FDA resources permit, agency reviewing officials will honor requests for such meetings

(a) Pre-investigational new drug (IND) meetings. Prior to the submission of the initial IND, the sponsor may request a meeting with FDA-reviewing officials. The primary purpose of this meeting is to review and reach agreement on the design of animal studies needed to initiate human testing. The meeting may also provide an opportunity for discussing the scope and design of phase 1 testing, plans for studying the drug product in pediatric populations, and the best approach for presentation and formatting of data in the IND.

(b) End-of-phase 1 meetings. When data from phase 1 clinical testing are available, the sponsor may again request a meeting with FDA-reviewing officials. The primary purpose of this meeting is to review and reach agreement on the design of phase 2 controlled clinical trials, with the goal that such testing will be adequate to provide sufficient data on the drug's safety and effectiveness to support a decision on its approvability for marketing, and to discuss the need for, as well as the design and timing of, studies of the drug in pediatric patients. For drugs for life-threatening diseases, FDA will provide its best judgment, at that time, whether pediatric studies will be required and whether their submission will be deferred until after approval. The procedures outlined in §312.47(b)(1) with respect to end-of-phase 2 conferences, including documentation of agreements reached, would also be used for end-of-phase 1 meetings.

[53 FR 41523, Oct. 21, 1988, as amended at 63 FR 66669, Dec. 2, 1998]

§312.83 Treatment protocols.

If the preliminary analysis of phase 2 test results appears promising, FDA may ask the sponsor to submit a treatment protocol to be reviewed under the procedures and criteria listed in §§312.34 and 312.35. Such a treatment protocol, if requested and granted, would normally remain in effect while the complete data necessary for a marketing application are being assembled by the sponsor and reviewed by FDA (unless grounds exist for clinical hold of ongoing protocols, as provided in §312.42(b)(3)(ii)).

§312.84 Risk-benefit analysis in review of marketing applications for drugs to treat life-threatening and severely-debilitating illnesses.

(a) FDA's application of the statutory standards for marketing approval shall recognize the need for a medical risk-benefit judgment in making the final decision on approvability. As part of this evaluation, consistent with the statement of purpose in §312.80, FDA will consider whether the benefits of the drug outweigh the known and potential risks of the drug and the need to answer remaining questions about risks and benefits of the drug, taking into consideration the severity of the disease and the absence of satisfactory alternative therapy.

(b) In making decisions on whether to grant marketing approval for products that have been the subject of an end-of-phase 1 meeting under §312.82, FDA will usually seek the advice of outside expert scientific consultants or advisory committees. Upon the filing of such a marketing application under

§314.101 or part 601 of this chapter, FDA will notify the members of the relevant standing advisory committee of the application's filing and its availability for review.

(c) If FDA concludes that the data presented are not sufficient for marketing approval, FDA will issue (for a drug) a not approvable letter pursuant to §314.120 of this chapter, or (for a biologic) a deficiencies letter consistent with the biological product licensing procedures. Such letter, in describing the deficiencies in the application, will address why the results of the research design agreed to under §312.82, or in subsequent meetings, have not provided sufficient evidence for marketing approval. Such letter will also describe any recommendations made by the advisory committee regarding the application.

(d) Marketing applications submitted under the procedures contained in this section will be subject to the requirements and procedures contained in part 314 or part 600 of this chapter, as well as those in this subpart.

§312.85 Phase 4 studies.

Concurrent with marketing approval, FDA may seek agreement from the sponsor to conduct certain postmarketing (phase 4) studies to delineate additional information about the drug's risks, benefits, and optimal use. These studies could include, but would not be limited to, studying different doses or schedules of administration than were used in phase 2 studies, use of the drug in other patient populations or other stages of the disease, or use of the drug over a longer period of time.

§312.86 Focused FDA regulatory research.

At the discretion of the agency, FDA may undertake focused regulatory research on critical rate-limiting aspects of the preclinical, chemical/manufacturing, and clinical phases of drug development and evaluation. When initiated, FDA will undertake such research efforts as a means for meeting a public health need in facilitating the development of therapies to treat life-threatening or severely debilitating illnesses.

§312.87 Active monitoring of conduct and evaluation of clinical trials.

For drugs covered under this section, the Commissioner and other agency officials will monitor the progress of the conduct and evaluation of clinical trials and be involved in facilitating their appropriate progress.

§312.88 Safeguards for patient safety.

All of the safeguards incorporated within parts 50, 56, 312, 314, and 600 of this chapter designed to ensure the safety of clinical testing and the safety of products following marketing approval apply to drugs covered by this section. This includes the requirements for informed consent (part 50 of this chapter) and institutional review boards (part 56 of this chapter). These safeguards further include the review of animal studies prior to initial human testing (§312.23), and the monitoring of adverse drug experiences through the requirements of IND safety reports (§312.32), safety update reports during agency review of a marketing application (§314.50 of this chapter), and postmarketing adverse reaction reporting (§314.80 of this chapter).

Subpart F—Miscellaneous

§312.110 Import and exportrequirements.

(a) Imports. An investigational new drug offered for import into the United States complies with the requirements of this part if it is subject to an IND that is in effect for it under §312.40 and: (1) The consignee in the United States is the sponsor of the IND; (2) the consignee is a qualified investigator named in the IND; or (3) the consignee is the domestic agent of a foreign sponsor, is responsible for the control and distribution of the investigational drug, and the IND identifies the consignee and describes what, if any, actions the consignee will take with respect to the investigational drug.

(b) Exports. An investigational new drug intended for export from the United States complies with the requirements of this part as follows:

(1) If an IND is in effect for the drug under §312.40 and each person who receives the drug is an investigator named in the application; or

(2) If FDA authorizes shipment of the drug for use in a clinical investigation. Authorization may be obtained as follows:

(i) Through submission to the International Affairs Staff (HFY-50), Associate Commissioner for Health Affairs, Food and Drug Administra-tion, 5600 Fishers Lane, Rockville, MD 20857, of a written request from the person that seeks to export the drug. A request must provide adequate information about the drug to satisfy FDA that the drug is appropriate for the proposed investigational use in humans, that the drug will be used for investigational purposes only, and that the drug may be legally used by that consignee in the importing country for the proposed investigational use. The request shall specify the quantity of the drug to be shipped per shipment and the frequency of expected shipments. If FDA authorizes exportation under this paragraph, the agency shall concurrently notify the government of the importing country of such authorization.

(ii) Through submission to the International Affairs Staff (HFY-50), Associate Commissioner for Health Affairs, Food and Drug Administra-tion, 5600 Fishers Lane, Rockville, MD 20857, of a formal request from an authorized official of the government of the country to which the drug is proposed to be shipped. A request must specify that the foreign government has adequate information about the drug and the proposed investigational use, that the drug will be used for investigational purposes only, and that the foreign government is satisfied that the drug may legally be used by the intended consignee in that country. Such a request shall specify the quantity of drug to be shipped per shipment and the frequency of expected shipments.

(iii) Authorization to export an investigational drug under paragraph (b)(2)(i) or (ii) of this section may be revoked by FDA if the agency finds that the conditions underlying its authorization are not longer met.

(3) This paragraph applies only where the drug is to be used for the purpose of clinical investigation.

(4) This paragraph does not apply to the export of new drugs (including biological products, antibiotic drugs, and insulin) approved or authorized for export under

section 802 of the act (21 U.S.C. 382) or section 351(h)(1)(A) of the Public Health Service Act (42 U.S.C. 262(h)(1)(A)).

[52 FR 8831, Mar. 19, 1987, as amended at 52 FR 23031, June 17, 1987; 64 FR 401, Jan. 5, 1999; 67 FR 9586, Mar. 4, 2002]

§312.120 Foreign clinical studies not conducted under an IND.

(a) Introduction. This section describes the criteria for acceptance by FDA of foreign clinical studies not conducted under an IND. In general, FDA accepts such studies provided they are well designed, well conducted, performed by qualified investigators, and conducted in accordance with ethical principles acceptable to the world community. Studies meeting these criteria may be utilized to support clinical investigations in the United States and/or marketing approval. Marketing approval of a new drug based solely on foreign clinical data is governed by §314.106.

(b) Data submissions. A sponsor who wishes to rely on a foreign clinical study to support an IND or to support an application for marketing approval shall submit to FDA the following information:

(1) A description of the investigator's qualifications;

(2) A description of the research facilities;

(3) A detailed summary of the protocol and results of the study, and, should FDA request, case records maintained by the investigator or additional background data such as hospital or other institutional records;

(4) A description of the drug substance and drug product used in the study, including a description of components, formulation, specifications, and bioavailability of the specific drug product used in the clinical study, if available; and

(5) If the study is intended to support the effectiveness of a drug product, information showing that the study is adequate and well controlled under §314.126.

(c) Conformance with ethical principles. (1) Foreign clinical research is required to have been conducted in accordance with the ethical principles stated in the "Declaration of Helsinki" (see paragraph (c)(4) of this section) or the laws and regulations of the country in which the research was conducted, whichever represents the greater protection of the individual.

(2) For each foreign clinical study submitted under this section, the sponsor shall explain how the research conformed to the ethical principles contained in the "Declaration of Helsinki" or the foreign country's standards, whichever were used. If the foreign country's standards were used, the sponsor shall explain in detail how those standards differ from the "Declaration of Helsinki" and how they offer greater protection.

(3) When the research has been approved by an independent review committee, the sponsor shall submit to FDA documentation of such review and approval, including the names and qualifications of the members of the committee. In this regard, a "review committee" means a committee composed of scientists and, where practicable, individuals who are otherwise qualified (e.g., other health professionals or laymen). The investigator may not vote on any aspect of the review of his or her protocol by a review committee.

(4) The "Declaration of Helsinki" states as follows:

Recommendations Guiding Physicians in Biomedical Research Involving Human Subjects

Introduction

It is the mission of the physician to safeguard the health of the people. His or her knowledge and conscience are dedicated to the fulfillment of this mission.

The Declaration of Geneva of the World Medical Association binds the physician with the words, "The health of my patient will be my first consideration," and the International Code of Medical Ethics declares that, "A physician shall act only in the patient's interest when providing medical care which might have the effect of weakening the physical and mental condition of the patient."

The purpose of biomedical research involving human subjects must be to improve diagnostic, therapeutic and prophylactic procedures and the understanding of the aetiology and pathogenesis of disease.

In current medical practice most diagnostic, therapeutic or prophylactic procedures involve hazards. This applies especially to biomedical research.

Medical progress is based on research which ultimately must rest in part on experimentation involving human subjects.

In the field of biomedical research a fundamental distinction must be recognized between medical research in which the aim is essentially diagnostic or therapeutic for a patient, and medical research, the essential object of which is purely scientific and without implying direct diagnostic or therapeutic value to the person subjected to the research.

Special caution must be exercised in the conduct of research which may affect the environment, and the welfare of animals used for research must be respected.

Because it is essential that the results of laboratory experiments be applied to human beings to further scientific knowledge and to help suffering humanity, the World Medical Association has prepared the following recommendations as a guide to every physician in biomedical research involving human subjects. They should be kept under review in the future. It must be stressed that the standards as drafted are only a guide to physicians all over the world. Physicians are not relieved from criminal, civil and ethical responsibilities under the laws of their own countries.

I. Basic Principles

1. Biomedical research involving human subjects must conform to generally accepted scientific principles and should be based on adequately performed laboratory and animal experimentation and on a thorough knowledge of the scientific literature.

2. The design and performance of each experimental procedure involving human subjects should be clearly formulated in an experimental protocol which should be transmitted for consideration, comment and guidance to a specially appointed committee independent of the investigator and the sponsor provided that this independent committee is in conformity with the laws and regulations of the country in which the research experiment is performed.

3. Biomedical research involving human subjects should be conducted only by scientifically qualified persons and under the supervision of a clinically competent medical person. The responsibility for the human subject must always rest with a medically qualified person and never rest on the subject of the research, even though the subject has given his or her consent.

4. Biomedical research involving human subjects cannot legitimately be carried out unless the importance of the objective is in proportion to the inherent risk to the subject.

5. Every biomedical research project involving human subjects should be preceded by careful assessment of predictable risks in comparison with foreseeable benefits to the subject or to others. Concern for the interests of the subject must always prevail over the interests of science and society.

6. The right of the research subject to safeguard his or her integrity must always be respected. Every precaution should be taken to respect the privacy of the subject and to minimize the impact of the study on the subject's physical and mental integrity and on the personality of the subject.

7. Physicians should abstain from engaging in research projects involving human subjects unless they are satisfied that the hazards involved are believed to be predictable. Physicians should cease any investigation if the hazards are found to outweigh the potential benefits.

8. In publication of the results of his or her research, the physician is obliged to preserve the accuracy of the results. Reports of experimentation not in accordance with the principles laid down in this Declaration should not be accepted for publication.

9. In any research on human beings, each potential subject must be adequately informed of the aims, methods, anticipated benefits and potential hazards of the study and the discomfort it may entail. He or she should be informed that he or she is at liberty to abstain from participation in the study and that he or she is free to withdraw his or her consent to participation at any time. The physician should then obtain the subject's freely-given informed consent, preferably in writing.

10. When obtaining informed consent for the research project the physician should be particularly cautious if the subject is in a dependent relationship to him or her or may consent under duress. In that case the informed consent should be obtained by a physician who is not engaged in the investigation and who is completely independent of this official relationship.

11. In case of legal incompetence, informed consent should be obtained from the legal guardian in accordance with national legislation. Where physical or mental incapacity makes it impossible to obtain informed consent, or when the subject is a minor, permission from the responsible relative replaces that of the subject in accordance with national legislation.

Whenever the minor child is in fact able to give a consent, the minor's consent must be obtained in addition to the consent of the minor's legal guardian.

12. The research protocol should always contain a statement of the ethical considerations involved and should indicate that the principles enunciated in the present Declaration are complied with.

II. Medical Research Combined with Professional Care (Clinical Research)

1. In the treatment of the sick person, the physician must be free to use a new diagnostic and therapeutic measure, if in his or her judgment it offers hope of saving life, reestablishing health or alleviating suffering.

2. The potential benefits, hazards and discomfort of a new method should be weighed against the advantages of the best current diagnostic and therapeutic methods.

3. In any medical study, every patient—including those of a control group, if any—should be assured of the best proven diagnostic and therapeutic method.

4. The refusal of the patient to participate in a study must never interfere with the physician-patient relationship.

5. If the physician considers it essential not to obtain informed consent, the specific reasons for this proposal should be stated in the experimental protocol for transmission to the independent committee (I, 2).

6. The physician can combine medical research with professional care, the objective being the acquisition of new medical knowledge, only to the extent that medical research is justified by its potential diagnostic or therapeutic value for the patient.

III. Non-Therapeutic Biomedical Research Involving Human Subjects (Non-Clinical Biomedical Research)

1. In the purely scientific application of medical research carried out on a human being, it is the duty of the physician to remain the protector of the life and health of that person on whom biomedical research is being carried out.

2. The subjects should be volunteers—either healthy persons or patients for whom the experimental design is not related to the patient's illness.

3. The investigator or the investigating team should discontinue the research if in his/her or their judgment it may, if continued, be harmful to the individual.

4. In research on man, the interest of science and society should never take precedence over considerations related to the well-being of the subject.

[52 FR 8831, Mar. 19, 1987, as amended at 52 FR 23031, June 17, 1987; 56 FR 22113, May 14, 1991; 64 FR 401, Jan. 5, 1999; 67 FR 9586, Mar. 4, 2002]

§312.130 Availability for public disclosure of data and information in an IND.

(a) The existence of an investigational new drug application will not be disclosed by FDA unless it has previously been publicly disclosed or acknowledged.

(b) The availability for public disclosure of all data and information in an investigational new drug application for a new drug will be handled in accordance with the provisions established in §314.430 for the confidentiality of data and information in applications submitted in part 314. The availability for public disclosure of all data and information in an investigational new drug application for a biological product will be governed by the provisions of §§601.50 and 601.51.

(c) Notwithstanding the provisions of §314.430, FDA shall disclose upon request to an individual to whom an investigational new drug has been given a copy of any IND safety report relating to the use in the individual.

(d) The availability of information required to be publicly disclosed for investigations involving an exception from informed consent under §50.24 of this chapter will be handled as follows: Persons wishing to request the publicly disclosable information in the IND that was required to be filed in Docket Number 95S-0158 in the Dockets Management Branch (HFA-305), Food and Drug Administration, 5630 Fishers Lane, rm. 1061, Rockville, MD 20852, shall submit a request under the Freedom of Information Act.

[52 FR 8831, Mar. 19, 1987. Redesignated at 53 FR 41523, Oct. 21, 1988, as amended at 61 FR 51530, Oct. 2, 1996; 64 FR 401, Jan. 5, 1999; 68 FR 24879, May 9, 2003]

§312.140 Address for correspondence.

(a) Except as provided in paragraph (b) of this section, a sponsor shall send an initial IND submission to the Central Document Room, Center for Drug Evaluation and Research, Food and Drug Administration, 5901–B Ammendale Rd., Beltsville, MD 20705–1266. On receiving the IND, FDA will inform the sponsor which one of the divisions in the Center for Drug Evaluation and Research or the Center for Biologics Evaluation and Research is responsible for the IND. Amendments, reports, and other correspondence relating to matters covered by the IND should be directed to the appropriate division. The outside wrapper of each submission shall state what is contained in the submission, for example, "IND Application", "Protocol Amendment", etc.

(b) Applications for the products listed below should be submitted to the Division of Biological Investigational New Drugs (HFB-230), Center for Biologics Evaluation and Research, Food and Drug Administration, 8800 Rockville Pike, Bethesda, MD 20892. (1) Products subject to the licensing provisions of the Public Health Service Act of July 1, 1944 (58 Stat. 682, as amended (42 U.S.C. 201 *et seq.*)) or subject to part 600; (2) ingredients packaged together with containers intended for the collection, processing, or storage of blood or blood components; (3) urokinase products; (4) plasma volume expanders and hydroxyethyl starch for leukapheresis; and (5) coupled antibodies, i.e., products that consist of an antibody component coupled with a drug or radionuclide component in which both components provide a pharmacological effect but the biological component determines the site of action.

(c) All correspondence relating to biological products for human use which are also radioactive drugs shall be submitted to the Division of Oncology and Radiopharmaceutical Drug Products (HFD–150), Center for Drug Evaluation and Research, Food and Drug Administration, 5600 Fishers Lane, Rockville, MD 20857, except that applications for coupled antibodies shall be submitted in accordance with paragraph (b) of this section.

(d) All correspondence relating to export of an investigational drug under §312.110(b)(2) shall be submitted to the International Affairs Staff (HFY–50), Office of Health Affairs, Food and Drug Administration, 5600 Fishers Lane, Rockville, MD 20857.

[52 FR 8831, Mar. 19, 1987, as amended at 52 FR 23031, June 17, 1987; 55 FR 11580, Mar. 29, 1990; 67 FR 9586, Mar. 4, 2002; 69 FR 13473, Mar. 23, 2004]

§312.145 Guidance documents.

(a) FDA has made available guidance documents under §10.115 of this chapter to help you to comply with certain requirements of this part.

(b) The Center for Drug Evaluation and Research (CDER) and the Center for Biologics Evaluation and Research (CBER) maintain lists of guidance documents that apply to the centers' regulations. The lists are maintained on the Internet and are published annually in the FEDERAL REGISTER. A request for a copy of the CDER list should be directed to the Office of Training and Communications, Division of Communications Management, Drug Information Branch (HFD-210), Center for Drug Evaluation and Research, Food and Drug Administration, 5600 Fishers Lane, Rockville, MD 20857. A request for a copy of the CBER list should be directed to the Office of Communication, Training, and Manufac-turers Assistance (HFM-40), Center for Biologics Evaluation and Research, Food and Drug Administration, 1401 Rockville Pike, Rockville, MD 20852-1448.

Subpart G—Drugs for Investigational Use in Laboratory Research Animals or In Vitro Tests

§312.160 Drugs for investigational use in laboratory research animals or in vitro tests.

(a) Authorization to ship. (1)(i) A person may ship a drug intended solely for tests in vitro or in animals used only for laboratory research purposes if it is labeled as follows:

"CAUTION: Contains a new drug for investigational use only in laboratory research animals, or for tests in vitro. Not for use in humans."

(ii) A person may ship a biological product for investigational in vitro diagnostic use that is listed in §312.2(b)(2)(ii) if it is labeled as follows:

"CAUTION: Contains a biological product for investigational in vitro diagnostic tests only."

(2) A person shipping a drug under paragraph (a) of this section shall use due diligence to assure that the consignee is regularly engaged in conducting such tests and that the shipment of the new drug will actually be used for tests in vitro or in animals used only for laboratory research.

(3) A person who ships a drug under paragraph (a) of this section shall maintain adequate records showing the name and post office address of the expert to whom the drug is shipped and the date, quantity, and batch or code mark of each shipment and delivery. Records of shipments under paragraph (a)(1)(i) of this section are to be maintained for a period of 2 years after the shipment. Records and reports of data and shipments under paragraph (a)(1)(ii) of this section are to be maintained in accordance with §312.57(b). The person who ships the drug shall upon request from any properly authorized officer or employee of the Food and Drug Administration, at reasonable times, permit such officer or employee to have access to and copy and verify records required to be maintained under this section.

(b) Termination of authorization to ship. FDA may terminate authorization to ship a drug under this section if it finds that:

(1) The sponsor of the investigation has failed to comply with any of the conditions for shipment established under this section; or

(2) The continuance of the investigation is unsafe or otherwise contrary to the public interest or the drug is used for purposes other than bona fide scientific investigation. FDA will notify the person shipping the drug of its finding and invite immediate correction. If correction is not immediately made, the person shall have an opportunity for a regulatory hearing before FDA pursuant to part 16.

(c) Disposition of unused drug. The person who ships the drug under paragraph (a) of this section shall assure the return of all unused supplies of the drug from individual investigators whenever the investigation discontinues or the investigation is terminated. The person who ships the drug may authorize in writing alternative disposition of unused supplies of the drug provided this alternative disposition does not expose humans to risks from the drug, either directly or indirectly (e.g., through food-producing animals). The shipper shall maintain records of any alternative disposition.

[52 FR 8831, Mar. 19, 1987, as amended at 52 FR 23031, June 17, 1987. Redesignated at 53 FR 41523, Oct. 21, 1988; 67 FR 9586, Mar. 4, 2002]

TITLE 45—PUBLIC WELFARE

Subtitle A—Department of Health and Human Services, General Administration
Subchapter A—General Administration

PART 46

Public Welfare

Subpart A—Basic HHS Policy for Protection of Human Research Subjects

Subpart B—Additional Protections for Pregnant Women, Human Fetuses and Neonates Involved in Research

Subpart C—Additional Protections Pertaining to Biomedical and Behavioral Research Involving Prisoners as Subjects

Subpart D—Additional Protections for Children Involved as Subjects in Research

Authority: 5 U.S.C. 301; 42 U.S.C. 289(a).

Editorial Note: The Department of Health and Human Services issued a notice of waiver regarding the requirements set forth in part 46, relating to protection of human subjects, as they pertain to demonstration projects, approved under section 1115 of the Social Security Act, which test the use of cost—sharing, such as deductibles, copayment and coinsurance, in the Medicaid program. For further information see 47 FR 9208, Mar. 4, 1982.

Subpart A—Basic HHS Policy for Protection of Human Research Subjects

Source: 56 FR 28012, 28022, June 18, 1991, unless otherwise noted.

§46.101 To what does this policy apply?

(a) Except as provided in paragraph (b) of this section, this policy applies to all research involving human subjects conducted, supported or otherwise subject to regulation by any federal department or agency which takes appropriate administrative action to make the policy applicable to such research. This includes research conducted by federal civilian employees or military personnel, except that each department or agency head may adopt such procedural modifications as may be appropriate from an administrative standpoint. It also includes research conducted, supported, or otherwise subject to regulation by the federal government outside the United States.

(1) Research that is conducted or supported by a federal department or agency, whether or not it is regulated as defined in §46.102(e), must comply with all sections of this policy.

(2) Research that is neither conducted nor supported by a federal department or agency but is subject to regulation as defined in §46.102(e) must be reviewed and approved, in compliance with §46.101, §46.102, and §46.107 through §46.117 of this policy, by an institutional review board (IRB) that operates in accordance with the pertinent requirements of this policy.

(b) Unless otherwise required by department or agency heads, research activities in which the only involvement of human subjects will be in one or more of the following categories are exempt from this policy:

(1) Research conducted in established or commonly accepted educational settings, involving normal educational practices, such as (i) research on regular and special education instructional strategies, or (ii) research on the effectiveness of or the comparison among instructional techniques, curricula, or classroom management methods.

(2) Research involving the use of educational tests (cognitive, diagnostic, aptitude, achievement), survey procedures, interview procedures or observation of public behavior, unless:

(i) Information obtained is recorded in such a manner that human subjects can be identified, directly or through identifiers linked to the subjects; and (ii) any disclosure of the human subjects' responses outside the research could reasonably place the subjects at risk of criminal or civil liability or be damaging to the subjects' financial standing, employability, or reputation.

(3) Research involving the use of educational tests (cognitive, diagnostic, aptitude, achievement), survey procedures, interview procedures, or observation of public behavior that is not exempt under paragraph (b)(2) of this section, if:

(i) The human subjects are elected or appointed public officials or candidates for public office; or (ii) federal statute(s) require(s) without exception that the confidentiality of the personally identifiable information will be maintained throughout the research and thereafter.

(4) Research, involving the collection or study of existing data, documents, records, pathological specimens, or diagnostic specimens, if these sources are publicly available or if the information is recorded by the investigator in such a manner that subjects cannot be identified, directly or through identifiers linked to the subjects.

(5) Research and demonstration projects which are conducted by or subject to the approval of department or agency heads, and which are designed to study, evaluate, or otherwise examine:

(i) Public benefit or service programs; (ii) procedures for obtaining benefits or services under those programs; (iii) possible changes in or alternatives to those programs or procedures; or (iv) possible changes in methods or levels of payment for benefits or services under those programs.

(6) Taste and food quality evaluation and consumer acceptance studies, (i) if wholesome foods without additives are consumed or (ii) if a food is consumed that contains a food ingredient at or below the level and for a use found to be safe, or agricultural chemical or environmental contaminant at or below the level found to be safe, by the Food and Drug Administration or approved by the Environmental Protection Agency or the Food Safety and Inspection Service of the U.S. Department of Agriculture.

(c) Department or agency heads retain final judgment as to whether a particular activity is covered by this policy.

(d) Department or agency heads may require that specific research activities or classes of research activities conducted, supported, or otherwise subject to regulation by the department or agency but not otherwise covered by this policy, comply with some or all of the requirements of this policy.

(e) Compliance with this policy requires compliance with pertinent federal laws or regulations which provide additional protections for human subjects.

(f) This policy does not affect any state or local laws or regulations which may otherwise be applicable and which provide additional protections for human subjects.

(g) This policy does not affect any foreign laws or regulations which may otherwise be applicable and which provide additional protections to human subjects of research.

(h) When research covered by this policy takes place in foreign countries, procedures normally followed in the foreign countries to protect human subjects may differ from those set forth in this policy. [An example is a foreign institution which complies with guidelines consistent with the World Medical Assembly Declaration (Declaration of Helsinki amended 1989) issued either by sovereign states or by an organization whose function for the protection of human research subjects is internationally recognized.] In these circumstances, if a department or agency head determines that the procedures prescribed by the institution afford protections that are at least equivalent to those provided in this policy, the department or agency head may approve the substitution of the foreign procedures in lieu of the procedural requirements provided in this policy. Except when otherwise required by statute, Executive Order, or the department or agency head, notices of these actions as they occur will be published in the Federal Register or will be otherwise published as provided in department or agency procedures.

(i) Unless otherwise required by law, department or agency heads may waive the applicability of some or all of the provisions of this policy to specific research activities or classes of research activities otherwise covered by this policy. Except when otherwise required by statute or Executive Order, the department or agency head shall forward advance notices of these actions to the Office for Protection from Research Risks, Department of Health and Human Services (HHS), and shall also publish them in the Federal Register or in such other manner as provided in department or agency procedures. [1]

1. Institutions with HHS-approved assurances on file will abide by provisions of title 45 CFR part 46 subparts A–D. Some of the other Departments and Agencies have incorporated all provisions of title 45 CFR part 46 into their policies and procedures as well. However, the exemptions at 45 CFR 46.101(b) do not apply to research involving prisoners, fetuses, pregnant women, or human in vitro fertilization, subparts B and C. The exemption at 45 CFR 46.101(b)(2), for research involving survey or interview procedures or observation of public behavior, does not apply to research with children, subpart D, except for research involving observations of public behavior when the investigator(s) do not participate in the activities being observed.

[56 FR 28012, 28022, June 18, 1991; 56 FR 29756, June 28, 1991]

§46.102 Definitions.

(a) Department or agency head means the head of any federal department or agency and any other officer or employee of any department or agency to whom authority has been delegated.

(b) Institution means any public or private entity or agency (including federal, state, and other agencies).

(c) Legally authorized representative means an individual or judicial or other body authorized under applicable law to consent on behalf of a prospective subject to the subject's participation in the procedure(s) involved in the research.

(d) Research means a systematic investigation, including research development, testing and evaluation, designed to develop or contribute to generalizable knowledge. Activities which meet this definition constitute research for purposes of this policy, whether or not they are conducted or supported under a program which is considered research for other purposes. For example, some demonstration and service programs may include research activities.

(e) Research subject to regulation, and similar terms are intended to encompass those research activities for which a federal department or agency has specific responsibility for regulating as a research activity, (for example, Investigational New Drug requirements administered by the Food and Drug Administration). It does not include research activities which are incidentally regulated by a federal department or agency solely as part of the department's or agency's broader responsibility to regulate certain types of activities whether research or non-research in nature (for example, Wage and Hour requirements administered by the Department of Labor).

(f) Human subject means a living individual about whom an investigator (whether professional or student) conducting research obtains

(1) Data through intervention or interaction with the individual, or

(2) Identifiable private information.

Intervention includes both physical procedures by which data are gathered (for example, venipuncture) and manipulations of the subject or the subject's environment that are performed for research purposes. Interaction includes communication or interpersonal contact between investigator and subject. Private information includes information about behavior that occurs in a context in which an individual can reasonably expect that no observation or recording is taking place, and information which has been provided for specific purposes by an individual and which the individual can reasonably expect will not be made public (for example, a medical record). Private information must be individually identifiable (i.e., the identity of the subject is or may readily be ascertained by the investigator or associated with the information) in order for obtaining the information to constitute research involving human subjects.

(g) IRB means an institutional review board established in accord with and for the purposes expressed in this policy.

(h) IRB approval means the determination of the IRB that the research has been reviewed and may be conducted at an institution within the constraints set forth by the IRB and by other institutional and federal requirements.

(i) Minimal risk means that the probability and magnitude of harm or discomfort anticipated in the research are not greater in and of themselves than those ordinarily encountered in daily life or during the performance of routine physical or psychological examinations or tests.

(j) Certification means the official notification by the institution to the supporting department or agency, in accordance with the requirements of this policy, that a research project or activity involving human subjects has been reviewed and approved by an IRB in accordance with an approved assurance.

§46.103 Assuring compliance with this policy—research conducted or supported by any Federal Department or Agency.

(a) Each institution engaged in research which is covered by this policy and which is conducted or supported by a federal department or agency shall provide written assurance satisfactory to the department or agency head that it will comply with the requirements set forth in this policy. In lieu of requiring submission of an assurance, individual department or agency heads shall accept the existence of a current assurance, appropriate for the research in question, on file with the Office for Protection from Research Risks, HHS, and approved for federalwide use by that office. When the existence of an HHS-approved assurance is accepted in lieu of requiring submission of an assurance, reports (except certification) required by this policy to be made to department and agency heads shall also be made to the Office for Protection from Research Risks, HHS.

(b) Departments and agencies will conduct or support research covered by this policy only if the institution has an assurance approved as provided in this section, and only if the institution has certified to the department or agency head that the research has been reviewed and approved by an IRB provided for in the assurance, and will be subject to continuing review by the IRB. Assurances applicable to federally supported or conducted research shall at a minimum include:

(1) A statement of principles governing the institution in the discharge of its responsibilities for protecting the rights and welfare of human subjects of research conducted at or sponsored by the institution, regardless of whether the research is subject to federal regulation. This may include an appropriate existing code, declaration, or statement of ethical principles, or a statement formulated by the institution itself. This requirement does not preempt provisions of this policy applicable to department- or agency-supported or regulated research and need not be applicable to any research exempted or waived under §46.101 (b) or (i).

(2) Designation of one or more IRBs established in accordance with the requirements of this policy, and for which provisions are made for meeting space and sufficient staff to support the IRB's review and recordkeeping duties.

(3) A list of IRB members identified by name; earned degrees; representative capacity; indications of experience such as board certifications, licenses, etc., sufficient to describe each member's chief anticipated contributions to IRB deliberations; and any employment or other relationship between each member and the institution; for example: full-time employee, part-time employee, member of governing panel or board, stockholder, paid or unpaid consultant. Changes in IRB membership shall be reported to the department or agency head, unless in accord with §46.103(a) of this policy, the existence of an HHS-approved assurance is accepted. In this case, change in IRB membership shall be reported to the Office for Protection from Research Risks, HHS.

(4) Written procedures which the IRB will follow (i) for conducting its initial and continuing review of research and for reporting its findings and actions to the investigator and the institution; (ii) for determining which projects require review more often than annually and which projects need verification from sources other than the investigators that no material changes have occurred since previous IRB review; and (iii) for ensuring prompt reporting to the IRB of proposed changes in a research activity, and for ensuring that such changes in approved research, during the period for which IRB approval has already been given, may not be initiated without IRB review and approval except when necessary to eliminate apparent immediate hazards to the subject.

(5) Written procedures for ensuring prompt reporting to the IRB, appropriate institutional officials, and the department or agency head of (i) any

unanticipated problems involving risks to subjects or others or any serious or continuing noncompliance with this policy or the requirements or determinations of the IRB and (ii) any suspension or termination of IRB approval.

(c) The assurance shall be executed by an individual authorized to act for the institution and to assume on behalf of the institution the obligations imposed by this policy and shall be filed in such form and manner as the department or agency head prescribes.

(d) The department or agency head will evaluate all assurances submitted in accordance with this policy through such officers and employees of the department or agency and such experts or consultants engaged for this purpose as the department or agency head determines to be appropriate. The department or agency head's evaluation will take into consideration the adequacy of the proposed IRB in light of the anticipated scope of the institution's research activities and the types of subject populations likely to be involved, the appropriateness of the proposed initial and continuing review procedures in light of the probable risks, and the size and complexity of the institution.

(e) On the basis of this evaluation, the department or agency head may approve or disapprove the assurance, or enter into negotiations to develop an approvable one. The department or agency head may limit the period during which any particular approved assurance or class of approved assurances shall remain effective or otherwise condition or restrict approval.

(f) Certification is required when the research is supported by a federal department or agency and not otherwise exempted or waived under §46.101 (b) or (i). An institution with an approved assurance shall certify that each application or proposal for research covered by the assurance and by §46.103 of this Policy has been reviewed and approved by the IRB. Such certification must be submitted with the application or proposal or by such later date as may be prescribed by the department or agency to which the application or proposal is submitted. Under no condition shall research covered by §46.103 of the Policy be supported prior to receipt of the certification that the research has been reviewed and approved by the IRB. Institutions without an approved assurance covering the research shall certify within 30 days after receipt of a request for such a certification from the department or agency, that the application or proposal has been approved by the IRB. If the certification is not submitted within these time limits, the application or proposal may be returned to the institution.

(Approved by the Office of Management and Budget under control number 9999–0020)

[56 FR 28012, 28022, June 18, 1991; 56 FR 29756, June 28, 1991]

§§46.104–46.106 [Reserved]

§46.107 IRB membership.

(a) Each IRB shall have at least five members, with varying backgrounds to promote complete and adequate review of research activities commonly conducted by the institution. The IRB shall be sufficiently qualified through the experience and expertise of its members, and the diversity of the members, including consideration of race, gender, and cultural backgrounds and sensitivity to such issues as community attitudes, to promote respect for its advice and counsel in safeguarding the rights and welfare of human subjects. In addition to possessing the professional competence necessary to review specific research activities, the IRB shall be able to ascertain the acceptability of proposed research in terms of institutional commitments and regulations, applicable law, and standards of professional conduct and practice. The IRB shall therefore include persons knowledgeable in these areas. If an IRB regularly reviews research that involves a vulnerable category of subjects, such as children, prisoners, pregnant women, or handicapped or mentally disabled persons, consideration shall be given to the inclusion of one or more individuals who are knowledgeable about and experienced in working with these subjects.

(b) Every nondiscriminatory effort will be made to ensure that no IRB consists entirely of men or entirely of women, including the institution's consideration of qualified persons of both sexes, so long as no selection is made to the IRB on the basis of gender. No IRB may consist entirely of members of one profession.

(c) Each IRB shall include at least one member whose primary concerns are in scientific areas and at least one member whose primary concerns are in nonscientific areas.

(d) Each IRB shall include at least one member who is not otherwise affiliated with the institution and who is not part of the immediate family of a person who is affiliated with the institution.

(e) No IRB may have a member participate in the IRB's initial or continuing review of any project in which the member has a conflicting interest, except to provide information requested by the IRB.

(f) An IRB may, in its discretion, invite individuals with competence in special areas to assist in the review of issues which require expertise beyond or in addition to that available on the IRB. These individuals may not vote with the IRB.

§46.108 IRB functions and operations.

In order to fulfill the requirements of this policy each IRB shall:

(a) Follow written procedures in the same detail as described in §46.103(b)(4) and, to the extent required by, §46.103(b)(5).

(b) Except when an expedited review procedure is used (see §46.110), review proposed research at convened meetings at which a majority of the members of the IRB are present, including at least one member whose primary concerns are in nonscientific areas. In order for the research to be approved, it shall receive the approval of a majority of those members present at the meeting.

§46.109 IRB review of research.

(a) An IRB shall review and have authority to approve, require modifications in (to secure approval), or disapprove all research activities covered by this policy.

(b) An IRB shall require that information given to subjects as part of informed consent is in accordance with §46.116. The IRB may require that information, in addition to that specifically mentioned in §46.116, be given to the subjects when in the IRB's judgment the information would meaningfully add to the protection of the rights and welfare of subjects.

(c) An IRB shall require documentation of informed consent or may waive documentation in accordance with §46.117.

(d) An IRB shall notify investigators and the institution in writing of its decision to approve or disapprove the proposed research activity, or of modifications required to secure IRB approval of the research activity. If the IRB decides to disapprove a research activity, it shall include in its written notification a statement of the reasons for its decision and give the investigator an opportunity to respond in person or in writing.

(e) An IRB shall conduct continuing review of research covered by this policy at intervals appropriate to the degree of risk, but not less than once per year, and shall have authority to observe or have a third party observe the consent process and the research.

(Approved by the Office of Management and Budget under control number 9999–0020)

§46.110 Expedited review procedures for certain kinds of research involving no more than minimal risk, and for minor changes in approved research.

(a) The Secretary, HHS, has established, and published as a Notice in the Federal Register, a list of categories of research that may be reviewed by the IRB through an expedited review procedure. The list will be amended, as appropriate after consultation with other departments and agencies, through periodic republication by the Secretary, HHS, in the Federal Register. A copy of the list is available from the Office for Protection from Research Risks, National Institutes of Health, HHS, Bethesda, Maryland 20892.

(b) An IRB may use the expedited review procedure to review either or both of the following:

(1) Some or all of the research appearing on the list and found by the reviewer(s) to involve no more than minimal risk,

(2) Minor changes in previously approved research during the period (of one year or less) for which approval is authorized.

Under an expedited review procedure, the review may be carried out by the IRB chairperson or by one or more experienced reviewers designated by the chairperson from among members of the IRB. In reviewing the research, the reviewers may exercise all of the authorities of the IRB except that the reviewers may not disapprove the research. A research activity may be disapproved only after review in accordance with the non-expedited procedure set forth in §46.108(b).

(c) Each IRB which uses an expedited review procedure shall adopt a method for keeping all members advised of research proposals which have been approved under the procedure.

(d) The department or agency head may restrict, suspend, terminate, or choose not to authorize an institution's or IRB's use of the expedited review procedure.

§46.111 Criteria for IRB approval of research.

(a) In order to approve research covered by this policy the IRB shall determine that all of the following requirements are satisfied:

(1) Risks to subjects are minimized: (i) By using procedures which are consistent with sound research design and which do not unnecessarily expose subjects to risk, and (ii) whenever appropriate, by using procedures already being performed on the subjects for diagnostic or treatment purposes.

(2) Risks to subjects are reasonable in relation to anticipated benefits, if any, to subjects, and the importance of the knowledge that may reasonably be expected to result. In evaluating risks and benefits, the IRB should consider only those risks and benefits that may result from the research (as distinguished from risks and benefits of therapies subjects would receive even if not participating in the research). The IRB should not consider possible long-range effects of applying knowledge gained in the research (for example, the possible effects of the research on public policy) as among those research risks that fall within the purview of its responsibility.

(3) Selection of subjects is equitable. In making this assessment the IRB should take into account the purposes of the research and the setting in which the research will be conducted and should be particularly cognizant of the special problems of research involving vulnerable populations, such as children, prisoners, pregnant women, mentally disabled persons, or economically or educationally disadvantaged persons.

(4) Informed consent will be sought from each prospective subject or the subject's legally authorized representative, in accordance with, and to the extent required by §46.116.

(5) Informed consent will be appropriately documented, in accordance with, and to the extent required by §46.117.

(6) When appropriate, the research plan makes adequate provision for monitoring the data collected to ensure the safety of subjects.

(7) When appropriate, there are adequate provisions to protect the privacy of subjects and to maintain the confidentiality of data.

(b) When some or all of the subjects are likely to be vulnerable to coercion or undue influence, such as children, prisoners, pregnant women, mentally disabled persons, or economically or educationally disadvantaged persons, additional safeguards have been included in the study to protect the rights and welfare of these subjects.

§46.112 Review by institution.

Research covered by this policy that has been approved by an IRB may be subject to further appropriate review and approval or disapproval by officials of the institution. However, those officials may not approve the research if it has not been approved by an IRB.

§46.113 Suspension or termination of IRB approval of research.

An IRB shall have authority to suspend or terminate approval of research that is not being conducted in accordance with the IRB's requirements or that has been associated with unexpected serious harm to subjects. Any suspension or termination of approval shall include a statement of the reasons for the IRB's action and shall be reported promptly to the investigator, appropriate institutional officials, and the department or agency head.

(Approved by the Office of Management and Budget under control number 9999–0020)

§46.114 Cooperative research.

Cooperative research projects are those projects covered by this policy which involve more than one institution. In the conduct of cooperative research projects, each institution is responsible for safeguarding the rights and welfare of human subjects and for complying with this policy. With the approval of the department or agency head, an institution participating in a cooperative project may enter into a joint review arrangement, rely upon the review of another qualified IRB, or make similar arrangements for avoiding duplication of effort.

§46.115 IRB records.

(a) An institution, or when appropriate an IRB, shall prepare and maintain adequate documentation of IRB activities, including the following:

(1) Copies of all research proposals reviewed, scientific evaluations, if any, that accompany the proposals, approved sample consent documents, progress reports submitted by investigators, and reports of injuries to subjects.

(2) Minutes of IRB meetings which shall be in sufficient detail to show attendance at the meetings; actions taken by the IRB; the vote on these actions including the number of members voting for, against, and abstaining; the basis for requiring changes in or disapproving research; and a written summary of the discussion of controverted issues and their resolution.

(3) Records of continuing review activities.

(4) Copies of all correspondence between the IRB and the investigators.

(5) A list of IRB members in the same detail as described is §46.103(b)(3).

(6) Written procedures for the IRB in the same detail as described in §46.103(b)(4) and §46.103(b)(5).

(7) Statements of significant new findings provided to subjects, as required by §46.116(b)(5).

(b) The records required by this policy shall be retained for at least 3 years, and records relating to research which is conducted shall be retained for at least 3 years after completion of the research. All records shall be accessible for inspection and copying by authorized representatives of the department or agency at reasonable times and in a reasonable manner.

(Approved by the Office of Management and Budget under control number 9999–0020)

§46.116 General requirements for informed consent.

Except as provided elsewhere in this policy, no investigator may involve a human being as a subject in research covered by this policy unless the investigator has obtained the legally effective informed consent of the subject or the subject's legally authorized representative. An investigator shall seek such consent only under circumstances that provide the prospective subject or the representative sufficient opportunity to consider whether or not to participate and that minimize the possibility of coercion or undue influence. The information that is given to the subject or the representative shall be in language understandable to the subject or the representative. No informed consent, whether oral or written, may include any exculpatory language through which the subject or the representative is made to waive or appear to waive any of the subject's legal rights, or releases or appears to release the investigator, the sponsor, the institution or its agents from liability for negligence.

(a) Basic elements of informed consent. Except as provided in paragraph (c) or (d) of this section, in seeking informed consent the following information shall be provided to each subject:

(1) A statement that the study involves research, an explanation of the purposes of the research and the expected duration of the subject's participation, a description of the procedures to be followed, and identification of any procedures which are experimental;

(2) A description of any reasonably foreseeable risks or discomforts to the subject;

(3) A description of any benefits to the subject or to others which may reasonably be expected from the research;

(4) A disclosure of appropriate alternative procedures or courses of treatment, if any, that might be advantageous to the subject;

(5) A statement describing the extent, if any, to which confidentiality of records identifying the subject will be maintained;

(6) For research involving more than minimal risk, an explanation as to whether any compensation and an explanation as to whether any medical treatments are available if injury occurs and, if so, what they consist of, or where further information may be obtained;

(7) An explanation of whom to contact for answers to pertinent questions about the research and research subjects' rights, and whom to contact in the event of a research-related injury to the subject; and

(8) A statement that participation is voluntary, refusal to participate will involve no penalty or loss of benefits to which the subject is otherwise entitled, and the subject may discontinue participation at

any time without penalty or loss of benefits to which the subject is otherwise entitled.

(b) Additional elements of informed consent. When appropriate, one or more of the following elements of information shall also be provided to each subject:

(1) A statement that the particular treatment or procedure may involve risks to the subject (or to the embryo or fetus, if the subject is or may become pregnant) which are currently unforeseeable;

(2) Anticipated circumstances under which the subject's participation may be terminated by the investigator without regard to the subject's consent;

(3) Any additional costs to the subject that may result from participation in the research;

(4) The consequences of a subject's decision to withdraw from the research and procedures for orderly termination of participation by the subject;

(5) A statement that significant new findings developed during the course of the research which may relate to the subject's willingness to continue participation will be provided to the subject; and

(6) The approximate number of subjects involved in the study.

(c) An IRB may approve a consent procedure which does not include, or which alters, some or all of the elements of informed consent set forth above, or waive the requirement to obtain informed consent provided the IRB finds and documents that:

(1) The research or demonstration project is to be conducted by or subject to the approval of state or local government officials and is designed to study, evaluate, or otherwise examine: (i) Public benefit of service programs; (ii) procedures for obtaining benefits or services under those programs; (iii) possible changes in or alternatives to those programs or procedures; or (iv) possible changes in methods or levels of payment for benefits or services under those programs; and

(2) The research could not practicably be carried out without the waiver or alteration.

(d) An IRB may approve a consent procedure which does not include, or which alters, some or all of the elements of informed consent set forth in this section, or waive the requirements to obtain informed consent provided the IRB finds and documents that:

(1) The research involves no more than minimal risk to the subjects;

(2) The waiver or alteration will not adversely affect the rights and welfare of the subjects;

(3) The research could not practicably be carried out without the waiver or alteration; and

(4) Whenever appropriate, the subjects will be provided with additional pertinent information after participation.

(e) The informed consent requirements in this policy are not intended to preempt any applicable federal, state, or local laws which require additional information to be disclosed in order for informed consent to be legally effective.

(f) Nothing in this policy is intended to limit the authority of a physician to provide emergency medical care, to the extent the physician is permitted to do so under applicable federal, state, or local law.

(Approved by the Office of Management and Budget under control number 9999–0020)

§46.117 Documentation of informed consent.

(a) Except as provided in paragraph (c) of this section, informed consent shall be documented by the use of a written consent form approved by the IRB and signed by the subject or the subject's legally authorized representative. A copy shall be given to the person signing the form.

(b) Except as provided in paragraph (c) of this section, the consent form may be either of the following:

(1) A written consent document that embodies the elements of informed consent required by §46.116. This form may be read to the subject or the subject's legally authorized representative, but in any event, the investigator shall give either the subject or the representative adequate opportunity to read it before it is signed; or

(2) A short form written consent document stating that the elements of informed consent required by §46.116 have been presented orally to the subject or the subject's legally authorized representative. When this method is used, there shall be a witness to the oral presentation. Also, the IRB shall approve a written summary of what is to be said to the subject or the representative. Only the short form itself is to be signed by the subject or the representative. However, the witness shall sign both the short form and a copy of the summary, and the person actually obtaining consent shall sign a copy of the summary. A copy of the summary shall be given to the subject or the representative, in addition to a copy of the short form.

(c) An IRB may waive the requirement for the investigator to obtain a signed consent form for some or all subjects if it finds either:

(1) That the only record linking the subject and the research would be the consent document and the principal risk would be potential harm resulting from a breach of confidentiality. Each subject will be asked whether the subject wants documentation linking the subject with the research, and the subject's wishes will govern; or

(2) That the research presents no more than minimal risk of harm to subjects and involves no procedures for which written consent is normally required outside of the research context.

In cases in which the documentation requirement is waived, the IRB may require the investigator to provide subjects with a written statement regarding the research.

(Approved by the Office of Management and Budget under control number 9999–0020)

§46.118 Applications and proposals lacking definite plans for involvement of human subjects.

Certain types of applications for grants, cooperative agreements, or contracts are submitted to departments or agencies with the knowledge that subjects may be involved within the period of support, but definite plans would not normally be set forth in the application or proposal. These include activities such as institutional type grants when selection of specific projects is the institution's responsibility; research training grants in which the activities involving subjects remain to be selected; and projects in which human subjects' involvement will depend upon completion of instruments, prior animal studies, or purification of compounds. These applications need not be reviewed by an IRB before an award may be made. However, except for research exempted or waived under §46.101 (b) or (i), no human subjects may be involved in any project supported by these awards until the project has been reviewed and approved by the IRB, as provided in this policy, and certification submitted, by the institution, to the department or agency.

§46.119 Research undertaken without the intention of involving human subjects.

In the event research is undertaken without the intention of involving human subjects, but it is later proposed to involve human subjects in the research, the research shall first be reviewed and approved by an IRB, as provided in this policy, a certification submitted, by the institution, to the department or agency, and final approval given to the proposed change by the department or agency.

§46.120 Evaluation and disposition of applications and proposals for research to be conducted or supported by a Federal Department or Agency.

(a) The department or agency head will evaluate all applications and proposals involving human subjects submitted to the department or agency through such officers and employees of the department or agency and such experts and consultants as the department or agency head determines to be appropriate. This evaluation will take into consideration the risks to the subjects, the adequacy of protection against these risks, the potential benefits of the research to the subjects and others, and the importance of the knowledge gained or to be gained.

(b) On the basis of this evaluation, the department or agency head may approve or disapprove the application or proposal, or enter into negotiations to develop an approvable one.

§46.121 [Reserved]

§46.122 Use of Federal funds.

Federal funds administered by a department or agency may not be expended for research involving human subjects unless the requirements of this policy have been satisfied.

§46.123 Early termination of research support: Evaluation of applications and proposals.

(a) The department or agency head may require that department or agency support for any project be terminated or suspended in the manner prescribed in applicable program requirements, when the department or agency head finds an institution has materially failed to comply with the terms of this policy.

(b) In making decisions about supporting or approving applications or proposals covered by this policy the department or agency head may take into account, in addition to all other eligibility requirements and program criteria, factors such as whether the applicant has been subject to a termination or suspension under paragarph (a) of this section and whether the applicant or the person or persons who would direct or has have directed the scientific and technical aspects of an activity has have, in the judgment of the department or agency head, materially failed to discharge responsibility for the protection of the rights and welfare of human subjects (whether or not the research was subject to federal regulation).

§46.124 Conditions.

With respect to any research project or any class of research projects the department or agency head may impose additional conditions prior to or at the time of approval when in the judgment of the department or agency head additional conditions are necessary for the protection of human subjects.

Subpart B—Additional Protections for Pregnant Women, Human Fetuses and Neonates Involved in Research

Source: 66 FR 56778, Nov. 13, 2001, unless otherwise noted.

§46.201 To what do these regulations apply?

(a) Except as provided in paragraph (b) of this section, this subpart applies to all research involving pregnant women, human fetuses, neonates of uncertain viability, or nonviable neonates conducted or supported by the Department of Health and Human Services (DHHS). This includes all research conducted in DHHS facilities by any person and all research conducted in any facility by DHHS employees.

(b) The exemptions at §46.101(b)(1) through (6) are applicable to this subpart.

(c) The provisions of §46.101(c) through (i) are applicable to this subpart. Reference to State or local laws in this subpart and in §46.101(f) is intended to include the laws of federally recognized American Indian and Alaska Native Tribal Governments.

(d) The requirements of this subpart are in addition to those imposed under the other subparts of this part.

§46.202 Definitions.

The definitions in §46.102 shall be applicable to this subpart as well. In addition, as used in this subpart:

(a) Dead fetus means a fetus that exhibits neither heartbeat, spontaneous respiratory activity, spontaneous movement of voluntary muscles, nor pulsation of the umbilical cord.

(b) Delivery means complete separation of the fetus from the woman by expulsion or extraction or any other means.

(c) Fetus means the product of conception from implantation until delivery.

(d) Neonate means a newborn.

(e) Nonviable neonate means a neonate after delivery that, although living, is not viable.

(f) Pregnancy encompasses the period of time from implantation until delivery. A woman shall be assumed to be pregnant if she exhibits any of the pertinent presumptive signs of pregnancy, such as missed menses, until the results of a pregnancy test are negative or until delivery.

(g) Secretary means the Secretary of Health and Human Services and any other officer or employee of the Department of Health and Human Services to whom authority has been delegated.

(h) Viable, as it pertains to the neonate, means being able, after delivery, to survive (given the benefit of available medical therapy) to the point of independently maintaining heartbeat and respiration. The Secretary may from time to time, taking into account medical advances, publish in the Federal Register guidelines to assist in determining whether a neonate is viable for purposes of this subpart. If a neonate is viable then it may be included in research only to the extent permitted and in accordance with the requirements of subparts A and D of this part.

§46.203 Duties of IRBs in connection with research involving pregnant women, fetuses, and neonates.

In addition to other responsibilities assigned to IRBs under this part, each IRB shall review research covered by this subpart and approve only research which satisfies the conditions of all applicable sections of this subpart and the other subparts of this part.

§46.204 Research involving pregnant women or fetuses.

Pregnant women or fetuses may be involved in research if all of the following conditions are met:

(a) Where scientifically appropriate, preclinical studies, including studies on pregnant animals, and clinical studies, including studies on nonpregnant women, have been conducted and provide data for assessing potential risks to pregnant women and fetuses;

(b) The risk to the fetus is caused solely by interventions or procedures that hold out the prospect of direct benefit for the woman or the fetus; or, if there is no such prospect of benefit, the risk to the fetus is not greater than minimal and the purpose of the research is the development of important biomedical knowledge which cannot be obtained by any other means;

(c) Any risk is the least possible for achieving the objectives of the research;

(d) If the research holds out the prospect of direct benefit to the pregnant woman, the prospect of a direct benefit both to the pregnant woman and the fetus, or no prospect of benefit for the woman nor the fetus when risk to the fetus is not greater than minimal and the purpose of the research is the development of important biomedical knowledge that cannot be obtained by any other means, her consent is obtained in accord with the informed consent provisions of subpart A of this part;

(e) If the research holds out the prospect of direct benefit solely to the fetus then the consent of the pregnant woman and the father is obtained in accord with the informed consent provisions of subpart A of this part, except that the father's consent need not be obtained if he is unable to consent because of unavailability, incompetence, or temporary incapacity or the pregnancy resulted from rape or incest.

(f) Each individual providing consent under paragraph (d) or (e) of this section is fully informed regarding the reasonably foreseeable impact of the research on the fetus or neonate;

(g) For children as defined in §46.402(a) who are pregnant, assent and permission are obtained in accord with the provisions of subpart D of this part;

(h) No inducements, monetary or otherwise, will be offered to terminate a pregnancy;

(i) Individuals engaged in the research will have no part in any decisions as to the timing, method, or procedures used to terminate a pregnancy; and

(j) Individuals engaged in the research will have no part in determining the viability of a neonate.

§46.205 Research involving neonates.

(a) Neonates of uncertain viability and nonviable neonates may be involved in research if all of the following conditions are met:

(1) Where scientifically appropriate, preclinical and clinical studies have been conducted and provide data for assessing potential risks to neonates.

(2) Each individual providing consent under paragraph (b)(2) or (c)(5) of this section is fully informed regarding the reasonably foreseeable impact of the research on the neonate.

(3) Individuals engaged in the research will have no part in determining the viability of a neonate.

(4) The requirements of paragraph (b) or (c) of this section have been met as applicable.

(b) Neonates of uncertain viability. Until it has been ascertained whether or not a neonate is viable, a neonate may not be involved in research covered by this subpart unless the following additional conditions are met:

(1) The IRB determines that:

(i) The research holds out the prospect of enhancing the probability of survival of the neonate to the point of viability, and any risk is the least possible for achieving that objective, or

(ii) The purpose of the research is the development of important biomedical knowledge which cannot be obtained by other means and there will be no added risk to the neonate resulting from the research; and

(2) The legally effective informed consent of either parent of the neonate or, if neither parent is able to consent because of unavailability, incompetence, or temporary incapacity, the legally effective informed consent of either parent's legally authorized representative is obtained in accord with subpart A of this part, except that the consent of the father or his legally authorized representative need not be obtained if the pregnancy resulted from rape or incest.

(c) Nonviable neonates. After delivery nonviable neonate may not be involved in research covered by this subpart unless all of the following additional conditions are met:

(1) Vital functions of the neonate will not be artificially maintained;

(2) The research will not terminate the heartbeat or respiration of the neonate;

(3) There will be no added risk to the neonate resulting from the research;

(4) The purpose of the research is the development of important biomedical knowledge that cannot be obtained by other means; and

(5) The legally effective informed consent of both parents of the neonate is obtained in accord with subpart A of this part, except that the waiver and alteration provisions of §46.116(c) and (d) do not apply. However, if either parent is unable to consent because of unavailability, incompetence, or temporary incapacity, the informed consent of one parent of a nonviable neonate will suffice to meet the requirements of this paragraph (c)(5), except that the consent of the father need not be obtained if the pregnancy resulted from rape or incest. The consent of a legally authorized representative of either or both of the parents of a nonviable neonate will not suffice to meet the requirements of this paragraph (c)(5).

(d) Viable neonates. A neonate, after delivery, that has been determined to be viable may be included in research only to the extent permitted by and in accord with the requirements of subparts A and D of this part.

§46.206 Research involving, after delivery, the placenta, the dead fetus or fetal material.

(a) Research involving, after delivery, the placenta; the dead fetus; macerated fetal material; or cells, tissue, or organs excised from a dead fetus, shall be conducted only in accord with any applicable Federal, State, or local laws and regulations regarding such activities.

(b) If information associated with material described in paragraph (a) of this section is recorded for research purposes in a manner that living individuals can be identified, directly or through identifiers linked to those individuals, those individuals are research subjects and all pertinent subparts of this part are applicable.

§46.207 Research not otherwise approvable which presents an opportunity to understand, prevent, or alleviate a serious problem affecting the health or welfare of pregnant women, fetuses, or neonates.

The Secretary will conduct or fund research that the IRB does not believe meets the requirements of §46.204 or § 46.205 only if:

(a) The IRB finds that the research presents a reasonable opportunity to further the understanding, prevention, or alleviation of a serious problem affecting the health or welfare of pregnant women, fetuses or neonates; and

(b) The Secretary, after consultation with a panel of experts in pertinent disciplines (for example: science, medicine, ethics, law) and following opportunity for public review and comment, including a public meeting announced in the Federal Register, has determined either:

(1) That the research in fact satisfies the conditions of §46.204, as applicable; or

(2) The following:

(i) The research presents a reasonable opportunity to further the understanding, prevention, or alleviation of a serious problem affecting the health or welfare of pregnant women, fetuses or neonates;

(ii) The research will be conducted in accord with sound ethical principles; and

(iii) Informed consent will be obtained in accord with the informed consent provisions of subpart A and other applicable subparts of this part.

Subpart C—Additional Protections Pertaining to Biomedical and Behavioral Research Involving Prisoners as Subjects

Source: 43 FR 53655, Nov. 16, 1978, unless otherwise noted.

§46.301 Applicability.

(a) The regulations in this subpart are applicable to all biomedical and behavioral research conducted or supported by the Department of Health and Human Services involving prisoners as subjects.

(b) Nothing in this subpart shall be construed as indicating that compliance with the procedures set forth herein will authorize research involving prisoners as subjects, to the extent such research is limited or barred by applicable State or local law.

(c) The requirements of this subpart are in addition to those imposed under the other subparts of this part.

§46.302 Purpose.

Inasmuch as prisoners may be under constraints because of their incarceration which could affect their ability to make a truly voluntary and uncoerced decision whether or not to participate as subjects in research, it is the purpose of this subpart to provide additional safeguards for the protection of prisoners involved in activities to which this subpart is applicable.

§46.303 Definitions.

As used in this subpart:

(a) Secretary means the Secretary of Health and Human Services and any other officer or employee of the Department of Health and Human Services to whom authority has been delegated.

(b) DHHS means the Department of Health and Human Services.

(c) Prisoner means any individual involuntarily confined or detained in a penal institution. The term is intended to encompass individuals sentenced to such an institution under a criminal or civil statute, individuals detained in other facilities by virtue of statutes or commitment procedures which provide alternatives to criminal prosecution or incarceration in a penal institution, and individuals detained pending arraignment, trial, or sentencing.

(d) Minimal risk is the probability and magnitude of physical or psychological harm that is normally encountered in the daily lives, or in the routine medical, dental, or psychological examination of healthy persons.

§46.304 Composition of Institutional Review Boards where prisoners are involved.

In addition to satisfying the requirements in §46.107 of this part, an Institutional Review Board, carrying out responsibilities under this part with respect to research covered by this subpart, shall also meet the following specific requirements:

(a) A majority of the Board (exclusive of prisoner members) shall have no association with the prison(s) involved, apart from their membership on the Board.

(b) At least one member of the Board shall be a prisoner, or a prisoner representative with appropriate background and experience to serve in that capacity, except that where a particular research project is reviewed by more than one Board only one Board need satisfy this requirement.

[43 FR 53655, Nov. 16, 1978, as amended at 46 FR 8386, Jan. 26, 1981]

§46.305 Additional duties of the Institutional Review Boards where prisoners are involved.

(a) In addition to all other responsibilities prescribed for Institutional Review Boards under this part, the Board shall review research covered by this subpart and approve such research only if it finds that:

(1) The research under review represents one of the categories of research permissible under §46.306(a)(2);

(2) Any possible advantages accruing to the prisoner through his or her participation in the research, when compared to the general living conditions, medical care, quality of food, amenities and opportunity for earnings in the prison, are not of such a magnitude that his or her ability to weigh the risks of the research against the value of such advantages in the limited choice environment of the prison is impaired;

(3) The risks involved in the research are commensurate with risks that would be accepted by nonprisoner volunteers;

(4) Procedures for the selection of subjects within the prison are fair to all prisoners and immune from arbitrary intervention by prison authorities or prisoners. Unless the principal investigator provides to the Board justification in writing for following some other procedures, control subjects must be selected randomly from the group of available prisoners who meet the characteristics needed for that particular research project;

(5) The information is presented in language which is understandable to the subject population;

(6) Adequate assurance exists that parole boards will not take into account a prisoner's participation in the research in making decisions regarding parole, and each prisoner is clearly informed in advance that participation in the research will have no effect on his or her parole; and

(7) Where the Board finds there may be a need for follow-up examination or care of participants after the end of their participation, adequate provision has been made for such examination or care, taking into account the varying lengths of individual prisoners' sentences, and for informing participants of this fact.

(b) The Board shall carry out such other duties as may be assigned by the Secretary.

(c) The institution shall certify to the Secretary, in such form and manner as the Secretary may require, that the duties of the Board under this section have been fulfilled.

§46.306 Permitted research involving prisoners.

(a) Biomedical or behavioral research conducted or supported by DHHS may involve prisoners as subjects only if:

(1) The institution responsible for the conduct of the research has certified to the Secretary that the Institutional Review Board has approved the research under §46.305 of this subpart; and

(2) In the judgment of the Secretary the proposed research involves solely the following:

(i) Study of the possible causes, effects, and processes of incarceration, and of criminal behavior, provided that the study presents no more than minimal risk and no more than inconvenience to the subjects;

(ii) Study of prisons as institutional structures or of prisoners as incarcerated persons, provided that the study presents no more than minimal risk and no more than inconvenience to the subjects;

(iii) Research on conditions particularly affecting prisoners as a class (for example, vaccine trials and other research on hepatitis which is much more prevalent in prisons than elsewhere; and research on social and psychological problems such as alcoholism, drug addiction and sexual assaults) provided that the study may proceed only after the Secretary has consulted with appropriate experts including experts in penology medicine and ethics, and published notice, in the

Federal Register, of his intent to approve such research; or

(iv) Research on practices, both innovative and accepted, which have the intent and reasonable probability of improving the health or well-being of the subject. In cases in which those studies require the assignment of prisoners in a manner consistent with protocols approved by the IRB to control groups which may not benefit from the research, the study may proceed only after the Secretary has consulted with appropriate experts, including experts in penology medicine and ethics, and published notice, in the Federal Register, of his intent to approve such research.

(b) Except as provided in paragraph (a) of this section, biomedical or behavioral research conducted or supported by DHHS shall not involve prisoners as subjects.

Subpart D—Additional Protections for Children Involved as Subjects in Research

Source: 48 FR 9818, Mar. 8, 1983, unless otherwise noted.

§46.401 To what do these regulations apply?

(a) This subpart applies to all research involving children as subjects, conducted or supported by the Department of Health and Human Services.

(1) This includes research conducted by Department employees, except that each head of an Operating Division of the Department may adopt such nonsubstantive, procedural modifications as may be appropriate from an administrative standpoint.

(2) It also includes research conducted or supported by the Department of Health and Human Services outside the United States, but in appropriate circumstances, the Secretary may, under paragraph (e) of §46.101 of Subpart A, waive the applicability of some or all of the requirements of these regulations for research of this type.

(b) Exemptions at §46.101(b)(1) and (b)(3) through (b)(6) are applicable to this subpart. The exemption at §46.101(b)(2) regarding educational tests is also applicable to this subpart. However, the exemption at §46.101(b)(2) for research involving survey or interview procedures or observations of public behavior does not apply to research covered by this subpart, except for research involving observation of public behavior when the investigator(s) do not participate in the activities being observed.

(c) The exceptions, additions, and provisions for waiver as they appear in paragraphs (c) through (i) of §46.101 of Subpart A are applicable to this subpart.

[48 FR 9818, Mar. 8, 1983; 56 FR 28032, June 18, 1991; 56 FR 29757, June 28, 1991]

§46.402 Definitions.

The definitions in §46.102 of Subpart A shall be applicable to this subpart as well. In addition, as used in this subpart:

(a) Children are persons who have not attained the legal age for consent to treatments or procedures involved in the research, under the applicable law of the jurisdiction in which the research will be conducted.

(b) Assent means a child's affirmative agreement to participate in research. Mere failure to object should not, absent affirmative agreement, be construed as assent.

(c) Permission means the agreement of parent(s) or guardian to the participation of their child or ward in research.

(d) Parent means a child's biological or adoptive parent.

(e) Guardian means an individual who is authorized under applicable State or local law to consent on behalf of a child to general medical care.

§46.403 IRB duties.

In addition to other responsibilities assigned to IRBs under this part, each IRB shall review research covered by this subpart and approve only research which satisfies the conditions of all applicable sections of this subpart.

§46.404 Research not involving greater than minimal risk.

HHS will conduct or fund research in which the IRB finds that no greater than minimal risk to children is presented, only if the IRB finds that adequate provisions are made for soliciting the assent of the children and the permission of their parents or guardians, as set forth in §46.408.

§46.405 Research involving greater than minimal risk but presenting the prospect of direct benefit to the individual subjects.

HHS will conduct or fund research in which the IRB finds that more than minimal risk to children is presented by an intervention or procedure that holds out the prospect of direct benefit for the individual subject, or by a monitoring procedure that is likely to contribute to the subject's well-being, only if the IRB finds that:

(a) The risk is justified by the anticipated benefit to the subjects;

(b) The relation of the anticipated benefit to the risk is at least as favorable to the subjects as that presented by available alternative approaches; and

(c) Adequate provisions are made for soliciting the assent of the children and permission of their parents or guardians, as set forth in §46.408.

§46.406 Research involving greater than minimal risk and no prospect of direct benefit to individual subjects, but likely to yield generalizable knowledge about the subject's disorder or condition.

HHS will conduct or fund research in which the IRB finds that more than minimal risk to children is presented by an intervention or procedure that does not hold out the prospect of direct benefit for the individual subject, or by a monitoring procedure which is not likely to contribute to the well-being of the subject, only if the IRB finds that:

(a) The risk represents a minor increase over minimal risk;

(b) The intervention or procedure presents experiences to subjects that are reasonably commensurate with those inherent in their actual or expected medical, dental, psychological, social, or educational situations;

(c) The intervention or procedure is likely to yield generalizable knowledge about the subjects' disorder or condition which is of vital importance for the understanding or amelioration of the subjects' disorder or condition; and

(d) Adequate provisions are made for soliciting assent of the children and permission of their parents or guardians, as set forth in §46.408.

§46.407 Research not otherwise approvable which presents an opportunity to understand, prevent, or alleviate a serious problem affecting the health or welfare of children.

HHS will conduct or fund research that the IRB does not believe meets the requirements of §46.404, §46.405, or §46.406 only if:

(a) The IRB finds that the research presents a reasonable opportunity to further the understanding, prevention, or alleviation of a serious problem affecting the health or welfare of children; and

(b) The Secretary, after consultation with a panel of experts in pertinent disciplines (for example: science, medicine, education, ethics, law) and following opportunity for public review and comment, has determined either:

(1) That the research in fact satisfies the conditions of §46.404, §46.405, or §46.406, as applicable, or

(2) The following:

(i) The research presents a reasonable opportunity to further the understanding, prevention, or alleviation of a serious problem affecting the health or welfare of children;

(ii) The research will be conducted in accordance with sound ethical principles;

(iii) Adequate provisions are made for soliciting the assent of children and the permission of their parents or guardians, as set forth in §46.408.

§46.408 Requirements for permission by parents or guardians and for assent by children.

(a) In addition to the determinations required under other applicable sections of this subpart, the IRB shall determine that adequate provisions are made for soliciting the assent of the children, when in the judgment of the IRB the children are capable of providing assent. In determining whether children are capable of assenting, the IRB shall take into account the ages, maturity, and psychological state of the children involved. This judgment may be made for all children to be involved in research under a particular protocol, or for each child, as the IRB deems appropriate. If the IRB determines that the capability of some or all of the children is so limited that they cannot reasonably be consulted or that the intervention or procedure involved in the research holds out a prospect of direct benefit that is important to the health or well-being of the children and is available only in the context of the research, the assent of the children is not a necessary condition for proceeding with the research. Even where the IRB determines that the subjects are capable of assenting, the IRB may still waive the assent requirement under circumstances in which consent may be waived in accord with §46.116 of Subpart A.

(b) In addition to the determinations required under other applicable sections of this subpart, the IRB shall determine, in accordance with and to the extent that consent is required by §46.116 of Subpart A, that adequate provisions are made for soliciting the permission of each child's parents or guardian. Where parental permission is to be obtained, the IRB may find that the permission of one parent is sufficient for research to be conducted under §46.404 or §46.405. Where research is covered by §§46.406 and 46.407 and permission is to be obtained from parents, both parents must give their permission unless one parent is deceased, unknown, incompetent, or not reasonably available, or when only one parent has legal responsibility for the care and custody of the child.

(c) In addition to the provisions for waiver contained in §46.116 of Subpart A, if the IRB determines that a research protocol is designed for conditions or for a subject population for which parental or guardian permission is not a reasonable requirement to protect the subjects (for example, neglected or abused children), it may waive the consent requirements in Subpart A of this part and paragraph (b) of this section, provided an appropriate mechanism for protecting the children who will participate as subjects in the research is substituted, and provided further that the waiver is not inconsistent with Federal, state or local law. The choice of an appropriate mechanism would depend upon the nature and purpose of the activities described in the protocol, the risk and anticipated benefit to the research subjects, and their age, maturity, status, and condition.

(d) Permission by parents or guardians shall be documented in accordance with and to the extent required by §46.117 of Subpart A.

(e) When the IRB determines that assent is required, it shall also determine whether and how assent must be documented.

§46.409 Wards.

(a) Children who are wards of the state or any other agency, institution, or entity can be included in research approved under §46.406 or §46.407 only if such research is:

(1) Related to their status as wards; or

(2) Conducted in schools, camps, hospitals, institutions, or similar settings in which the majority of children involved as subjects are not wards.

(b) If the research is approved under paragraph (a) of this section, the IRB shall require appointment of an advocate for each child who is a ward, in addition to any other individual acting on behalf of the child as guardian or in loco parentis. One individual may serve as advocate for more than one child. The advocate shall be an individual who has the background and experience to act in, and agrees to act in, the best interests of the child for the duration of the child's participation in the research and who is not associated in any way (except in the role as advocate or member of the IRB) with the research, the investigator(s), or the guardian organization.

Form FDA 1572

DEPARTMENT OF HEALTH AND HUMAN SERVICES PUBLIC HEALTH SERVICE FOOD AND DRUG ADMINISTRATION **STATEMENT OF INVESTIGATOR** ***TITLE 21, CODE OF FEDERAL REGULATIONS (CRF) Part 312)*** (See instructions on reverse side.)	Form Approved: OMB No. 0910-004 Expiration Date: June 30, 1992 *See OMB Statement on Reverse* Note: No investigator may participate in an investigation until her/she provides the sponsor with a completed, signed Statement of investigator. Form FDA 1572 (21 CFR 312.53)).

1. NAME AND ADDRESS OF INVESTIGATOR.

2. EDUCATION, TRAINING AND EXPERIENCE THAT QUALIFIES THE INVESTIGATOR AS AN EXPERT IN THE CLINICAL INVESTIGATION OF THE DRUG FOR TH USE UNDER INVESTIGATION. ONE OF THE FOLLOWING IS ATTACHED:

☐ CURRICULUM VITAE ☐ OTHER STATEMENT OF QUALIFICATIONS

3. NAME AND ADDRESS OF ANY MEDICAL SCHOOL, HOSPITAL OR OTHER RESEARCH FACILITY WHERE THE CLINICAL INVESTIGATION(S) WILL BE CONDUCTED.

4. NAME AND ADDRESS OF ANY CLINICAL LABORATORY FACILITIES TO BE USED IN THE STUDY.

5. NAME AND ADDRESS OF THE INSTITUTIONAL REVIEW BOARD (IRB) THAT IS RESPONSIBLE FOR REVIEW AND APPROVAL OF THE STUDY(IES).

6. NAME(S) OF THE SUBINVESTIGATORS (e.g. research fellows, residents, associates) WHO WILL BE ASSISTING THE INVESTIGATOR IN THE CONDUCT OF THE INVESTIGATION(S).

7. NAME AND CODE NUMBER, IF ANY, OF THE PROTOCOL(S) IN THE IND FOR THE STUDY(IES) TO BE CONDUCTED BY THE INVESTIGATOR.

FORM FDA 1572 (12/91) PREVIOUS EDITION IS OBSOLETE.

8. ATTACH THE FOLLOWING CLINICAL PROTOCOL INFORMATION:

☐ FOR PHASE 1 INVESTIGATIONS, A GENERAL OUTLINE OF THE PLANNED INVESTIGATION INCLUDING THE ESTIMATED DURATION OF THE STUDY AND THE MAXIMUM NUMBER OF SUBJECTS THAT WILL BE INVOLVED.

☐ FOR PHASE 2 OR 3 INVESTIGATIONS, AN OUTLINE OF THE STUDY PROTOCOL INCLUDING AN APPROXIMATION OF THE NUMBER OF SUBJECTS TO BE TREATED WITH THE DRUG AND THE NUMBER TO BE EMPLOYED AS CONTROLS IF ANY: THE CLINICAL USES TO BE INVESTIGATED: CHARACTERISTICS OF SUBJECTS BY AGE, SEX AND CONDITION; THE KIND OF CLINICAL OBSERVATIONS AND LABORATORY TESTS TO BE CONDUCTED: THE ESTIMATED DURATION OF THE STUDY; AND COPIES OR A DESCRIPTION OF CASE REPORT FORMS TO BE USED.

9. COMMITMENTS:

I agree to conduct the study(ies) in accordance with the relevant, current protocol(s) and will only make changes in a protocol after notifying the sponsor, except when necessary to protect the safety, rights, or welfare of subjects.

I agree to personally conduct or supervise the described investigation(s).

I agree to inform any patients, or any persons used as controls, that the drugs are being used for investigational purposes and I will ensure that the requirements relating to obtaining informed consent in 21 CFR Part 50 and institutional review board (IRB) review and approval in 21 CFR Part 56 are met.

I agree to report to the sponsor adverse experiences that occur in the course of the investigation(s) in accordance with 21 CFR 312.64.

I have read and understand the information in the investigator's brochure, including the potential risks and side effects of the drug.

I agree to ensure that all associates, colleagues, and employees assisting in the conduct of the study(ies) are informed about their obligations in meeting the above commitments.

I agree to maintain adequate and accurate records in accordance with 21 CFR 312 62 and to make those records available for inspection in accordance with 21 CFR 312 68.

I will ensure that an IRB that complies with the requirements of 21 CFR Part 56 will be responsible for the initial and continuing review and approval of the clinical investigation. I also agree to promptly report to the IRB all changes in the research activity and all unanticipated problems involving risks to human subjects or others. Additionally, I will not make any changes in the research without IRB approval, except where necessary to eliminate apparent immediate hazards to human subjects.

I agree to comply with all other requirements regarding the obligations of clinical investigators and all other pertinent requirements in 21 CFR Part 312.

INSTRUCTIONS FOR COMPLETING FORM FDA 1572 STATEMENT OF INVESTIGATOR:

1. Complete all sections. Attach a separate page if additional space is needed.
2. Attach curriculum vitae or other statement of qualifications as described in Section 2.
3. Attach protocol outline as described in Section 8.
4. Sign and date below.
5. FORWARD THE COMPLETED FORM AND ATTACHMENTS TO THE SPONSOR. The sponsor will incorporate this information along with other technical data into an Investigational New Drug Application (IND). INVESTIGATORS SHOULD NOT SEND THIS FORM DIRECTLY TO THE FOOD AND DRUG ADMINISTRATION.

10. SIGNATURE OF INVESTIGATOR	11. DATE

Public reporting burden for this collection of information is estimated to average 1 hour per response, including the time for reviewing instructions, searching existing data sources, gathering and maintaining the data needed, and completing reviewing the collection of information. Send comments regarding this burden estimate or any other aspect of this collection of information, including suggestions for reducing this burden to:

Reports Clearance Officer, PHS
Hubert H. Humphrey Building, Room 721-B
200 Independence Avenue, S.W.
Washington, DC 20201
Attn: PRA

and to:

Office of Management and Budget
Paperwork Reduction Project (0910-0014)
Washington, DC 20503

Please DO NOT RETURN this application to either of these addresses.

APPENDIX f

Harmonized Tripartite Guideline for Good Clinical Practice

Introduction

Good Clinical Practice (GCP) is an international ethical and scientific quality standard for designing, conducting, recording and reporting trials that involve the participation of human subjects. Compliance with this standard provides public assurance that the rights, safety and well-being of trial subjects are protected, consistent with the principles that have their origin in the Declaration of Helsinki, and that the clinical trial data are credible.

The objective of this ICH GCP Guideline is to provide a unified standard for the European Union (EU), Japan and the United States to facilitate the mutual acceptance of clinical data by the regulatory authorities in these jurisdictions. The guideline was developed with consideration of the current good clinical practices of the European Union, Japan, and the United States, as well as those of Australia, Canada, the Nordic countries and the World Health Organization (WHO). This guideline should be followed when generating clinical trial data that are intended to be submitted to regulatory authorities. The principles established in this guideline may also be applied to other clinical investigations that may have an impact on the safety and well-being of human subjects.

1. Glossary

1.1 *Adverse Drug Reaction* (ADR). In the pre-approval clinical experience with a new medicinal product or its new usages, particularly as the therapeutic dose(s) may not be established: all noxious and unintended responses to a medicinal product related to any dose should be considered adverse drug reactions. The phrase responses to a medicinal product means that a causal relationship between a medicinal product and an adverse event is at least a reasonable possibility, i.e. the relationship cannot be ruled out. Regarding marketed medicinal products: a response to a drug which is noxious and unintended and which occurs at doses normally used in man for prophylaxis, diagnosis, or therapy of diseases or for modification of physiological function (see the ICH Guideline for Clinical Safety Data Management: Definitions and Standards for Expedited Reporting).

1.2 *Adverse Event* (AE). Any untoward medical occurrence in a patient or clinical investigation subject administered a pharmaceutical product and which does not necessarily have a causal relationship with this treatment. An adverse event (AE) can therefore be any unfavorable and unintended sign (including an abnormal laboratory finding), symptom, or disease temporally associated with the use of a medicinal (investigational) product, whether or not related to the medicinal (investigational) product (see the ICH Guideline for Clinical Safety Data Management: Definitions and Standards for Expedited Reporting).

1.3 *Amendment* (to the protocol). See Protocol Amendment.

1.4 *Applicable Regulatory Requirement*(s). Any law(s) and regulation(s) addressing the conduct of clinical trials of investigational products.

1.5 *Approval* (in relation to Institutional Review Boards). The affirmative decision of the IRB that the clinical trial has been reviewed and may be conducted at the institution site within the constraints set forth by the IRB, the institution, Good Clinical Practice (GCP), and the applicable regulatory requirements.

1.6 *Audit.* A systematic and independent examination of trial related activities and documents to determine whether the evaluated trial related activities were conducted, and the data were recorded, analyzed and accurately reported according to the protocol, sponsor's standard operating procedures (SOPs), Good Clinical Practice (GCP), and the applicable regulatory requirement(s).

1.7 *Audit Certificate.* A declaration of confirmation by the auditor that an audit has taken place.

1.8 *Audit Report.* A written evaluation by the sponsor's auditor of the results of the audit..

1.9 *Audit Trail.* Documentation that allows reconstruction of the course of events.

1.10 *Blinding/Masking.* A procedure in which one or more parties to the trial are kept unaware of the treatment assignment(s). Single-blinding usually refers to the subject(s) being unaware, and double-blinding usually refers to the subject(s), investigator(s), monitor, and, in some cases, data analyst(s) being unaware of the treatment assignment(s).

1.11 *Case Report Form* (CRF). A printed, optical, or electronic document designed to record all of the protocol required information to be reported to the sponsor on each trial subject.

1.12 *Clinical Trial/Study.* Any investigation in human subjects intended to discover or verify the clinical, pharmacological and/or other pharmacodynamic effects of an investigational product(s), and/or to identify any adverse reactions to an investigational product(s), and/or to study absorption, distribution, metabolism, and excretion of an investigational product(s) with the object of ascertaining its safety and/or efficacy. The terms clinical trial and clinical study are synonymous.

1.13 *Clinical Trial/Study Report.* A written description of a trial/study of any therapeutic, prophylactic, or diagnostic agent conducted in human subjects, in which the clinical and statistical description, presentations, and analyses are fully integrated into a single report (see the ICH Guideline for Structure and Content of Clinical Study Reports).

1.14 *Comparator* (Product). An investigational or marketed product (i.e., active control), or placebo, used as a reference in a clinical trial.

1.15 *Compliance* (in relation to trials). Adherence to all the trial-related requirements, Good Clinical Practice (GCP) requirements, and the applicable regulatory requirements.

1.16 *Confidentiality.* Prevention of disclosure, to other than authorized individuals, of a sponsor's proprietary information or of a subject's identity.

1.17 *Contract.* A written, dated, and signed agreement between two or more involved parties that sets out any arrangements on delegation and distribution of tasks and obligations and, if appropriate, on financial matters. The protocol may serve as the basis of a contract.

1.18 *Coordinating Committee.* A committee that a sponsor may organize to coordinate the conduct of a multicentre trial.

1.19 *Coordinating Investigator.* An investigator assigned the responsibility for the coordination of investigators at different centers participating in a multicentre trial.

1.20 *Contract Research Organization* (CRO). A person or an organization (commercial, academic, or other) contracted by the sponsor to perform one or more of a sponsor's trial-related duties and functions.

1.21 *Direct Access.* Permission to examine, analyze, verify, and reproduce any records and reports that are important to evaluation of a clinical trial. Any party (e.g., domestic and foreign regulatory authorities, sponsor's monitors and auditors) with direct access should take all reasonable precautions within the constraints of the applicable regulatory requirement(s) to maintain the confidentiality of subjects' identities and sponsor's proprietary information.

1.22 *Documentation.* All records, in any form (including, but not limited to, written, electronic, magnetic, and optical records, and scans, x-rays, and electrocardiograms) that describe or record the methods, conduct, and/or results of a trial, the factors affecting a trial, and the actions taken.

1.23 *Essential Documents.* Documents which individually and collectively permit evaluation of the conduct of a study and the quality of the data produced (see 8. Essential Documents for the Conduct of a Clinical Trial).

1.24 Good Clinical Practice (GCP)
A standard for the design, conduct, performance, monitoring, auditing, recording, analyses, and reporting of clinical trials that provides assurance that the data and reported results are credible and accurate, and that the rights, integrity, and confidentiality of trial subjects are protected.

1.25 *Independent Data-Monitoring Committee* (IDMC) (Data and Safety Monitoring Board, Monitoring Committee, Data Monitoring Committee). An independent data-monitoring committee that may be established by the sponsor to assess at intervals the progress of a clinical trial, the safety data, and the critical efficacy endpoints, and to recommend to the sponsor whether to continue, modify, or stop a trial.

1.26 *Impartial Witness.* A person, who is independent of the trial, who cannot be unfairly influenced by people involved with the trial, who attends the informed consent process if the subject or the subject's legally acceptable representative cannot read, and who reads the informed consent form and any other written information supplied to the subject

1.27 *Independent Ethics Committee* (IEC). An independent body (a review board or a committee, institutional, regional, national, or supranational), constituted of medical professionals and non-medical members, whose responsibility it is to ensure the protection of the rights, safety and well-being of human subjects involved in a trial and to provide public assurance of that protection, by, among other things, reviewing and approving/providing favorable opinion on, the trial protocol, the suitability of the investigator(s), facilities, and the methods and material to be used in obtaining and documenting informed consent of the trial subjects. The legal status, composition, function, operations and regulatory requirements pertaining to Independent Ethics Committees may differ among countries, but should allow the Independent Ethics Committee to act in agreement with GCP as described in this guideline.

1.28 *Informed Consent.* A process by which a subject voluntarily confirms his or her willingness to participate in a particular trial, after having been informed of all aspects of the trial that are relevant to the subject's decision to participate. Informed consent is documented by means of a written, signed and dated informed consent form.

1.29 *Inspection.* The act by a regulatory authority(ies) of conducting an official review of documents, facilities, records, and any other resources that are deemed by the authority(ies) to be related to the clinical trial and that may be located at the site of the trial, at the sponsor's and/or contract research organization's (CRO's) facilities, or at other establishments deemed appropriate by the regulatory authority(ies).

1.30 *Institution* (medical) Any public or private entity or agency or medical or dental facility where clinical trials are conducted.

1.31 *Institutional Review Board* (IRB)
An independent body constituted of medical, scientific, and non-scientific members, whose responsibility is to ensure the protection of the rights, safety and well-being of human subjects involved in a trial by, among other things, reviewing, approving, and providing continuing review of trial protocol and amendments and of the methods and material to be used in obtaining and documenting informed consent of the trial subjects.

1.32 *Interim Clinical Trial/Study Report.* A report of intermediate results and their evaluation based on analyses performed during the course of a trial.

1.33 *Investigational Product.* A pharmaceutical form of an active ingredient or placebo being tested or used as a reference in a clinical trial, including a product with a marketing authorization when used or assembled (formulated or packaged) in a way different from the approved form, or when used for an unapproved indication, or when used to gain further information about an approved use.

1.34 *Investigator.* A person responsible for the conduct of the clinical trial at a trial site. If a trial is conducted by a team of individuals at a trial site, the investigator is the responsible leader of the team and may be called the principal investigator. See also Subinvestigator.

1.35 *Investigator/Institution.* An expression meaning "the investigator and/or institution, where required by the applicable regulatory requirements".

1.36 *Investigator's Brochure.* A compilation of the clinical and nonclinical data on the investigational product(s) which is relevant to the study of the investigational product(s) in human subjects (see 7. Investigator's Brochure).

1.37 *Legally Acceptable Representative.* An individual or juridical or other body authorized under applicable law to consent, on behalf of a prospective subject, to the subject's participation in the clinical trial.

1.38 *Monitoring.* The act of overseeing the progress of a clinical trial, and of ensuring that it is conducted, recorded, and reported in accordance with the protocol, Standard Operating Procedures (SOPs), Good Clinical Practice (GCP), and the applicable regulatory requirement(s).

1.39 *Monitoring Report.* A written report from the monitor to the sponsor after each site visit and/or other trial-related communication according to the sponsor's SOPs.

1.40 *Multicentre Trial.* A clinical trial conducted according to a single protocol but at more than one site, and therefore, carried out by more than one investigator.

1.41 *Nonclinical Study.* Biomedical studies not performed on human subjects.

1.42 *Opinion.* (in relation to Independent Ethics Committee). The judgement and/or the advice provided by an Independent Ethics Committee (IEC).

1.43 *Original Medical Record.* See Source Documents.

1.44 *Protocol.* A document that describes the objective(s), design, methodology, statistical considerations, and organization of a trial. The protocol usually also gives the background and rationale for the trial, but these could be provided in other protocol referenced documents. Throughout the ICH GCP Guideline the term protocol refers to protocol and protocol amendments.

1.45 *Protocol Amendment.* A written description of a change(s) to or formal clarification of a protocol.

1.46 *Quality Assurance* (QA). All those planned and systematic actions that are established to ensure that the trial is performed and the data are generated, documented (recorded), and reported in compliance with Good Clinical Practice (GCP) and the applicable regulatory requirement(s).

1.47 *Quality Control* (QC). The operational techniques and activities undertaken within the quality assurance system to verify that the requirements for quality of the trial-related activities have been fulfilled.

1.48 *Randomization.* The process of assigning trial subjects to treatment or control groups using an element of chance to determine the assignments in order to reduce bias.

1.49 *Regulatory Authorities.* Bodies having the power to regulate. In the ICH GCP guideline the expression Regulatory Authorities includes the authorities that review submitted clinical data and those that conduct inspections (see 1.29). These bodies are sometimes referred to as competent authorities.

1.50 *Serious Adverse Event* (SAE) or *Serious Adverse Drug Reaction* (Serious ADR). Any untoward medical occurrence that at any dose:

- results in death,
- is life-threatening,
- requires inpatient hospitalization or prolongation of existing hospitalization,
- results in persistent or significant disability/incapacity,

or

- is a congenital anomaly/birth defect

(see the ICH Guideline for Clinical Safety Data Management: Definitions and Standards for Expedited Reporting).

1.51 *Source Data.* All information in original records and certified copies of original records of clinical findings, observations, or other activities in a clinical trial necessary for the reconstruction and evaluation of the trial. Source data are contained in source documents (original records or certified copies).

1.52 *Source Documents.* Original documents, data, and records (e.g., hospital records, clinical and office charts, laboratory notes, memoranda, subjects' diaries or evaluation checklists, pharmacy dispensing records, recorded data from automated instruments, copies or transcriptions certified after verification as being accurate copies, microfiches, photographic negatives, microfilm or magnetic media, x-rays, subject files, and records kept at the pharmacy, at the laboratories and at medico-technical departments involved in the clinical trial).

1.53 *Sponsor*. An individual, company, institution, or organization which takes responsibility for the initiation, management, and/or financing of a clinical trial.

1.54 *Sponsor-Investigator*. An individual who both initiates and conducts, alone or with others, a clinical trial, and under whose immediate direction the investigational product is administered to, dispensed to, or used by a subject. The term does not include any person other than an individual (e.g., it does not include a corporation or an agency). The obligations of a sponsor-investigator include both those of a sponsor and those of an investigator.

1.55 *Standard Operating Procedures* (SOPs). Detailed, written instructions to achieve uniformity of the performance of a specific function.

1.56 *Subinvestigator*. Any individual member of the clinical trial team designated and supervised by the investigator at a trial site to perform critical trial-related procedures and/or to make important trial-related decisions (e.g., associates, residents, research fellows). See also Investigator.

1.57 *Subject/Trial Subject*. An individual who participates in a clinical trial, either as a recipient of the investigational product(s) or as a control.

1.58 *Subject Identification Code*. A unique identifier assigned by the investigator to each trial subject to protect the subject's identity and used in lieu of the subject's name when the investigator reports adverse events and/or other trial related data.

1.59 *Trial Site*. The location(s) where trial-related activities are actually conducted.

1.60 *Unexpected Adverse Drug Reaction*. An adverse reaction, the nature or severity of which is not consistent with the applicable product information (e.g., Investigator's Brochure for an unapproved investigational product or package insert/summary of product characteristics for an approved product) (see the ICH Guideline for Clinical Safety Data Management: Definitions and Standards for Expedited Reporting).

1.61 *Vulnerable Subjects*. Individuals whose willingness to volunteer in a clinical trial may be unduly influenced by the expectation, whether justified or not, of benefits associated with participation, or of a retaliatory response from senior members of a hierarchy in case of refusal to participate. Examples are members of a group with a hierarchical structure, such as medical, pharmacy, dental, and nursing students, subordinate hospital and laboratory personnel, employees of the pharmaceutical industry, members of the armed forces, and persons kept in detention. Other vulnerable subjects include patients with incurable diseases, persons in nursing homes, unemployed or impoverished persons, patients in emergency situations, ethnic minority groups, homeless persons, nomads, refugees, minors, and those incapable of giving consent.

1.62 *Well-being* (of the trial subjects). The physical and mental integrity of the subjects participating in a clinical trial.

2. The Principles of ICH GCP

2.1 Clinical trials should be conducted in accordance with the ethical principles that have their origin in the Declaration of Helsinki, and that are consistent with GCP and the applicable regulatory requirement(s).

2.2 Before a trial is initiated, foreseeable risks and inconveniences should be weighed against the anticipated benefit for the individual trial subject and society. A trial should be initiated and continued only if the anticipated benefits justify the risks.

2.3 The rights, safety, and well-being of the trial subjects are the most important considerations and should prevail over interests of science and society.

2.4 The available nonclinical and clinical information on an investigational product should be adequate to support the proposed clinical trial.

2.5 Clinical trials should be scientifically sound, and described in a clear, detailed protocol.

2.6 A trial should be conducted in compliance with the protocol that has received prior institutional review board (IRB)/independent ethics committee (IEC) approval/favorable opinion.

2.7 The medical care given to, and medical decisions made on behalf of, subjects should always be the responsibility of a qualified physician or, when appropriate, of a qualified dentist.

2.8 Each individual involved in conducting a trial should be qualified by education, training, and experience to perform his or her respective task(s).

2.9 Freely given informed consent should be obtained from every subject prior to clinical trial participation.

2.10 All clinical trial information should be recorded, handled, and stored in a way that allows its accurate reporting, interpretation and verification.

2.11 The confidentiality of records that could identify subjects should be protected, respecting the privacy and confidentiality rules in accordance with the applicable regulatory requirement(s).

2.12 Investigational products should be manufactured, handled, and stored in accordance with applicable good manufacturing practice (GMP). They should be used in accordance with the approved protocol.

2.13 Systems with procedures that assure the quality of every aspect of the trial should be implemented.

3. Institutional Review Board/Independent Ethics Committee (IRB/IEC)

3.1 Responsibilities

3.1.1 An IRB/IEC should safeguard the rights, safety, and well-being of all trial subjects. Special attention should be paid to trials that may include vulnerable subjects.

3.1.2 The IRB/IEC should obtain the following documents:
Trial protocol(s)/amendment(s), written informed consent form(s) and consent form updates that the investigator proposes for use in the trial, subject recruitment procedures (e.g. advertisements), written information to be provided to subjects, Investigator's Brochure (IB), available safety information, information about payments and compensation available to subjects, the investigator's current curriculum vitae and/or other documentation evidencing qualifications, and any other documents that the IRB/IEC may need to fulfil its responsibilities.

The IRB/IEC should review a proposed clinical trial within a reasonable time and document its views in writing, clearly identifying the trial, the documents reviewed and the dates for the following:

- approval/favorable opinion;
- modifications required prior to its approval/favorable opinion;
- disapproval/negative opinion; and
- termination/suspension of any prior approval/favorable opinion.

3.1.3 The IRB/IEC should consider the qualifications of the investigator for the proposed trial, as documented by a current curriculum vitae and/or by any other relevant documentation the IRB/IEC requests.

3.1.4 The IRB/IEC should conduct continuing review of each ongoing trial at intervals appropriate to the degree of risk to human subjects, but at least once per year.

3.1.5 The IRB/IEC may request more information than is outlined in paragraph 4.8.10 be given to subjects when, in the judgement of the IRB/IEC, the additional information would add meaningfully to the protection of the rights, safety and/or well-being of the subjects.

3.1.6 When a non-therapeutic trial is to be carried out with the consent of the subject's legally acceptable representative (see 4.8.12, 4.8.14), the IRB/IEC should determine that the proposed protocol and/or other document(s) adequately addresses relevant ethical concerns and meets applicable regulatory requirements for such trials.

3.1.7 Where the protocol indicates that prior consent of the trial subject or the subject's legally acceptable representative is not possible (see 4.8.15), the IRB/IEC should determine that the proposed protocol and/or other document(s) adequately addresses relevant ethical concerns and meets applicable regulatory requirements for such trials (i.e. in emergency situations).

3.1.8 The IRB/IEC should review both the amount and method of payment to subjects to assure that neither presents problems of coercion or undue influence on the trial subjects. Payments to a subject should be prorated and not wholly contingent on completion of the trial by the subject.

3.1.9 The IRB/IEC should ensure that information regarding payment to subjects, including the methods, amounts, and schedule of payment to trial subjects, is set forth in the written informed consent form and any other information to be provided to subjects. The way payment will be prorated should be specified.

3.2 Composition, Functions and Operations

3.2.1 The IRB/IEC should consist of a reasonable number of members, who collectively have the qualifications and experience to review and evaluate the science, medical aspects, and ethics of the proposed trial. It is recommended that the IRB/IEC should include:

a. At least five members.
b. At least one member whose primary area of interest is in a nonscientific area.
c. At least one member who is independent of the institution/trial site.

Only those IRB/IEC members who are independent of the investigator and the sponsor of the trial should vote/provide opinion on a trial-related matter. A list of IRB/IEC members and their qualifications should be maintained.

3.2.2 The IRB/IEC should perform its functions according to written operating procedures, should maintain written records of its activities and minutes of its meetings, and should comply with GCP and with the applicable regulatory requirement(s).

3.2.3 An IRB/IEC should make its decisions at announced meetings at which at least a quorum, as stipulated in its written operating procedures, is present.

3.2.4 Only members who participate in the IRB/IEC review and discussion should vote/provide their opinion and/or advise.

3.2.5 The investigator may provide information on any aspect of the trial, but should not participate in the deliberations of the IRB/IEC or in the vote/opinion of the IRB/IEC.

3.2.6 An IRB/IEC may invite nonmembers with expertise in special areas for assistance.

3.3 Procedures

The IRB/IEC should establish, document in writing, and follow its procedures, which should include:

3.3.1 Determining its composition (names and qualifications of the members) and the authority under which it is established.

3.3.2 Scheduling, notifying its members of, and conducting its meetings.

3.3.3 Conducting initial and continuing review of trials.

3.3.4 Determining the frequency of continuing review, as appropriate.

3.3.5 Providing, according to the applicable regulatory requirements, expedited review and approval/favorable opinion of minor change(s) in ongoing trials that have the approval/favorable opinion of the IRB/IEC.

3.3.6 Specifying that no subject should be admitted to a trial before the IRB/IEC issues its written approval/favorable opinion of the trial.

3.3.7 Specifying that no deviations from, or changes of, the protocol should be initiated without prior written IRB/IEC approval/favorable opinion of an appropriate amendment, except when necessary to eliminate immediate hazards to the subjects or when the change(s) involves only logistical or administrative aspects of the trial (e.g., change of monitor(s), telephone number(s)) (see 4.5.2).

3.3.8 Specifying that the investigator should promptly report to the IRB/IEC:

a. Deviations from, or changes of, the protocol to eliminate immediate hazards to the trial subjects (see 3.3.7, 4.5.2, 4.5.4).

b. Changes increasing the risk to subjects and/or affecting significantly the conduct of the trial (see 4.10.2).
c. All adverse drug reactions (ADRs) that are both serious and unexpected.
d. New information that may affect adversely the safety of the subjects or the conduct of the trial.

3.3.9 Ensuring that the IRB/IEC promptly notify in writing the investigator/institution concerning:
a. Its trial-related decisions/opinions.
b. The reasons for its decisions/opinions.
c. Procedures for appeal of its decisions/opinions.

3.4 Records

The IRB/IEC should retain all relevant records (e.g., written procedures, membership lists, lists of occupations/affiliations of members, submitted documents, minutes of meetings, and correspondence) for a period of at least 3 years after completion of the trial and make them available upon request from the regulatory authority(ies). The IRB/IEC may be asked by investigators, sponsors or regulatory authorities to provide its written procedures and membership lists.

4. Investigator

4.1 Investigator's Qualifications and Agreements

4.1.1 The investigator(s) should be qualified by education, training, and experience to assume responsibility for the proper conduct of the trial, should meet all the qualifications specified by the applicable regulatory requirement(s), and should provide evidence of such qualifications through up-to-date curriculum vitae and/or other relevant documentation requested by the sponsor, the IRB/IEC, and/or the regulatory authority(ies).

4.1.2 The investigator should be thoroughly familiar with the appropriate use of the investigational product(s), as described in the protocol, in the current Investigator's Brochure, in the product information and in other information sources provided by the sponsor.

4.1.3 The investigator should be aware of, and should comply with, GCP and the applicable regulatory requirements.

4.1.4 The investigator/institution should permit monitoring and auditing by the sponsor, and inspection by the appropriate regulatory authority(ies)..

4.1.5 The investigator should maintain a list of appropriately qualified persons to whom the investigator has delegated significant trial-related duties.

4.2 Adequate Resources

4.2.1 The investigator should be able to demonstrate (e.g., based on retrospective data) a potential for recruiting the required number of suitable subjects within the agreed recruitment period.

4.2.2 The investigator should have sufficient time to properly conduct and complete the trial within the agreed trial period.

4.2.3 The investigator should have available an adequate number of qualified staff and adequate facilities for the foreseen duration of the trial to conduct the trial properly and safely.

4.2.4 The investigator should ensure that all persons assisting with the trial are adequately informed about the protocol, the investigational product(s), and their trial-related duties and functions.

4.3 Medical Care of Trial Subjects

4.3.1 A qualified physician (or dentist, when appropriate), who is an investigator or a sub-investigator for the trial, should be responsible for all trial-related medical (or dental) decisions.

4.3.2 During and following a subject's participation in a trial, the investigator/institution should ensure that adequate medical care is provided to a subject for any adverse events, including clinically significant laboratory values, related to the trial. The investigator/institution should inform a subject when medical care is needed for intercurrent illness(es) of which the investigator becomes aware.

4.3.3 It is recommended that the investigator inform the subject's primary physician about the subject's participation in the trial if the subject has a primary physician and if the subject agrees to the primary physician being informed.

4.3.4 Although a subject is not obliged to give his/her reason(s) for withdrawing prematurely from a trial, the investigator should make a reasonable effort to ascertain the reason(s), while fully respecting the subject's rights.

4.4 Communication with IRB/IEC

4.4.1 Before initiating a trial, the investigator/institution should have written and dated approval/favorable opinion from the IRB/IEC for the trial protocol, written informed consent form, consent form updates, subject recruitment procedures (e.g., advertisements), and any other written information to be provided to subjects.

4.4.2 As part of the investigator's/institution's written application to the IRB/IEC, the investigator/institution should provide the IRB/IEC with a current copy of the Investigator's Brochure. If the Investigator's Brochure is updated during the trial, the investigator/institution should supply a copy of the updated Investigator's Brochure to the IRB/IEC.

4.4.3 During the trial the investigator/institution should provide to the IRB/IEC all documents subject to review..

4.5 Compliance with Protocol

4.5.1 The investigator/institution should conduct the trial in compliance with the protocol agreed to by the sponsor and, if required, by the regulatory authority(ies) and which was given approval/favorable opinion by the IRB/IEC. The investigator/institution and the sponsor should sign the protocol, or an alternative contract, to confirm agreement.

4.5.2 The investigator should not implement any deviation from, or changes of the protocol without agreement by the sponsor and prior review and documented approval/favorable opinion from the IRB/IEC of an amendment, except where necessary to eliminate an immediate hazard(s) to trial subjects, or when the change(s) involves only logistical or administrative aspects of the trial (e.g., change in monitor(s), change of telephone number(s)).

4.5.3 The investigator, or person designated by the investigator, should document and explain any deviation from the approved protocol.

4.5.4 The investigator may implement a deviation from, or a change of, the protocol to eliminate an immediate hazard(s) to trial subjects without prior IRB/IEC approval/favorable opinion. As soon as possible, the implemented deviation or change, the reasons for it, and, if appropriate, the proposed protocol amendment(s) should be submitted:

a. to the IRB/IEC for review and approval/favorable opinion,
b. to the sponsor for agreement and, if required,
c. to the regulatory authority(ies).

4.6 Investigational Product(s)

4.6.1 Responsibility for investigational product(s) accountability at the trial site(s) rests with the investigator/institution.

4.6.2 Where allowed/required, the investigator/institution may/should assign some or all of the investigator's/institution's duties for investigational product(s) accountability at the trial site(s) to an appropriate pharmacist or another appropriate individual who is under the supervision of the investigator/institution..

4.6.3 The investigator/institution and/or a pharmacist or other appropriate individual, who is designated by the investigator/institution, should maintain records of the product's delivery to the trial site, the inventory at the site, the use by each subject, and the return to the sponsor or alternative disposition of unused product(s). These records should include dates, quantities, batch/serial numbers, expiration dates (if applicable), and the unique code numbers assigned to the investigational product(s) and trial subjects. Investigators should maintain records that document adequately that the subjects were provided the doses specified by the protocol and reconcile all investigational product(s) received from the sponsor.

4.6.4 The investigational product(s) should be stored as specified by the sponsor (see 5.13.2 and 5.14.3) and in accordance with applicable regulatory requirement(s).

4.6.5 The investigator should ensure that the investigational product(s) are used only in accordance with the approved protocol.

4.6.6 The investigator, or a person designated by the investigator/institution, should explain the correct use of the investigational product(s) to each subject and should check, at intervals appropriate for the trial, that each subject is following the instructions properly.

4.7 Randomization Procedures and Unblinding

The investigator should follow the trial's randomization procedures, if any, and should ensure that the code is broken only in accordance with the protocol. If the trial is blinded, the investigator should promptly document and explain to the sponsor any premature unblinding (e.g., accidental unblinding, unblinding due to a serious adverse event) of the investigational product(s).

4.8 Informed Consent of Trial Subjects

4.8.1 In obtaining and documenting informed consent, the investigator should comply with the applicable regulatory requirement(s), and should adhere to GCP and to the ethical principles that have their origin in the Declaration of Helsinki. Prior to the beginning of the trial, the investigator should have the IRB/IEC's written approval/favorable opinion of the written informed consent form and any other written information to be provided to subjects.

4.8.2 The written informed consent form and any other written information to be provided to subjects should be revised whenever important new information becomes available that may be relevant to the subject's consent. Any revised written informed consent form, and written information should receive the IRB/IEC's approval/favorable opinion in advance of use. The subject or the subject's legally acceptable representative should be informed in a timely manner if new information becomes available that may be relevant to the subject's willingness to continue participation in the trial. The communication of this information should be documented.

4.8.3 Neither the investigator, nor the trial staff, should coerce or unduly influence a subject to participate or to continue to participate in a trial.

4.8.4 None of the oral and written information concerning the trial, including the written informed consent form, should contain any language that causes the subject or the subject's legally acceptable representative to waive or to appear to waive any legal rights, or that releases or appears to release the investigator, the institution, the sponsor, or their agents from liability for negligence.

4.8.5 The investigator, or a person designated by the investigator, should fully inform the subject or, if the subject is unable to provide informed consent, the subject's legally acceptable representative, of all pertinent aspects of the trial including the written information and the approval/favorable opinion by the IRB/IEC.

4.8.6 The language used in the oral and written information about the trial, including the written informed consent form, should be as non-technical as practical and should be understandable to the subject or the subject's legally acceptable representative and the impartial witness, where applicable.

4.8.7 Before informed consent may be obtained, the investigator, or a person designated by the investigator, should provide the subject or the subject's legally acceptable representative ample time and opportunity to inquire details of the trial and to decide whether or not to participate in the trial. All questions about the trial should be answered to the satisfaction of the subject or the subject's legally acceptable representative.

4.8.8 Prior to a subject's participation in the trial, the written informed consent form should be signed and personally dated by the subject or by the subject's legally acceptable representative, and by the person who conducted the informed consent discussion.

4.8.9 If a subject is unable to read or if a legally acceptable representative is unable to read, an impartial witness should be present during the entire informed consent discussion. After the written informed consent form and any other written information to be provided to subjects, is read and explained to the subject or the subject's legally acceptable representative, and after the subject or the subject's legally acceptable representative has orally consented to the subject's participation in the trial and, if capable of doing so, has signed and personally dated the informed consent form, the witness should sign and personally date the consent form. By signing the consent form, the witness attests that the information in the consent form and any other written information was accurately explained to, and apparently understood by, the subject or the subject's legally acceptable representative, and that informed consent was freely given by the subject or the subject's legally acceptable representative.

4.8.10 Both the informed consent discussion and the written informed consent form and any other written information to be provided to subjects should include explanations of the following:

a. That the trial involves research.
b. The purpose of the trial.
c. The trial treatment(s) and the probability for random assignment to each treatment.
d. The trial procedures to be followed, including all invasive procedures.
e. The subject's responsibilities.
f. Those aspects of the trial that are experimental.
g. The reasonably foreseeable risks or inconveniences to the subject and, when applicable, to an embryo, fetus, or nursing infant.
h. The reasonably expected benefits. When there is no intended clinical benefit to the subject, the subject should be made aware of this.
i. The alternative procedure(s) or course(s) of treatment that may be available to the subject, and their important potential benefits and risks.
j. The compensation and/or treatment available to the subject in the event of trial-related injury.
k. The anticipated prorated payment, if any, to the subject for participating in the trial.
l. The anticipated expenses, if any, to the subject for participating in the trial.
m. That the subject's participation in the trial is voluntary and that the subject may refuse to participate or withdraw from the trial, at any time, without penalty or loss of benefits to which the subject is otherwise entitled.
n. That the monitor(s), the auditor(s), the IRB/IEC, and the regulatory authority(ies) will be granted direct access to the subject's original medical records for verification of clinical trial procedures and/or data, without violating the confidentiality of the subject, to the extent permitted by the applicable laws and regulations and that, by signing a written informed consent form, the subject or the subject's legally acceptable representative is authorizing such access.
o. That records identifying the subject will be kept confidential and, to the extent permitted by the applicable laws and/or regulations, will not be made publicly available. If the results of the trial are published, the subject's identity will remain confidential.
p. That the subject or the subject's legally acceptable representative will be informed in a timely manner if information becomes available that may be relevant to the subject's willingness to continue participation in the trial.

q. The person(s) to contact for further information regarding the trial and the rights of trial subjects, and whom to contact in the event of trial-related injury.
r. The foreseeable circumstances and/or reasons under which the subject's participation in the trial may be terminated.
s. The expected duration of the subject's participation in the trial.
t. The approximate number of subjects involved in the trial.

4.8.11 Prior to participation in the trial, the subject or the subject's legally acceptable representative should receive a copy of the signed and dated written informed consent form and any other written information provided to the subjects. During a subject's participation in the trial, the subject or the subject's legally acceptable representative should receive a copy of the signed and dated consent form updates and a copy of any amendments to the written information provided to subjects.

4.8.12 When a clinical trial (therapeutic or non-therapeutic) includes subjects who can only be enrolled in the trial with the consent of the subject's legally acceptable representative (e.g., minors, or patients with severe dementia), the subject should be informed about the trial to the extent compatible with the subject's understanding and, if capable, the subject should sign and personally date the written informed consent.

4.8.13 Except as described in 4.8.14, a non-therapeutic trial (i.e. a trial in which there is no anticipated direct clinical benefit to the subject), should be conducted in subjects who personally give consent and who sign and date the written informed consent form.

4.8.14 Non-therapeutic trials may be conducted in subjects with consent of a legally acceptable representative provided the following conditions are fulfilled:

a. The objectives of the trial can not be met by means of a trial in subjects who can give informed consent personally.
b. The foreseeable risks to the subjects are low.
c. The negative impact on the subject's well-being is minimized and low.
d. The trial is not prohibited by law.
e. The approval/favorable opinion of the IRB/IEC is expressly sought on the inclusion of such subjects, and the written approval/favorable opinion covers this aspect. Such trials, unless an exception is justified, should be conducted in patients having a disease or condition for which the investigational product is intended. Subjects in these trials should be particularly closely monitored and should be withdrawn if they appear to be unduly distressed.

4.8.15 In emergency situations, when prior consent of the subject is not possible, the consent of the subject's legally acceptable representative, if present, should be requested. When prior consent of the subject is not possible, and the subject's legally acceptable representative is not available, enrolment of the subject should require measures described in the protocol and/or elsewhere, with documented approval/favorable opinion by the IRB/IEC, to protect the rights, safety and well-being of the subject and to ensure compliance with applicable regulatory requirements. The subject or the subject's legally acceptable representative should be informed about the trial as soon as possible and consent to continue and other consent as appropriate (see 4.8.10) should be requested.

4.9 Records and Reports

4.9.1 The investigator should ensure the accuracy, completeness, legibility, and timeliness of the data reported to the sponsor in the CRFs and in all required reports.

4.9.2 Data reported on the CRF, that are derived from source documents, should be consistent with the source documents or the discrepancies should be explained.

4.9.3 Any change or correction to a CRF should be dated, initialed, and explained (if necessary) and should not obscure the original entry (i.e. an audit trail should be maintained); this applies to both written and electronic changes or corrections (see 5.18.4 (n)). Sponsors should provide guidance to investigators and/or the investigators' designated representatives on making such corrections. Sponsors should have written procedures to assure that changes or corrections in CRFs made by sponsor's designated representatives are documented, are necessary, and are endorsed by the investigator. The investigator should retain records of the changes and corrections.

4.9.4 The investigator/institution should maintain the trial documents as specified in Essential Documents for the Conduct of a Clinical Trial (see 8.) and as required by the applicable regulatory requirement(s). The investigator/institution should take measures to prevent accidental or premature destruction of these documents.

4.9.5 Essential documents should be retained until at least 2 years after the last approval of a marketing application in an ICH region and until there are no pending or contemplated marketing applications in an ICH region or at least 2 years have elapsed since the formal discontinuation of clinical development of the investigational product. These documents should be retained for a longer period however if required by the applicable regulatory requirements or by an agreement with the sponsor. It is the responsibility of the sponsor to inform the investigator/institution as to when these documents no longer need to be retained (see 5.5.12).

4.9.6 The financial aspects of the trial should be documented in an agreement between the sponsor and the investigator/institution.

4.9.7 Upon request of the monitor, auditor, IRB/IEC, or regulatory authority, the investigator/institution should make available for direct access all requested trial-related records.

4.10 Progress Reports

4.10.1 The investigator should submit written summaries of the trial status to the IRB/IEC annually, or more frequently, if requested by the IRB/IEC.

4.10.2 The investigator should promptly provide written reports to the sponsor, the IRB/IEC (see 3.3.8) and, where applicable, the institution on any changes significantly affecting the conduct of the trial, and/or increasing the risk to subjects.

4.11 Safety Reporting

4.11.1 All serious adverse events (SAEs) should be reported immediately to the sponsor except for those SAEs that the protocol or other document (e.g., Investigator's Brochure) identifies as not needing immediate reporting. The immediate reports should be followed promptly by detailed, written reports. The immediate and follow-up reports should identify subjects by unique code numbers assigned to the trial subjects rather than by the subjects' names, personal identification numbers, and/or addresses. The investigator should also comply with the applicable regulatory requirement(s) related to the reporting of unexpected serious adverse drug reactions to the regulatory authority(ies) and the IRB/IEC.

4.11.2 Adverse events and/or laboratory abnormalities identified in the protocol as critical to safety evaluations should be reported to the sponsor according to the reporting requirements and within the time periods specified by the sponsor in the protocol.

4.11.3 For reported deaths, the investigator should supply the sponsor and the IRB/IEC with any additional requested information (e.g., autopsy reports and terminal medical reports).

4.12 Premature Termination or Suspension of a Trial

If the trial is prematurely terminated or suspended for any reason, the investigator/institution should promptly inform the trial subjects, should assure appropriate therapy and follow-up for the subjects, and, where required by the applicable regulatory requirement(s), should inform the regulatory authority(ies). In addition:

4.12.1 If the investigator terminates or suspends a trial without prior agreement of the sponsor, the investigator should inform the institution where applicable, and the investigator/institution should promptly inform the sponsor and the IRB/IEC, and should provide the sponsor and the IRB/IEC a detailed written explanation of the termination or suspension.

4.12.2 If the sponsor terminates or suspends a trial (see 5.21), the investigator should promptly inform the institution where applicable and the investigator/institution should promptly inform the IRB/IEC and provide the IRB/IEC a detailed written explanation of the termination or suspension.

4.12.3 If the IRB/IEC terminates or suspends its approval/favorable opinion of a trial (see 3.1.2 and 3.3.9), the investigator should inform the institution where applicable and the investigator/institution should promptly notify the sponsor and provide the sponsor with a detailed written explanation of the termination or suspension.

4.13 Final Report(s) by Investigator
Upon completion of the trial, the investigator, where applicable, should inform the institution; the investigator/institution should provide the IRB/IEC with a summary of the trial's outcome, and the regulatory authority(ies) with any reports required.

5. Sponsor

5.1 Quality Assurance and Quality Control

5.1.1 The sponsor is responsible for implementing and maintaining quality assurance and quality control systems with written SOPs to ensure that trials are conducted and data are generated, documented (recorded), and reported in compliance with the protocol, GCP, and the applicable regulatory requirement(s).

5.1.2 The sponsor is responsible for securing agreement from all involved parties to ensure direct access (see 1.21) to all trial related sites, source data/documents , and reports for the purpose of monitoring and auditing by the sponsor, and inspection by domestic and foreign regulatory authorities.

5.1.3 Quality control should be applied to each stage of data handling to ensure that all data are reliable and have been processed correctly.
5.1.4 Agreements, made by the sponsor with the investigator/institution and any other parties involved with the clinical trial, should be in writing, as part of the protocol or in a separate agreement.

5.2 Contract Research Organization (CRO)

5.2.1 A sponsor may transfer any or all of the sponsor's trial-related duties and functions to a CRO, but the ultimate responsibility for the quality and integrity of the trial data always resides with the sponsor. The CRO should implement quality assurance and quality control.

5.2.2 Any trial-related duty and function that is transferred to and assumed by a CRO should be specified in writing.

5.2.3 Any trial-related duties and functions not specifically transferred to and assumed by a CRO are retained by the sponsor.

5.2.4 All references to a sponsor in this guideline also apply to a CRO to the extent that a CRO has assumed the trial related duties and functions of a sponsor.

5.3 Medical Expertise

The sponsor should designate appropriately qualified medical personnel who will be readily available to advise on trial related medical questions or problems. If necessary, outside consultant(s) may be appointed for this purpose.

5.4 Trial Design

5.4.1 The sponsor should utilize qualified individuals (e.g. biostatisticians, clinical pharmacologists, and physicians) as appropriate, throughout all stages of the trial process, from designing the protocol and CRFs and planning the analyses to analyzing and preparing interim and final clinical trial reports.

5.4.2 For further guidance: Clinical Trial Protocol and Protocol Amendment(s) (see 6.), the ICH Guideline for Structure and Content of Clinical Study Reports, and other appropriate ICH guidance on trial design, protocol and conduct.

5.5 Trial Management, Data Handling, and Record Keeping

5.5.1 The sponsor should utilize appropriately qualified individuals to supervise the overall conduct of the trial, to handle the data, to verify the data, to conduct the statistical analyses, and to prepare the trial reports.

5.5.2 The sponsor may consider establishing an independent data-monitoring committee (IDMC) to assess the progress of a clinical trial, including the safety data and the critical efficacy endpoints at intervals, and to recommend to the sponsor whether to continue, modify, or stop a trial. The IDMC should have written operating procedures and maintain written records of all its meetings.

5.5.3 When using electronic trial data handling and/or remote electronic trial data systems, the sponsor should:

a. Ensure and document that the electronic data processing system(s) conforms to the sponsor's established requirements for completeness, accuracy, reliability, and consistent intended performance (i.e. validation).
b. Maintains SOPs for using these systems.

c. Ensure that the systems are designed to permit data changes in such a way that the data changes are documented and that there is no deletion of entered data (i.e. maintain an audit trail, data trail, edit trail).
d. Maintain a security system that prevents unauthorized access to the data.
e. Maintain a list of the individuals who are authorized to make data changes (see 4.1.5 and 4.9.3).
f. Maintain adequate backup of the data.
g. Safeguard the blinding, if any (e.g. maintain the blinding during data entry and processing).

5.5.4 If data are transformed during processing, it should always be possible to compare the original data and observations with the processed data.

5.5.5 The sponsor should use an unambiguous subject identification code (see 1.58) that allows identification of all the data reported for each subject

5.5.6 The sponsor, or other owners of the data, should retain all of the sponsor-specific essential documents pertaining to the trial (see 8. Essential Documents for the Conduct of a Clinical Trial).

5.5.7 The sponsor should retain all sponsor-specific essential documents in conformance with the applicable regulatory requirement(s) of the country(ies) where the product is approved, and/or where the sponsor intends to apply for approval(s).

5.5.8 If the sponsor discontinues the clinical development of an investigational product (i.e. for any or all indications, routes of administration, or dosage forms), the sponsor should maintain all sponsor-specific essential documents for at least 2 years after formal discontinuation or in conformance with the applicable regulatory requirement(s).

5.5.9 If the sponsor discontinues the clinical development of an investigational product, the sponsor should notify all the trial investigators/institutions and all the regulatory authorities.
5.5.10 Any transfer of ownership of the data should be reported to the appropriate authority(ies), as required by the applicable regulatory requirement(s).

5.5.11 The sponsor specific essential documents should be retained until at least 2 years after the last approval of a marketing application in an ICH region and until there are no pending or contemplated marketing applications in an ICH region or at least 2 years have elapsed since the formal discontinuation of clinical development of the investigational product. These documents should be retained for a longer period however if required by the applicable regulatory requirement(s) or if needed by the sponsor.

5.5.12 The sponsor should inform the investigator(s)/institution(s) in writing of the need for record retention and should notify the investigator(s)/institution(s) in writing when the trial related records are no longer needed.

5.6 Investigator Selection

5.6.1 The sponsor is responsible for selecting the investigator(s)/institution(s). Each investigator should be qualified by training and experience and should have adequate resources (see 4.1, 4.2) to properly conduct the trial for which the investigator is selected. If organization of a coordinating committee and/or selection of coordinating investigator(s) are to be utilized in multicentre trials, their organization and/or selection are the sponsor's responsibility.

5.6.2 Before entering an agreement with an investigator/institution to conduct a trial, the sponsor should provide the investigator(s)/institution(s) with the protocol and an up-to-date Investigator's Brochure, and should provide sufficient time for the investigator/institution to review the protocol and the information provided.

5.6.3 The sponsor should obtain the investigator's/institution's agreement:

a. to conduct the trial in compliance with GCP, with the applicable regulatory requirement(s) (see 4.1.3), and with the protocol agreed to by the sponsor and given approval/favorable opinion by the IRB/IEC (see 4.5.1);
b. to comply with procedures for data recording/reporting.
c. to permit monitoring, auditing and inspection (see 4.1.4) and
d. to retain the trial related essential documents until the sponsor informs the investigator/institution these documents are no longer needed (see 4.9.4 and 5.5.12). The sponsor and the investigator/institution should sign the protocol, or an alternative document, to confirm this agreement.

5.7 Allocation of Responsibilities

Prior to initiating a trial, the sponsor should define, establish, and allocate all trial-related duties and functions.

5.8 Compensation to Subjects and Investigators

5.8.1 If required by the applicable regulatory requirement(s), the sponsor should provide insurance or should indemnify (legal and financial coverage) the investigator/the institution against claims arising from the trial, except for claims that arise from malpractice and/or negligence.

5.8.2 The sponsor's policies and procedures should address the costs of treatment of trial subjects in the event of trial-related injuries in accordance with the applicable regulatory requirement(s).

5.8.3 When trial subjects receive compensation, the method and manner of compensation should comply with applicable regulatory requirement(s).

5.9 Financing

The financial aspects of the trial should be documented in an agreement between the sponsor and the investigator/institution.

5.10 Notification/Submission to Regulatory Authority(ies)

Before initiating the clinical trial(s), the sponsor (or the sponsor and the investigator, if required by the applicable regulatory requirement(s)) should submit any required application(s) to the appropriate authority(ies) for review, acceptance, and/or permission (as required by the applicable regulatory requirement(s)) to begin the trial(s). Any notification/submission should be dated and contain sufficient information to identify the protocol.

5.11 Confirmation of Review by IRB/IEC

5.11.1 The sponsor should obtain from the investigator/institution:

a. The name and address of the investigator's/institution's IRB/IEC.
b. A statement obtained from the IRB/IEC that it is organized and operates according to GCP and the applicable laws and regulations.
c. Documented IRB/IEC approval/favorable opinion and, if requested by the sponsor, a current copy of protocol, written informed consent form(s) and any other written information to be provided to subjects, subject recruiting procedures, and documents related to payments and compensation available to the subjects, and any other documents that the IRB/IEC may have requested.

5.11.2 If the IRB/IEC conditions its approval/favorable opinion upon change(s) in any aspect of the trial, such as modification(s) of the protocol, written informed consent form and any other written information to be provided to subjects, and/or other procedures, the sponsor should obtain from the investigator/institution a copy of the modification(s) made and the date approval/favorable opinion was given by the IRB/IEC.

5.11.3 The sponsor should obtain from the investigator/institution documentation and dates of any IRB/IEC reapprovals/re-evaluations with favorable opinion, and of any withdrawals or suspensions of approval/favorable opinion.

5.12 Information on Investigational Product(s)

5.12.1 When planning trials, the sponsor should ensure that sufficient safety and efficacy data from nonclinical studies and/or clinical trials are available to support human exposure by the route, at the dosages, for the duration, and in the trial population to be studied.

5.12.2 The sponsor should update the Investigator's Brochure as significant new information becomes available (see 7. Investigator's Brochure).

5.13 Manufacturing, Packaging, Labeling, and Coding Investigational Product(s)

5.13.1 The sponsor should ensure that the investigational product(s) (including active comparator(s) and placebo, if applicable) is characterized as appropriate to the stage of development of the product(s), is manufactured in accordance with any applicable GMP, and is coded and labeled in a manner that protects the blinding, if applicable. In addition, the labeling should comply with applicable regulatory requirement(s).

5.13.2 The sponsor should determine, for the investigational product(s), acceptable storage temperatures, storage conditions (e.g. protection from light), storage times, reconstitution fluids and procedures, and devices for product infusion, if any. The sponsor should inform all involved parties (e.g. monitors, investigators, pharmacists, storage managers) of these determinations.

5.13.3 The investigational product(s) should be packaged to prevent contamination and unacceptable deterioration during transport and storage.

5.13.4 In blinded trials, the coding system for the investigational product(s) should include a mechanism that permits rapid identification of the product(s) in case of a medical emergency, but does not permit undetectable breaks of the blinding.

5.13.5 If significant formulation changes are made in the investigational or comparator product(s) during the course of clinical development, the results of any additional studies of the formulated product(s) (e.g. stability, dissolution rate, bioavailability) needed to assess whether these changes would significantly alter the pharmacokinetic profile of the product should be available prior to the use of the new formulation in clinical trials.

5.14 Supplying and Handling Investigational Product(s)

5.14.1 The sponsor is responsible for supplying the investigator(s)/institution(s) with the investigational product(s).

5.14.2 The sponsor should not supply an investigator/institution with the investigational product(s) until the sponsor obtains all required documentation (e.g. approval/favorable opinion from IRB/IEC and regulatory authority(ies)).

5.14.3 The sponsor should ensure that written procedures include instructions that the investigator/institution should follow for the handling and storage of investigational product(s) for the trial and documentation thereof.

The procedures should address adequate and safe receipt, handling, storage, dispensing, retrieval of unused product from subjects, and return of unused investigational product(s) to the sponsor (or alternative disposition if authorized by the sponsor and in compliance with the applicable regulatory requirement(s)).

5.14.4 The sponsor should:

a. Ensure timely delivery of investigational product(s) to the investigator(s).
b. Maintain records that document shipment, receipt, disposition, return, and destruction of the investigational product(s) (see 8. Essential Documents for the Conduct of a Clinical Trial).
c. Maintain a system for retrieving investigational products and documenting this retrieval (e.g. for deficient product recall, reclaim after trial completion, expired product reclaim).
d. Maintain a system for the disposition of unused investigational product(s) and for the documentation of this disposition.

5.14.5 The sponsor should:

a. Take steps to ensure that the investigational product(s) are stable over the period of use.
b. Maintain sufficient quantities of the investigational product(s) used in the trials to reconfirm specifications, should this become necessary, and maintain records of batch sample analyses and characteristics. To the extent stability permits, samples should be retained either until the analyses of the trial data are complete or as required by the applicable regulatory requirement(s), whichever represents the longer retention period.

5.15 Record Access

5.15.1 The sponsor should ensure that it is specified in the protocol or other written agreement that the investigator(s)/institution(s) provide direct access to source data/documents for trial-related monitoring, audits, IRB/IEC review, and regulatory inspection.

5.15.2 The sponsor should verify that each subject has consented, in writing, to direct access to his/her original medical records for trial-related monitoring, audit, IRB/IEC review, and regulatory inspection.

5.16 Safety Information

5.16.1 The sponsor is responsible for the ongoing safety evaluation of the investigational product(s).

5.16.2 The sponsor should promptly notify all concerned investigator(s)/institution(s) and the regulatory authority(ies) of findings that could affect adversely the safety of subjects, impact the conduct of the trial, or alter the IRB/IEC's approval/favorable opinion to continue the trial.

5.17 Adverse Drug Reaction Reporting

5.17.1 The sponsor should expedite the reporting to all concerned investigator(s)/institutions(s), to the IRB(s)/IEC(s), where required, and to the regulatory authority(ies) of all adverse drug reactions (ADRs) that are both serious and unexpected.

5.17.2 Such expedited reports should comply with the applicable regulatory requirement(s) and with the ICH Guideline for Clinical Safety Data Management: Definitions and Standards for Expedited Reporting.

5.17.3 The sponsor should submit to the regulatory authority(ies) all safety updates and periodic reports, as required by applicable regulatory requirement(s).

5.18 Monitoring

5.18.1 Purpose

The purposes of trial monitoring are to verify that:

a. The rights and well-being of human subjects are protected.
b. The reported trial data are accurate, complete, and verifiable from source documents.
c. The conduct of the trial is in compliance with the currently approved protocol/amendment(s), with GCP, and with the applicable regulatory requirement(s).

5.18.2 Selection and Qualifications of Monitors

a. Monitors should be appointed by the sponsor.
b. Monitors should be appropriately trained, and should have the scientific and/or clinical knowledge needed to monitor the trial adequately. A monitor's qualifications should be documented.
c. Monitors should be thoroughly familiar with the investigational product(s), the protocol, written informed consent form and any other written information to be provided to subjects, the sponsor's SOPs, GCP, and the applicable regulatory requirement(s).

5.18.3 *Extent and Nature of Monitoring.* The sponsor should ensure that the trials are adequately monitored. The sponsor should determine the appropriate extent and nature of monitoring. The determination of the extent and nature of monitoring should be based on considerations such as the objective, purpose, design, complexity, blinding, size, and endpoints of the trial. In general there is a need for on-site monitoring, before, during, and after the trial; however in exceptional circumstances the sponsor may determine that central monitoring in conjunction with procedures such as investigators' training and meetings, and extensive written guidance can assure appropriate conduct of the trial in accordance with GCP. Statistically controlled sampling may be an acceptable method for selecting the data to be verified.

5.18.4 *Monitor's Responsibilities.* The monitor(s) in accordance with the sponsor's requirements should ensure that the trial is conducted and documented properly by carrying out the following activities when relevant and necessary to the trial and the trial site:

a. Acting as the main line of communication between the sponsor and the investigator.
b. Verifying that the investigator has adequate qualifications and resources (see 4.1, 4.2, 5.6) and remain adequate throughout the trial period, that facilities, including laboratories, equipment, and staff, are adequate to safely and properly conduct the trial and remain adequate throughout the trial period.
c. Verifying, for the investigational product(s):
    i. That storage times and conditions are acceptable, and that supplies are sufficient throughout the trial.
    ii. That the investigational product(s) are supplied only to subjects who are eligible to receive it and at the protocol specified dose(s).
    iii. That subjects are provided with necessary instruction on properly using, handling, storing, and returning the investigational product(s).
    iv. That the receipt, use, and return of the investigational product(s) at the trial sites are controlled and documented adequately.
    v. That the disposition of unused investigational product(s) at the trial sites complies with applicable regulatory requirement(s) and is in accordance with the sponsor.
d. Verifying that the investigator follows the approved protocol and all approved amendment(s), if any.
e. Verifying that written informed consent was obtained before each subject's participation in the trial.
f. Ensuring that the investigator receives the current Investigator's Brochure, all documents, and all trial supplies needed to conduct the trial properly and to comply with the applicable regulatory requirement(s).
g. Ensuring that the investigator and the investigator's trial staff are adequately informed about the trial.
h. Verifying that the investigator and the investigator's trial staff are performing the specified trial functions, in accordance with the protocol and any other written agreement between the sponsor and the investigator/institution, and have not delegated these functions to unauthorized individuals.
i. Verifying that the investigator is enrolling only eligible subjects.
j. Reporting the subject recruitment rate.
k. Verifying that source documents and other trial records are accurate, complete, kept up-to-date and maintained.

l. Verifying that the investigator provides all the required reports, notifications, applications, and submissions, and that these documents are accurate, complete, timely, legible, dated, and identify the trial.
m. Checking the accuracy and completeness of the CRF entries, source documents and other trial-related records against each other. The monitor specifically should verify that:
   i. The data required by the protocol are reported accurately on the CRFs and are consistent with the source documents.
   ii. Any dose and/or therapy modifications are well documented for each of the trial subjects.
   iii. Adverse events, concomitant medications and intercurrent illnesses are reported in accordance with the protocol on the CRFs.
   iv. Visits that the subjects fail to make, tests that are not conducted, and examinations that are not performed are clearly reported as such on the CRFs.
   v. All withdrawals and dropouts of enrolled subjects from the trial are reported and explained on the CRFs.
n. Informing the investigator of any CRF entry error, omission, or illegibility. The monitor should ensure that appropriate corrections, additions, or deletions are made, dated, explained (if necessary), and initialed by the investigator or by a member of the investigator's trial staff who is authorized to initial CRF changes for the investigator. This authorization should be documented.
o. Determining whether all adverse events (AEs) are appropriately reported within the time periods required by GCP, the protocol, the IRB/IEC, the sponsor, and the applicable regulatory requirement(s).
p. Determining whether the investigator is maintaining the essential documents (see 8. Essential Documents for the Conduct of a Clinical Trial).
q. Communicating deviations from the protocol, SOPs, GCP, and the applicable regulatory requirements to the investigator and taking appropriate action designed to prevent recurrence of the detected deviations.

5.18.5 *Monitoring Procedures.* The monitor(s) should follow the sponsor's established written SOPs as well as those procedures that are specified by the sponsor for monitoring a specific trial.

5.18.6 *Monitoring Report*

a. The monitor should submit a written report to the sponsor after each trial-site visit or trial-related communication.
b. Reports should include the date, site, name of the monitor, and name of the investigator or other individual(s) contacted.
c. Reports should include a summary of what the monitor reviewed and the monitor's statements concerning the significant findings/facts, deviations and deficiencies, conclusions, actions taken or to be taken and/or actions recommended to secure compliance.

d. The review and follow-up of the monitoring report with the sponsor should be documented by the sponsor's designated representative.

5.19 Audit

If or when sponsors perform audits, as part of implementing quality assurance, they should consider:

5.19.1 *Purpose.* The purpose of a sponsor's audit, which is independent of and separate from routine monitoring or quality control functions, should be to evaluate trial conduct and compliance with the protocol, SOPs, GCP, and the applicable regulatory requirements.

5.19.2 Selection and Qualification of Auditors

a. The sponsor should appoint individuals, who are independent of the clinical trials/systems, to conduct audits.
b. The sponsor should ensure that the auditors are qualified by training and experience to conduct audits properly. An auditor's qualifications should be documented.

5.19.3 Auditing Procedures

a. The sponsor should ensure that the auditing of clinical trials/systems is conducted in accordance with the sponsor's written procedures on what to audit, how to audit, the frequency of audits, and the form and content of audit reports.
b. The sponsor's audit plan and procedures for a trial audit should be guided by the importance of the trial to submissions to regulatory authorities, the number of subjects in the trial, the type and complexity of the trial, the level of risks to the trial subjects, and any identified problem(s).
c. The observations and findings of the auditor(s) should be documented.
d. To preserve the independence and value of the audit function, the regulatory authority(ies) should not routinely request the audit reports. Regulatory authority(ies) may seek access to an audit report on a case by case basis when evidence of serious GCP non-compliance exists, or in the course of legal proceedings.
e. When required by applicable law or regulation, the sponsor should provide an audit certificate.

5.20 Noncompliance

5.20.1 Noncompliance with the protocol, SOPs, GCP, and/or applicable regulatory requirement(s) by an investigator/institution, or by member(s) of the sponsor's staff should lead to prompt action by the sponsor to secure compliance.

5.20.2 If the monitoring and/or auditing identifies serious and/or persistent noncompliance on the part of an investigator/institution, the sponsor should terminate the investigator's/institution's participation in the trial. When an investigator's/institution's participation is terminated because of noncompliance, the sponsor should notify promptly the regulatory authority(ies).

5.21 Premature Termination or Suspension of a Trial

If a trial is prematurely terminated or suspended, the sponsor should promptly inform the investigators/institutions, and the regulatory authority(ies) of the termination or suspension and the reason(s) for the termination or suspension. The IRB/IEC should also be informed promptly and provided the reason(s) for the termination or suspension by the sponsor or by the investigator/institution, as specified by the applicable regulatory requirement(s).

5.22 Clinical Trial/Study Reports

Whether the trial is completed or prematurely terminated, the sponsor should ensure that the clinical trial reports are prepared and provided to the regulatory agency(ies) as required by the applicable regulatory requirement(s). The sponsor should also ensure that the clinical trial reports in marketing applications meet the standards of the ICH Guideline for Structure and Content of Clinical Study Reports. (NOTE: The ICH Guideline for Structure and Content of Clinical Study Reports specifies that abbreviated study reports may be acceptable in certain cases.)

5.23 Multicentre Trials

For multicentre trials, the sponsor should ensure that:

5.23.1 All investigators conduct the trial in strict compliance with the protocol agreed to by the sponsor and, if required, by the regulatory authority(ies), and given approval/favorable opinion by the IRB/IEC.

5.23.2 The CRFs are designed to capture the required data at all multicentre trial sites. For those investigators who are collecting additional data, supplemental CRFs should also be provided that are designed to capture the additional data.

5.23.3 The responsibilities of coordinating investigator(s) and the other participating investigators are documented prior to the start of the trial.

5.23.4 All investigators are given instructions on following the protocol, on complying with a uniform set of standards for the assessment of clinical and laboratory findings, and on completing the CRFs.

5.23.5 Communication between investigators is facilitated.

6. Clinical Trial Protocol and Protocol Amendment(s)

The contents of a trial protocol should generally include the following topics. However, site specific information may be provided on separate protocol page(s), or addressed in a separate agreement, and some of the information listed below may be contained in other protocol referenced documents, such as an Investigator's Brochure.

6.1 General Information

6.1.1 Protocol title, protocol identifying number, and date. Any amendment(s) should also bear the amendment number(s) and date(s).

6.1.2 Name and address of the sponsor and monitor (if other than the sponsor).

6.1.3 Name and title of the person(s) authorized to sign the protocol and the protocol amendment(s) for the sponsor.

6.1.4 Name, title, address, and telephone number(s) of the sponsor's medical expert (or dentist when appropriate) for the trial.

6.1.5 Name and title of the investigator(s) who is (are) responsible for conducting the trial, and the address and telephone number(s) of the trial site(s).

6.1.6 Name, title, address, and telephone number(s) of the qualified physician (or dentist, if applicable), who is responsible for all trial-site related medical (or dental) decisions (if other than investigator). 6.1.7 Name(s) and address(es) of the clinical laboratory(ies) and other medical and/or technical department(s) and/or institutions involved in the trial.

6.2 Background Information

6.2.1 Name and description of the investigational product(s).

6.2.2 A summary of findings from nonclinical studies that potentially have clinical significance and from clinical trials that are relevant to the trial.

6.2.3 Summary of the known and potential risks and benefits, if any, to human subjects.

6.2.4 Description of and justification for the route of administration, dosage, dosage regimen, and treatment period(s).

6.2.5 A statement that the trial will be conducted in compliance with the protocol, GCP and the applicable regulatory requirement(s).

6.2.6 Description of the population to be studied.

6.2.7 References to literature and data that are relevant to the trial, and that provide background for the trial.

6.3 Trial Objectives and Purpose

A detailed description of the objectives and the purpose of the trial.

6.4 Trial Design

The scientific integrity of the trial and the credibility of the data from the trial depend substantially on the trial design. A description of the trial design, should include:

6.4.1 A specific statement of the primary endpoints and the secondary endpoints, if any, to be measured during the trial.

6.4.2 A description of the type/design of trial to be conducted (e.g. double-blind, placebo-controlled, parallel design) and a schematic diagram of trial design, procedures and stages.

6.4.3 A description of the measures taken to minimize/avoid bias, including:

a. Randomization.
b. Blinding.

6.4.4 A description of the trial treatment(s) and the dosage and dosage regimen of the investigational product(s). Also include a description of the dosage form, packaging, and labeling of the investigational product(s).

6.4.5 The expected duration of subject participation, and a description of the sequence and duration of all trial periods, including follow-up, if any.

6.4.6 A description of the "stopping rules" or "discontinuation criteria" for individual subjects, parts of trial and entire trial.

6.4.7 Accountability procedures for the investigational product(s), including the placebo(s) and comparator(s), if any.

6.4.8 Maintenance of trial treatment randomization codes and procedures for breaking codes.

6.4.9 The identification of any data to be recorded directly on the CRFs (i.e. no prior written or electronic record of data), and to be considered to be source data.

6.5 Selection and Withdrawal of Subjects

6.5.1 Subject inclusion criteria.

6.5.2 Subject exclusion criteria.

6.5.3 Subject withdrawal criteria (i.e. terminating investigational product treatment/trial treatment) and procedures specifying:

a. When and how to withdraw subjects from the trial/investigational product treatment.
b. The type and timing of the data to be collected for withdrawn subjects.
c. Whether and how subjects are to be replaced.
d. The follow-up for subjects withdrawn from investigational product treatment/trial treatment.

6.6 Treatment of Subjects

6.6.1 The treatment(s) to be administered, including the name(s) of all the product(s), the dose(s), the dosing schedule(s), the route/mode(s) of administration, and the treatment period(s), including the follow-up period(s) for subjects for each investigational product treatment/trial treatment group/arm of the trial.

6.6.2 Medication(s)/treatment(s) permitted (including rescue medication) and not permitted before and/or during the trial.

6.6.3 Procedures for monitoring subject compliance.

6.7 Assessment of Efficacy

6.7.1 Specification of the efficacy parameters.

6.7.2 Methods and timing for assessing, recording, and analyzing of efficacy parameters.

6.8 Assessment of Safety

6.8.1 Specification of safety parameters.

6.8.2 The methods and timing for assessing, recording, and analyzing safety parameters.

6.8.3 Procedures for eliciting reports of and for recording and reporting adverse event and intercurrent illnesses.

6.8.4 The type and duration of the follow-up of subjects after adverse events.

6.9 Statistics

6.9.1 A description of the statistical methods to be employed, including timing of any planned interim analysis(ses).

6.9.2 The number of subjects planned to be enrolled. In multicentre trials, the numbers of enrolled subjects projected for each trial site should be specified. Reason for choice of sample size, including reflections on (or calculations of) the power of the trial and clinical justification.

6.9.3 The level of significance to be used.

6.9.4 Criteria for the termination of the trial.

6.9.5 Procedure for accounting for missing, unused, and spurious data.

6.9.6 Procedures for reporting any deviation(s) from the original statistical plan (any deviation(s) from the original statistical plan should be described and justified in protocol and/or in the final report, as appropriate).

6.9.7 The selection of subjects to be included in the analyses (e.g. all randomized subjects, all dosed subjects, all eligible subjects, evaluable subjects).

6.10 Direct Access to Source Data/Documents

The sponsor should ensure that it is specified in the protocol or other written agreement that the investigator(s)/institution(s) will permit trial-related monitoring, audits, IRB/IEC review, and regulatory inspection(s), providing direct access to source data/documents.

6.11 Quality Control and Quality Assurance

6.12 Ethics

Description of ethical considerations relating to the trial.

6.13 Data Hand ling and Record Keeping

6.14 Financing and Insurance

Financing and insurance if not addressed in a separate agreement.

6.15 Publication Policy

Publication policy, if not addressed in a separate agreement.

6.16 Supplements

(NOTE: Since the protocol and the clinical trial/study report are closely related, further relevant information can be found in the ICH Guideline for Structure and Content of Clinical Study Reports.).

7. Investigator's Brochure

7.1 Introduction

The Investigator's Brochure (IB) is a compilation of the clinical and nonclinical data on the investigational product(s) that are relevant to the study of the product(s) in human subjects. Its purpose is to provide the investigators and others involved in the trial with the information to facilitate their understanding of the rationale for, and their compliance with, many key features of the protocol, such as the dose, dose frequency/interval, methods of administration: and safety monitoring procedures. The IB also provides insight to support the clinical management of the study subjects during the course of the clinical trial. The information should be presented in a concise, simple, objective, balanced, and non-promotional form that enables a clinician, or potential investigator, to understand it and make his/her own unbiased risk-benefit assessment of the appropriateness of the proposed trial. For this reason, a medically qualified person should generally participate in the editing of an IB, but the contents of the IB should be approved by the disciplines that generated the described data.

This guideline delineates the minimum information that should be included in an IB and provides suggestions for its layout. It is expected that the type and extent of information available will vary with the stage of development of the investigational product. If the investigational product is marketed and its pharmacology is widely understood by medical practitioners, an extensive IB may not be necessary. Where permitted by regulatory authorities, a basic product information brochure, package leaflet, or labeling may be an appropriate alternative, provided that it includes current, comprehensive, and detailed information on all aspects of the investigational product that might be of importance to the investigator. If a marketed product is being studied for a new use (i.e., a new indication), an IB specific to that new use should be prepared. The IB should be reviewed at least annually and revised as necessary in compliance with a sponsor's written procedures. More frequent revision may be appropriate depending on the stage of development and the generation of relevant new information. However, in accordance with Good Clinical Practice, relevant new information may be so important that it should be communicated to the investigators, and possibly to the Institutional Review Boards (IRBs)/Independent Ethics Committees (IECs) and/or regulatory authorities before it is included in a revised IB.

Generally, the sponsor is responsible for ensuring that an up-to-date IB is made available to the investigator(s) and the investigators are responsible for providing the up-to-date IB to the responsible IRBs/IECs. In the case of an investigator sponsored trial, the sponsor-investigator should determine whether a brochure is available from the commercial manufacturer. If the investigational product is provided by the sponsor-investigator, then he or she should provide the necessary information to the trial personnel. In cases where preparation of a formal IB is impractical, the sponsor-investigator should provide, as a substitute, an expanded background information section in the trial protocol that contains the minimum current information described in this guideline.

7.2 General Considerations

The IB should include:

7.2.1 *Title Page.* This should provide the sponsor's name, the identity of each investigational product (i.e., research number, chemical or approved generic name, and trade name(s) where legally permissible and desired by the sponsor), and the release date. It is also suggested that an edition number, and a reference to the number and date of the edition it supersedes, be provided. An example is given in Appendix 1.

7.2.2 *Confidentiality Statement.* The sponsor may wish to include a statement instructing the investigator/recipients to treat the IB as a confidential document for the sole information and use of the investigator's team and the IRB/IEC.

7.3 Contents of the Investigator's Brochure

The IB should contain the following sections, each with literature references where appropriate:

7.3.1 *Table of Contents.* An example of the Table of Contents is given in Appendix 2

7.3.2 *Summary.* A brief summary (preferably not exceeding two pages) should be given, highlighting the significant physical, chemical, pharmaceutical, pharmacological, toxicological, pharmacokinetic, metabolic, and clinical information available that is relevant to the stage of clinical development of the investigational product.

7.3.3 *Introduction.* A brief introductory statement should be provided that contains the chemical name (and generic and trade name(s) when approved) of the investigational product(s), all active ingredients, the investigational product (s) pharmacological class and its expected position within this class (e.g. advantages), the rationale for performing research with the investigational product(s), and the anticipated prophylactic, therapeutic, or diagnostic indication(s). Finally, the introductory statement should provide the general approach to be followed in evaluating the investigational product.

7.3.4 *Physical, Chemical, and Pharmaceutical Properties and Formulation.* A description should be provided of the investigational product substance(s) (including the chemical and/or structural formula(e)), and a brief summary should be given of the relevant physical, chemical, and pharmaceutical properties. To permit appropriate safety measures to be taken in the course of the trial, a description of the formulation(s) to be used, including excipients, should be provided and justified if clinically relevant. Instructions for the storage and handling of the dosage form(s) should also be given. Any structural similarities to other known compounds should be mentioned.

7.3.5 *Nonclinical Studies.* Introduction: The results of all relevant nonclinical pharmacology, toxicology, pharmacokinetic, and investigational product metabolism studies should be provided in summary form. This summary should address the methodology used, the results, and a discussion of the relevance of the findings to the investigated therapeutic and the possible unfavorable and unintended effects in humans.

The information provided may include the following, as appropriate, if known/available:

- Species tested
- Number and sex of animals in each group
- Unit dose (e.g., milligram/kilogram (mg/kg))
- Dose interval
- Route of administration
- Duration of dosing
- Information on systemic distribution
- Duration of post-exposure follow-up
- Results, including the following aspects:
- Nature and frequency of pharmacological or toxic effects
- Severity or intensity of pharmacological or toxic effects
- Time to onset of effects
- Reversibility of effects
- Duration of effects
- Dose response

Tabular format/listings should be used whenever possible to enhance the clarity of the presentation. The following sections should discuss the most important findings from the studies, including the dose response of observed effects, the relevance to humans, and any aspects to be studied in humans. If applicable, the effective and nontoxic dose findings in the same animal species should be compared (i.e., the therapeutic index should be discussed). The relevance of this information to the proposed human dosing should be addressed. Whenever possible, comparisons should be made in terms of blood/tissue levels rather than on a mg/kg basis.

a. *Nonclinical Pharmacology.* A summary of the pharmacological aspects of the investigational product and, where appropriate, its significant metabolites studied in animals, should be included. Such a summary should incorporate studies that assess potential therapeutic activity (e.g. efficacy models, receptor binding, and specificity) as well as those that assess safety (e.g., special studies to assess pharmacological actions other than the intended therapeutic effect(s)).
b. *Pharmacokinetics and Product Metabolism in Animals.* A summary of the pharmacokinetics and biological transformation and disposition of the investigational product in all species studied should be given. The discussion of the findings should address the absorption and the local and systemic bioavailability of the investigational product and its metabolites, and their relationship to the pharmacological and toxicological findings in animal species.

c. *Toxicology.* A summary of the toxicological effects found in relevant studies conducted in different animal species should be described under the following headings where appropriate:

- Single dose
- Repeated dose
- Carcinogenicity
- Special studies (e.g. irritancy and sensitization)
- Reproductive toxicity
- Genotoxicity (mutagenicity)

7.3.6 *Effects in Humans.* Introduction: A thorough discussion of the known effects of the investigational product(s) in humans should be provided, including information on pharmacokinetics, metabolism, pharmacodynamics, dose response, safety, efficacy, and other pharmacological activities. Where possible, a summary of each completed clinical trial should be provided. Information should also be provided regarding results of any use of the investigational product(s) other than from in clinical trials, such as from experience during marketing.

a. *Pharmacokinetics and Product Metabolism in Humans.* A summary of information on the pharmacokinetics of the investigational product(s) should be presented, including the following, if available:
   - Pharmacokinetics (including metabolism, as appropriate, and absorption, plasma protein binding, distribution, and elimination).
   - Bioavailability of the investigational product (absolute, where possible, and/or relative) using a reference dosage form.
   - Population subgroups (e.g., gender, age, and impaired organ function).
   - Interactions (e.g., product-product interactions and effects of food).
   - Other pharmacokinetic data (e.g., results of population studies performed within clinical trial(s).

b. *Safety and Efficacy.* A summary of information should be provided about the investigational product's/products' (including metabolites, where appropriate) safety, pharmacodynamics, efficacy, and dose response that were obtained from preceding trials in humans (healthy volunteers and/or patients). The implications of this information should be discussed. In cases where a number of clinical trials have been completed, the use of summaries of safety and efficacy across multiple trials by indications in subgroups may provide a clear presentation of the data. Tabular summaries of adverse drug reactions for all the clinical trials (including those for all the studied indications) would be useful. Important differences in adverse drug reaction patterns/incidences across indications or subgroups should be discussed. The IB should provide a description of the possible risks and adverse drug reactions to be anticipated on the basis of prior experiences with the product under investigation and with related products. A description should also be provided of the precautions or special monitoring to be done as part of the investigational use of the product(s).

c. *Marketing Experience.* The IB should identify countries where the investigational product has been marketed or approved. Any significant information arising from the marketed use should be summarized (e.g., formulations, dosages, routes of administration, and adverse product reactions). The IB should also identify all the countries where the investigational product did not receive approval/registration for marketing or was withdrawn from marketing/registration.

7.3.7 *Summary of Data and Guidance for the Investigator.* This section should provide an overall discussion of the nonclinical and clinical data, and should summarize the information from various sources on different aspects of the investigational product(s), wherever possible. In this way, the investigator can be provided with the most informative interpretation of the available data and with an assessment of the implications of the information for future clinical trials. Where appropriate, the published reports on related products should be discussed. This could help the investigator to anticipate adverse drug reactions or other problems in clinical trials.

The overall aim of this section is to provide the investigator with a clear understanding of the possible risks and adverse reactions, and of the specific tests, observations, and precautions that may be needed for a clinical trial. This understanding should be based on the available physical, chemical, pharmaceutical, pharmacological, toxicological, and clinical information on the investigational product(s). Guidance should also be provided to the clinical investigator on the recognition and treatment of possible overdose and adverse drug reactions that is based on previous human experience and on the pharmacology of the investigational product.

7.4 APPENDIX 1:

Title Page (Example)

SPONSOR'S NAME
Product:
Research Number:
Name(s): Chemical, Generic (if approved)
Trade Name(s) (if legally permissible and desired by the sponsor)
INVESTIGATOR'S BROCHURE
Edition Number:
Release Date:
Replaces Previous Edition Number:
Date:

7.5 APPENDIX 2:

Table of Contents of Investigator's Brochure (Example)

Confidentiality Statement (optional)
Signature Page (optional)
1 Table of Contents
2 Summary
3 Introduction
4 Physical, Chemical, and Pharmaceutical Properties and Formulation
5 Nonclinical Studies
 5.1 Nonclinical Pharmacology
 5.2 Pharmacokinetics and Product Metabolism in Animals
 5.3 Toxicology
6 Effects in Humans
 6.1 Pharmacokinetics and Product Metabolism in Humans
 6.2 Safety and Efficacy
 6.3 Marketing Experience
7 Summary of Data and Guidance for the Investigator
NB: References on (These references should be found at the end of each chapter)
 1 Publications
 2 Reports
Appendices (if any).

8. Essential Documents for the Conduct of a Clinical Trial

8.1 Introduction

Essential Documents are those documents which individually and collectively permit evaluation of the conduct of a trial and the quality of the data produced. These documents serve to demonstrate the compliance of the investigator, sponsor and monitor with the standards of Good Clinical Practice and with all applicable regulatory requirements. Essential Documents also serve a number of other important purposes. Filing essential documents at the investigator/institution and sponsor sites in a timely manner can greatly assist in the successful management of a trial by the investigator, sponsor and monitor. These documents are also the ones which are usually audited by the sponsor's independent audit function and inspected by the regulatory authority (ies) as part of the process to confirm the validity of the trial conduct and the integrity of data collected. The minimum list of essential documents which has been developed follows. The various documents are grouped in three sections according to the stage of the trial during which they will normally be generated: 1) before the clinical phase of the trial commences, 2) during the clinical conduct of the trial, and 3) after completion or termination of the trial. A description is given of the purpose of each document, and whether it should be filed in either the investigator/institution or sponsor files, or both. It is acceptable to combine some of the documents, provided the individual elements are readily identifiable. Trial master files should be established at the beginning of the trial, both at the investigator/institution's site and at the sponsor's office. A final close-out of a trial can only be done when the monitor has reviewed both investigator/institution and sponsor files and confirmed that all necessary documents are in the appropriate files.

Any or all of the documents addressed in this guideline may be subject to, and should be available for, audit by the sponsor's auditor and inspection by the regulatory authority(ies).

8.2 before the clinical phase of the trial commences

During this planning stage the following documents should be generated and should be on file before the trial formally starts

	Title of Document/Purpose	Located in the files of	
		Invest/ Site	**Sponsor**
8.2.1	**Investigator's Brochure** To document that relevant and current scientific information about the investigational product has been provided to the investigator	X	X
8.2.2	**Signed Protocol, Amendments, If Any, & Sample CRF** To document investigator and sponsor agreement to the protocol/amendment(s) and crf	X	X
8.2.3	**Info. Given to Trial Subject**	X	X
	– *Informed Consent Form* Including all applicable translations) to document the informed consent.	X	X
	– *Any Other Written Information* To document that subjects will be given appropriate written information (content and wording) to support their ability to give fully informed consent.	X	X
	– *Advertisement For Subject Recruitment* (if used) to document that recruitment measures are appropriate and not coercive.	X	X
8.2.4	**Financial Aspects of the Trial** To document the financial agreement between the investigator/institution and the sponsor for the trial	X	X

	Title of Document/Purpose	Located in the files of: Invest/ Site	Sponsor
8.2.5	**Insurance Statement** (where required) to document that compensation to subject(s) for trial-related injury will be available	X	X
8.2.6	**Signed Agreement Between Involved Parties** To document agreements. E.g.: Investigator/ institution & sponsor – investigator/institution & cro – sponsor & cro –investigator/institution & authority(ies)*	X	X
8.2.7	**Dated, Documented Approval/Favorable Opinion of IRB/IEC of the Following:** – *Protocol and Any Amendments* – *CRF (If Applicable)* – *Informed Consent Form(s)* – *Any Other Written Information to be Provided to the Subject(s)* – *Advertisement For Subject Recruitment (If Used)* – *Subject Compensation (If Any)* – *Any Other Documents Given Approval/Favorable Opinion* To document that the trial has been subject to IRB/IEC review and given approval/favorable opinion. To identify the version number and date of the document(s)	X	X
8.2.8	**IRB/Independent Ethics Committee Composition** To document that the irb/iec is constituted in Agreement with GCP	X	X
8.2.9	**Regulatory Authority(ies) Authorization/Approval/ Notification of Protocol** (Where Required) To document appropriate authorisation/approval/ notification by the regulatory authority(ies) has been obtained prior to initiation of the trial in compliance with the applicable regulatory requirement(s)	X	X

	Title of Document/Purpose	Located in the files of: Invest/Site	Sponsor
8.2.10	**Curriculum Vitae and/or Other Relevant Documents Evidencing Qualifications of Investigator(s) and Sub-Investigator(s)** To document qualifications and eligibility to conduct trial and/or provide medical supervision of subjects	X	X
8.2.11	**Normal Value(s)/Range(s) For Medical/ Laboratory/Technical Procedure(s) and/or Test(s) Included in the Protocol** To document normal values and/or ranges of thetests	X	X
8.2.12	**Medical/Laboratory/Technical ProceduresTests** – *Certification or* – *Accreditation or* – *Established Quality Control and/or External Quality Assessment or* – *Other Validation** To document competence of facility to perform required test(s) , and support reliability of results	X	X
8.2.13	**Sample of Label(s) Attached to Investigational Product Container(s)** To document compliance with applicable labeling regulations and appropriateness of instructions provided to the subjects	X	X
8.2.14	**Instructions For Handling of Investigational Product(s) and Trial-Related Materials (If Not Included in Protocol or Investigator's Brochure)** To document instructions needed to ensure proper storage, packaging, dispensing and disposition of investigational products and trial- related materials	X	X
8.2.15	**Shipping Records For Investigational Product(s) and Trial-Related Materials** To document shipment dates, batch numbers and method of shipment of investigational product(s) and trial-related materials. Allows tracking of product batch, review of shipping conditions, and accountability	X	X

	Title of Document/Purpose	Located in the files of: Invest/ Site	Sponsor
8.2.16	**Certificate(s) of Analysis of Investigational Product(s) Shipped** To document identity, purity, and strength of investigational product(s) to be used in the trial		X
8.2.17	**Decoding Procedures For Blinded Trials** To document how, in case of an emergency, identity of blinded investigational product can be revealed without breaking the blind for the remaining subjects' treatment	X	X**
8.2.18	**Master Randomization List** To document method for randomization of trial subjects		X**
8.2.19	**Pre-Trial Monitoring Report** To document that the site is suitable for the trial (may be combined with 8.2.20)	X	X
8.2.20	**Trial Initiation Monitoring Report** To document that trial procedures were reviewed with the investigator and the investigator's trial staff (may be combined with 8.2.19)	X	X

8.3 during the clinical conduct of the trial

In addition to having on file the above documents, the following should be added to the files during the trial as evidence that all new relevant information is documented as it becomes available.

	Title of Document/Purpose	Located in the files of: Invest/ Site	Sponsor
8.3.1	**Investigator's Brochure Updates** To document that investigator is informed in a timely manner of relevant information as it becomes available	X	X

	Title of Document/Purpose	Located in the files of Invest/ Site	Located in the files of Sponsor
8.3.2	**Any Revision to:** – *Protocol/Amendment(s) and CRF* – *Informed Consent Form* – *Any Other Written Information Provided to Subjects* – *Advertisement For Subject Recruitment (If Used)* To document revisions of these trial related documents that take effect during trial	X	X
8.3.3	**Dated, Documented Approval/Favorable Opinion of IRB/IEC of the Following:** – *Protocol Amendment(s)* – *Revision(s) of:* – *Informed Consent Form* – *Any Other Written Information to be Provided to the Subject* – *Advertisement For Subject Recruitment* – *Any Other Documents Given Approval/Favorable Opinion* – *Continuing Review of Trial** To document that the amendment(s) and/or revision(s) have been subject to irb/iec review and were given approval/favourable opinion. To identify the version number and date of the document(s).	X	X
8.3.4	**Regulatory Authority(ies) Authorizations/Approvals/ Notifications Where Required For:** – *Protocol Amendment(s) and Other Documents* To document compliance with applicable regulatory requirements.	X	X
8.3.5	**CVs For New Investigator(s) and/or Sub-Investigator(s)** see 8.2.10.	X	X
8.3.6	**Updates to Normal Value(s)/Range(s) For Medical/Laboratory/Technical Procedure(s)/ Test(s) Included in the Protocol** To document normal values and ranges that are revised during the trial (see 8.2.11).	X	X

	Title of Document/Purpose	Located in the files of Invest/ Site	Located in the files of Sponsor
8.3.7	**Updates of Medical/Laboratory/Technical Procedures/Tests** – *Certification or* – *Accreditation or* – *Established Quality Control and/or External Quality Assessment or* – *Other Validation (Where Required)* To document that tests remain adequate throughout the trial period (see 8.2.12).	X	X
8.3.8	**Documentation of Investigational Product(s) and Trial-Related Materials Shipment** (see 8.2.15.)	X	X
8.3.9	**Certificate(s) of Analysis For New Batches of Investigational Products** (see 8.2.16)		X
8.3.10	**Monitoring Visit Reports** To document site visits by, and findings of, the monitor	X	X
8.3.11	**Relevant Communications Other Than Site Visits** – *Letters* – *Meeting Notes* – *Notes of Telephone Calls* To document any agreements or significant discussions regarding trial administration, protocol violations, trial conduct, adverse event(ae) reporting.	X	X
8.3.12	**Signed Informed Consent Forms** To document that consent is obtained in accordance with gcp and protocol and dated prior to participation of each subject in trial. Also to document direct access permission (see 8.2.3).	X	X

	Title of Document/Purpose	Located in the files of Invest/ Site	Located in the files of Sponsor
8.3.13	**Source Documents** To document the existence of the subject and substantiate integrity of trial data collected. To include original documents related to the trial, to medical treatment, and history of subject	X	X
8.3.14	**Signed, Dated and Completed Case Report Forms (CRF)** To document that the investigator or authorized member of the investigator's staff confirms the observations recorded	X copy	X orig.
8.3.15	**Documentation of CRF Corrections** To document all changes/additions or corrections made to crf after initial data were recorded	X copy	X orig.
8.3.16	**Notification By Originating Investigator to Sponsor of Serious Adverse Events and Related Reports** Notification by originating investigator to sponsor of serious adverse events and related reports in accordance with 4.11	X	X
8.3.17	**Notification By Sponsor and/or Investigator, If Needed, to Regulatory Authority(ies) and IRB(s)/IEC(s) of Unexpected Serious Adverse Drug Reactions and of Other Safety Information** Notification by sponsor and/or investigator, where applicable, to regulatory authorities and irb(s)/iec(s) of unexpected serious adverse drug reactions in accordance with 5.17 and 4.11.1 and of other safety information in accordance with 5.16.2 and 4.11.2.	X*	X
8.3.18	**Notification By Sponsor to Investigators of Safety Information** Notification by sponsor to investigators of safety information in accordance with 5.16.2.	X	X

	Title of Document/Purpose	Located in the files of Invest/ Site	Sponsor
8.3.19	**Interim or Annual Reports to IRB/IEC and Authority(ies)** Interim or annual reports provided to irb/iec in accordance with 4.10 and to authority(ies) in accordance with 5.17.3.	X	X*
8.3.20	**Subject Screening Log** To document identification of subjects who entered pre-trial screening.	X	X
8.3.21	**Subject Identification Code List** To document that investigator/institution keeps a confidential list of names of all subjects allocated to trial numbers on enrolling in the trial. Allows investigator/institution to reveal identity of any subject.	X	X*
8.3.22	**Subject Enrolment Log** To document chronological enrolment of subjects by trial number.	X	
8.3.23	**Investigational Products Accountability atthe Site** To document that investigational product(s) have been used according to the protocol.	X	X
8.3.24	**Signature Sheet** To document signatures and initials of all persons authorised to make entries and/or corrections on CRFs.	X	X
8.3.25	**Record of Retained Body Fluids/Tissue Samples (If Any)** To document location and identification of retained samples if assays need to be repeated.	X	X

8.4 after completion or termination of the trial

After completion or termination of the trial, all of the documents identified in sections 8.2 and 8.3 should be in the file together with the following

		Located in the files of	
	Title of Document/Purpose	**Invest/ Site**	**Sponsor**
8.4.1	**Investigational Product(s) Accountability at the Site** To document that the investigational product(s) have been used according to the protocol. To documents the final accounting of investigational product(s) received at the site, dispensed to subjects, returned by the subjects, and returned to sponsor.	X	X
8.4.2	**Documentation of Investigational Product Destruction** To document destruction of unused investigational products by sponsor or at site.	X***	X
8.4.3	**Completed Subject Identification Code List** To permit identification of all subjects enrolled in the trial in case follow-up is required. List should be kept in a confidential manner and for agreed upon time.	X	X
8.4.4	**Audit Certificate (if available)** to document that audit was performed.	X	X
8.4.5	**Final Trial Close-Out Monitoring Report** To document that all activities required for trial close-out are completed, and copies of essential documents are held in the appropriate files.	X	X
8.4.6	**Treatment Allocation and Decoding Documentation** Returned to sponsor to document any decoding that may have occurred.	X	X
8.4.7	**Final Report By Investigator to IRB/IEC Where Required, and Where Applicable, to the Regulatory Authority(ies)** To document completion of the trial.	X	X

	Title of Document/Purpose	**Located in the files of** Invest/Site	Sponsor
8.4.8	**Clinical Study Report** To document results and interpretation of trial.	X*	X

* if applicable/required
** third party if applicable
*** if destroyed at the site

APPENDIX g

Examination

1. The purpose of an IRB is to:
   a. Inform study subjects about the protocol and drug.
   b. Protect the rights and welfare of human subjects of research.
   c. Ensure that sponsors are meeting FDA regulations.
   d. Write easily understood consent forms.
   e. Ensure that only innovative new drugs are studied.

2. The investigator must obtain IRB approval of the study and the consent form:
   a. Before the study has been completed.
   b. Before enrolling any patients in the study.
   c. Before receiving any grant money for the study.
   d. Within one month of starting the study.
   e. Before the first patient has completed the study.

3. The IRB must inform the investigator the study has been approved by:
   a. Written notification saying it has been approved.
   b. A visit or phone call from the IRB chairperson.
   c. A preliminary call followed by written minutes of the meeting.
   d. The IRB informs the sponsor, who in turn informs the investigator by shipping drug.
   e. The IRB informs the institution administration, who then informs the investigator.

4. For initial approval of proposed research, the investigator must submit to the IRB:
   a. A protocol synopsis and the investigator brochure.
   b. The informed consent and a protocol synopsis.
   c. The full protocol.
   d. The full protocol and the informed consent.
   e. The investigator brochure.

5. Any proposed advertising for the study:
   a. Must be submitted to the IRB and approved before it can be used.
   b. Can be used as long as the IRB has approved a similar ad in the past.
   c. Must be submitted to the IRB for information, but is not approved.
   d. Must come from the sponsor, since the sponsor pays for it.
   e. Must be submitted before the study can start.

6. Any amendment that ______________ must be approved by the IRB prior to implementation.
   a. Increases the risk to subjects.
   b. Decreases the number of subjects.
   c. Changes the protocol in any way.
   d. All of the above.
   e. None of the above.

7. Which of the following are necessary to waive consent?
   a. Subject is unable to give consent.
   b. No time or unable to contact next of kin.
   c. Life-threatening condition.
   d. No other treatment available.
   e. None of the above.
   f. All of the above.

8. The investigator's signature must be on the consent form.
   a. True.
   b. False.

9. The process by which a subject voluntarily confirms his or her willingness to participate in a clinical trial is known as:
   a. HIPAA authorization.
   b. IRB approval.
   c. Legally authorized agreement.
   d. Intent to treat.
   e. Informed consent.

10. Informed consent is documented by:
    a. A written, signed and dated informed consent form.
    b. A witness signature.
    c. The IRB chairperson.
    d. The investigator.
    e. The subject's legally authorized representative.

11. Which signatures are required by regulation to be on the consent form?
    a. The investigator.
    b. The subject.
    c. The investigator and the subject.
    d. The subject and a witness.
    e. The investigator, the subject and a witness.

12. ICH guidelines provide a unified standard for ______________ clinical trials involving human subjects.
    a. Designing.
    b. Conducting.
    c. Recording.
    d. Reporting.
    e. All of the above.

13. What are the two main themes covered by the formal ICH definition of "Good Clinical Practice"?
    a. Rights and well-being of study subjects and compliance with regulations.
    b. Rights and well-being of study subjects and credibility of the data.
    c. Compliance with regulations and credibility of the data.
    d. Compliance with the regulations and the formal marketing approval process.
    e. Credibility of the data and international consistency.

14. GCPs are derived from all of the following except:
    a. Safety surveillance systems.
    b. Federal regulations.
    c. Ethical codes.
    d. ICH guidelines.
    e. Official guidance documents.

15. Non-clinical studies refer to studies that do not involve:
    a. Animal testing.
    b. Drugs.
    c. Human subjects.
    d. Toxicology parameters.
    e. Safety.

16. In which development phase might normal, healthy volunteers be given a new drug?
    a. Phase I.
    b. Phase II.
    c. Phase III.
    d. Phase IIIB.
    e. Phase IV.

17. Large multicenter studies are usually done in:
    a. Phase I.
    b. Phase II.
    c. Phase III.
    d. Phase IIIB.
    e. Phase IV.

18. One of the primary purposes of a Phase II study is to:
    a. Demonstrate long-term safety and efficacy.
    b. Gather information on additional indications for the drug.
    c. Demonstrate efficacy within the established safe dose range.
    d. Familiarize physicians with the drug.

19. By regulation, an investigator must keep records relating to:
    a. Disposition of the study drug.
    b. Case histories.
    c. Case report forms.
    d. Signed informed consent forms.
    e. All of the above.

20. Most sponsors will expect an investigative site to keep all study records for:
    a. Fifteen years.
    b. Three years.
    c. Five years.
    d. Until the sponsor says they may be destroyed.
    e. Two years after the last subject finished treatment.

21. Which of the following should be kept separately from other study documents?
    a. Signed consent forms.
    b. Grant information.
    c. IND safety reports.
    d. IRB communications.
    e. Screening logs.

22. A source document is any document where:
    a. Lab values are shown.
    b. HIPAA authorization was received.
    c. Data are first recorded.
    d. A subject's name is shown.
    e. Sponsor access to the document is not allowed.

23. Standard operating procedures (SOPs) are essential for:
    a. Standardizing processes.
    b. Ensuring that regulatory requirements are met.
    c. Training new personnel.
    d. Managing workload.
    e. All the above.

24. SOPs are:
    a. Written descriptions of how tasks are to be performed.
    b. Legally binding on employees.
    c. Usually provided by the sponsor.
    d. Required by regulation.
    e. All of the above.

25. Once an SOP is in place, it should never be changed.
    a. True.
    b. False.

26. In general, a sponsor will not place a study at a site without:
    a. An on-site IRB.
    b. A study coordinator.
    c. An assurance that the study will enroll at least a given number of subjects.
    d. An assurance that there will be no staff turnover during the study.
    e. At least one sub-investigator who is a physician.

27. A competing study can be one that is ongoing in:
    a. The site.
    b. The same clinic or hospital.
    c. The community.
    d. Only a and b above.
    e. a, b and c above.

28. Some of the questions an investigator and a CRC should ask when assessing protocol feasibility at their site include all the following except:
    a. Will the sponsor pay at least 30% of the grant in advance?
    b. Have we worked with this sponsor before and was the partnership successful?
    c. Is the number of subjects to be enrolled realistic?
    d. Is the study scientifically sound?
    e. Is the IRB apt to have problems with any aspects of this protocol?

29. Most sponsors operate on which kind of basis when it comes to grant payments?
    a. Twenty percent up front.
    b. The entire grant paid in one up-front payment.
    c. Fee-for-service.
    d. Payment for each subject when the subject completes the trial.
    e. Payment upon request from the investigator.

30. Financial disclosure applies to:
    a. Only the investigator.
    b. The investigator and the CRC.
    c. Anyone at the site who is involved in the trial.
    d. Only those people listed on the 1572.
    e. The investigator, the CRC and the pharmacist.

31. Investigator meetings are a requirement for any multicenter study with six or more sites.
    a. True.
    b. False.

32. Study initiation meetings are usually held:
    a. At least two months before the study starts.
    b. After the site has received all study materials and is ready to start enrollment.
    c. After the first two subjects have been enrolled.
    d. Before the investigator meeting.
    e. At the sponsor's place of business.

33. One of the most difficult aspects of doing clinical trials is:
    a. Following the protocol.
    b. Finding a good coordinator.
    c. Recruiting sufficient subjects.
    d. Working with the pharmacy.
    e. Obtaining a high enough grant.

34. The FDA considers advertising for study subjects to be:
    a. Part of the consent process.
    b. Necessary for all trials.
    c. Acceptable only in phase I trials.
    d. Never appropriate with vulnerable populations of subjects.
    e. Acceptable only in print media, as opposed to radio and television ads.

35. Payments to subjects in clinical trials should:
    a. Never be done.
    b. Be done only for phase I trials.
    c. Be one only with prior IRB approval.
    d. Be done only once, at the end of the subject's trial involvement.
    e. Never be more than $100 for completing a study.

36. Potential reasons to discontinue a subject in a trial are:
    a. The subject is not compliant with study procedures.
    b. The subject has intolerable medical events during treatment.
    c. Pregnancy.
    d. a and b above.
    e. a, b and c above.

37. Visit windows are:
    a. Always plus and minus 2 days.
    b. Determined by the investigator.
    c. The number of days around a specific date that the patient may come in for a study visit.
    d. The number of visits included in a protocol.
    e. A percentage of the total days in a protocol divided by the number of visits.

38. Patient compliance with study drug dosing is a statistical issue, so site personnel do not have to be concerned about it.
    a. True.
    b. False.

39. Which of the following should not be included in a protocol?
    a. A description of the objectives and purpose of the study.
    b. The inclusion and exclusion criteria for study subject.
    c. The design of the study.
    d. The amount of the grant per subject.
    e. The investigator's responsibilities.

40. Case report forms are usually completed by:
    a. The investigator.
    b. The CRC.
    c. The CRA.
    d. The subject.
    e. The sponsor.

41. In general, corrections to case report forms should be made by:
    a. The CRA.
    b. The data entry person.
    c. The CRC or the investigator.
    d. Only the investigator.
    e. The person who finds the error.

42. It is a regulatory requirement to have a source document for every data item collected on case report forms.
    a. True.
    b. False.

43. The most common reason for a study to be closed at a site is:
    a. The study is complete.
    b. The drug was found to be ineffective.
    c. There were safety problems with the drug.
    d. Lack of enrollment.
    e. Falsification of data.

44. By regulation, investigators are required to make a final study report to:
    a. The FDA and the sponsor.
    b. The sponsor and the IRB.
    c. The institution.
    d. The sponsor, the IRB and the FDA.
    e. The sponsor.

45. There are two main reasons that a sponsor might audit a study site. They are:
    a. The IRB has requested a sponsor audit.
    b. To ensure that the site is complying with the regulations and protocol.
    c. There is evidence that the site is out of compliance and the sponsor wants to verify whether or not this is true.
    d. a and b above.
    e. b and c above.

46. The FDA _______________ sponsor audit reports of a study site.
    a. Does not have routine access to
    b. Does have routine access to
    c. Will always receive a copy of
    d. Should receive from the investigator a copy of
    e. Will never see

47. Which of the following is not one of the purposes of an FDA study-related or investigator-related audit?
    a. To determine the validity of the data.
    b. To determine the integrity of the data.
    c. To determine that the drug was properly manufactured.
    d. To assess adherence to regulations and guidelines.
    e. To determine that the rights and safety of subjects were properly protected.

48. In study-related audits by the FDA, the studies audited are usually:
    a. Just starting to enroll.
    b. About half done, but still enrolling new subjects.
    c. Ongoing, but closed to new enrollment.
    d. Closed.
    e. Phase IIIB studies.

49. The two main aspects of a study that will be looked at by the FDA during an audit are:
    a. Study conduct and study data.
    b. Study conduct and recruitment methods.
    c. Study data and statistical methodology.
    d. Drug storage conditions and pharmacy records.
    e. a and d above.

50. There are three classifications that result from an FDA audit. The one that means that deviations from the regulations were found but that they were not serious, is:
    a. VAI.
    b. NAI.
    c. OAI.
    d. BIMO-2.
    e. EIR.

Answer Key

1. b
2. b
3. a
4. d
5. a
6. a
7. f
8. b
9. e
10. a
11. b
12. e
13. b
14. a
15. c
16. a
17. c
18. c
19. e
20. d
21. b
22. c
23. e
24. a
25. b
26. b
27. e
28. a
29. c
30. d
31. b
32. b
33. c
34. a
35. c
36. e
37. c
38. b
39. d
40. b
41. c
42. b
43. a
44. b
45. e
46. a
47. c
48. d
49. a
50. a

ABOUT THOMSON CENTERWATCH

Thomson CenterWatch is a Boston-based publishing and information services company that focuses on the clinical trials industry and is a business of The Thomson Corporation. We provide a variety of information services used by pharmaceutical and biotechnology companies, CROs, SMOs and investigative sites involved in the management and conduct of clinical trials. CenterWatch also provides educational materials for clinical research professionals, health professionals and health consumers. We provide market research and market intelligence services that many major companies have retained to help develop new business strategies, to guide the implementation of new clinical research-related initiatives and to assist in due diligence activities. Some of our top publications and services are described on the next several pages. For a comprehensive listing with detailed information about our publications and services, please visit our web site at **www.centerwatch.com**. You can also contact us at (800) 765-9647 for subscription and order information.

CenterWatch Training and Education Manuals

The Investigator's Guide to Clinical Research, 3rd edition

This 250-page step-by-step manual is filled with tips, instructions and insights for health professionals interested in conducting clinical trials. *The Investigator's Guide* is designed to help the novice clinical investigator get involved in conducting clinical trials. The guide is also a valuable resource for experienced investigative sites looking for ways to improve and increase their involvement and success in clinical research. Developed in accordance with ACCME, readers can apply for CME credits. An exam is provided online.

How to Find & Secure Clinical Grants

This 28-page guidebook is an ideal resource for healthcare professionals interested in conducting clinical trials. The guidebook provides tips and insights for new and experienced investigative sites to compete more effectively for clinical study grants.

A Guide to Patient Recruitment and Retention

This 250+ page manual is designed to help clinical research professionals improve the effectiveness of their patient recruitment and retention efforts. Written by Diana Anderson, Ph.D., with contributions from 18 industry experts and thought leaders, this guide offers real world, practical recruitment and retention strategies, tactics and metrics. It is considered an invaluable resource for educating professionals who manage and conduct clinical research about ways to plan and execute effective patient recruitment and retention efforts.

The CRA's Guide to Monitoring Clinical Research

This 400-page CE-accredited book is an ideal resource for novice and experienced CRAs, as well as professionals interested in pursuing a career as study monitors. *The CRA's Guide* covers important topics along with updated regulations, guidelines and worksheets, including resources such as: 21 CFR Parts 50, 54, 56 & 312 Guidelines, various checklists (monitoring visit, site evaluation, informed consent) and a study documentation file verification log. This manual will be routinely referenced throughout the CRA's career. Developed in acccordance with ANCC, readers can apply for Nursing Contact Hours. An exam is provided online.

eClinical Trials: Planning and Implementation

This invaluable resource is designed to assist biopharmaceutical companies, CROs and investigative sites in understanding, planning and implementing electronic clinical trial (eCT) technology solutions to accelerate and improve their research operations. Written by highly respected thought leaders in the field today, this 180+ page book describes and addresses the concepts and complexities of managing and conducting an optimal eCT, while offering practical guidance, facts and advice on implementing eCT technologies.

Protecting Study Volunteers in Research, Third Edition
The third edition of our top-selling manual addresses current and emerging issues that are critical to our system of human subject protection oversight and now includes an entire chapter on how to implement the HIPAA Privacy Rule in research. The book is designed to help organizations provide the highest standards of safe and ethical treatment of study volunteers. Developed in accordance with the essentials and standards of the ACCME, readers can apply for up to 7.5 CME credits. Developed in accordance with the essentials and standards of the ANCCC, readers can apply for up to 9 Nursing Contact Hours. An exam is provided with each manual.

Evaluating the Informed Consent Process
This 12-page booklet reviews the results of a recent survey conducted among more than 1,500 study volunteers. This booklet presents firsthand experiences from study volunteers and offers valuable insights, facts and data on the informed consent process and how this process works.

Online Directories and Sourcebooks

The Drugs in Clinical Trials Database
This database is a comprehensive web-based, searchable resource offering detailed profiles of new investigational treatments in phase I through III clinical trials. Updated daily, this online and searchable directory provides information on more than 2,000 drugs for more than 800 indications worldwide in a well-organized and easy-to-reference format. Search results may be downloaded to Excel for further sorting and analysis. Detailed profile information is provided for each drug along with a separate section on pediatric treatments. *The Drugs in Clinical Trials Database* is an ideal online resource for industry professionals to use for monitoring the performance of drugs in clinical trials; tracking competitors' development activity; identifying development partners; and identifying clinical study grant opportunities.

The eDirectory of the Clinical Trials Industry
Previously available as a printed directory, the new *eDirectory* is a comprehensive, online, searchable and downloadable database featuring detailed contact and profile information on 1,500+ organizations involved in the clinical trials industry. Company profiles can be searched by keyword, company name, city, state, phase focus, therapeutic specialties and services offered. Search results can be downloaded to an Excel spreadsheet for further sorting and analysis.

Profiles of Service Providers on the CenterWatch Clinical Trials Listing Service™

The CenterWatch web site (**www.centerwatch.com**) attracts tens of thousands of sponsor and CRO company representatives every month who are looking for experienced service providers and investigative sites to manage and conduct their clinical trials. No registration is required. Sponsors and CROs use this online directory free of charge. The CenterWatch web site offers all contract service providers—both CROs and investigative sites—the opportunity to present more information than any other Internet-based service available. This service is an ideal way to secure new contracts and clinical study grants.

An Industry in Evolution, 4th edition

This 250-page sourcebook provides extensive qualitative and quantitative information documenting clinical trial industry trends and benchmarked practices. The material—charts, statistics and analytical reports—is presented in an easy-to-reference format. This important and valuable resource is used for developing business strategies and plans, for preparing presentations and for conducting business and market intelligence.

CenterWatch Compilation Reports Series

These topic-specific reports provide comprehensive, in-depth features, original research and analyses and fact-based company/institution business and financial profiles. Reports are available on Site Management Organizations, Academic Medical Centers, Contract Research Organizations, and Investigative Sites. Spanning nearly seven years of in-depth coverage and analyses, these reports provide valuable insights into company strategies, market dynamics and successful business practices. Ideal for business planning and for market intelligence/market research activities.

CenterWatch Shopper!

The *Shopper*! focuses on specific products and services and presents them in a compelling format designed to make it easier for you to compare them and to select the best options for your business needs. Experts and thought leaders contribute tips and pointers to assist you in considering and evaluating various product and service offerings.

CenterWatch Patient Education Resources

As part of ongoing reforms in human subject protection oversight, institutional and independent IRBs and research centers are actively identifying educational programs and assessment mechanisms to use with their study volunteers. These initiatives are of particular interest among those IRBs that are applying for voluntary accreditation with the Association for the Accreditation of Human Research Protection Programs (AAHRPP) and the National Committee for Quality Assurance (NCQA). CenterWatch offers a variety of educational communications for use by IRB and clinical research professionals.

Informed Consent™: A Guide to the Risks and Benefits of Volunteering for Clinical Trials

This comprehensive 300-page reference resource is designed to assist patients and health consumers in understanding the clinical trial process and their rights and recourse as study volunteers. Based on extensive review and input from bioethicists and regulatory and industry experts, the guide provides facts, insights and case examples designed to assist individuals in making informed decisions about participating in clinical trials. The guide is an ideal educational reference that research and IRB professionals can use to review with their study volunteers, to address volunteer questions and concerns, and to further build relationships with the patient community. Professionals also refer to this guide for assistance in responding to the media.

Volunteering for a Clinical Trial: Your Guide to Participating in Research Studies

This easy-to-read, six-page patient education brochure is designed for research centers to provide consistent, professional and unbiased educational information for their potential clinical study subjects. The brochure is IRB-approved and is used by sponsors, CROs and investigative sites to help set patient expectations about participating in clinical trials. *Volunteering for a Clinical Trial* can be distributed in a variety of ways including direct mailings to patients, displays in waiting rooms or as handouts to guide discussions. The brochure can be customized with company logos and custom information.

A Word from Study Volunteers: Opinions and Experiences of Clinical Trial Participants

This straightforward and easy-to-read ten-page pamphlet reviews the results of a survey conducted among more than 1,200 clinical research volunteers. This brochure presents first-hand experiences from clinical trial volunteers. It offers valuable insights for individuals interested in participating in a clinical trial. The brochure can be customized with company logos and custom information.

Understanding the Informed Consent Process

An easy-to-read, eight-page brochure designed specifically for study volunteers that provides valuable information and facts about the informed consent process, and reviews the volunteer's "Bill of Rights."

The CenterWatch Clinical Trials Listing Service™

Now in its ninth year of operation, *The CenterWatch Clinical Trials Listing Service™* provides the largest and most comprehensive listing of industry- and government-sponsored clinical trials on the Internet. In 2003, the CenterWatch web site—along with numerous coordinated online and print affiliations—reached more than 10 million Americans. *The CenterWatch Clinical Trials Listing Service™* provides an international listing of more than 42,000 ongoing and IRB-approved phase I–IV clinical trials.

CenterWatch Newsletters

The CenterWatch Monthly

Our award-winning monthly newsletter provides pharmaceutical and biotechnology companies, CROs, SMOs, academic institutions, research centers and the investment community with in-depth business news and insights, feature articles on trends and clinical research practices, original market intelligence and analysis, as well as grant lead information for investigative sites.

CWWeekly

This weekly newsletter, available as a fax or in electronic format, reports on the top stories and breaking news in the clinical trials industry. Each week the newsletter includes business headlines, financial information, market intelligence, drug pipeline and clinical trial results.

JobWatch

This web-based resource at **www.centerwatch.com**, complemented by a print publication, provides comprehensive listings of career and educational opportunities in the clinical trials industry, including a searchable resume database service. Companies use *JobWatch* regularly to identify qualified clinical research professionals and career and educational services.

CenterWatch Content and Information Services

Market Intelligence Reports and Services

With nearly a decade of experience gathering original data and writing about all aspects of the clinical research enterprise, the CenterWatch Market Intelligence Department is uniquely positioned to provide a wide range of market research services designed to assist organizations in making more informed strategic business decisions that impact their clinical research activities. Our clients include major biopharmaceutical companies, CROs and contract service providers, site networks, investment analysts and management consulting firms. CenterWatch brings unprecedented industry knowledge, extensive industry-wide relationships and expertise gathering, analyzing and presenting primary and secondary quantitative and qualitative data. Along with our custom research projects for clients, CenterWatch also facilitates on-site management forums designed to explore critical business trends and their implications. These sessions offer a wealth of data and a unique opportunity for senior professionals to think about business problems in new ways.

TrialWatch Site-Identification Service

Several hundred sponsor and CRO companies use the *TrialWatch* service to identify prospective investigative sites to conduct their upcoming clinical trials. Every month, companies post bulletins of their phase I–IV development programs that are actively seeking clinical investigators. These bulletins are included in *The CenterWatch Monthly*—our flagship monthly publication that reaches as many as 25,000 experienced investigators every month. Use of the *TrialWatch* service is FREE.

Content License Services

CenterWatch offers both database content and static text under license. All CenterWatch content can be seamlessly integrated into your company Internet, Intranet or Extranet web site(s) with or without frames. Our database offerings include: *The Clinical Trials Listing Service*™, *Clinical Trial Results*, *The Drugs in Clinical Trials Database*, *Newly Approved Drugs*, *The eDirectory of the Clinical Trials Industry*, and *CW-Mobile* for Wireless OS® Devices. Our static text offerings include: an editorial feature on background information on clinical trials and a glossary of clinical trial terminology.

Continuing Medical Education (CME) Symposia

Continuing medical education (CME) symposia feature a variety of useful and practical topics for clinical research investigators, study coordinators, CRAs, clinical research scientists, physicians and allied health professionals. Thomson CenterWatch has developed flexible, turnkey programs that can be integrated into investigator educational settings in order to promote higher levels of compliance and study conduct performance.

NOTES